Ima... Urology

Simon Bott • Uday Patel • Bob Djavan
Peter Carroll
Editors

Images in Urology

Diagnosis and Management

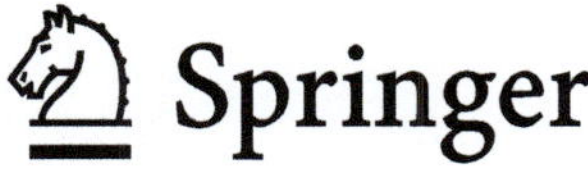

Editors
Simon Bott, M.D., F.R.C.S. (Urol) F.E.B.U
Department of Urology
Frimley Park Hospital
Camberley, Surrey
UK

Uday Patel, M.B.Ch.B., M.R.C.P., F.R.C.R
Department of Radiology
St George's Hospital
London
UK

Bob Djavan, M.D., Ph.D
Minimally Invasive and Prostate Centre
Department of Urology
New York
University Hospital
New York
USA

Peter Carroll, M.D., M.P.H
Helen Diller Family Comprehensive
Cancer Centre
Department of Urology
San Francisco, CA
USA

ISBN 978-1-4471-6893-5 ISBN 978-0-85729-769-3 (eBook)
DOI 10.1007/978-0-85729-769-3
Springer London Dordrecht Heidelberg New York

British Library Cataloguing in Publication Data
A catalogue record for this book is available from the British Library

Printed on acid-free paper

Springer is part of Springer Science+Business Media (www.springer.com)

Preface

The urological image and its role in the management of patients has evolved dramatically over time; the oldest surviving images are Australian Aboriginal cave paintings dating back to at least 10,000 BC. However, these images demonstrate ritual rather than therapeutic acts, portraying circumcision as an adolescent rite of passage. Further paintings showing ritual circumcision were discovered in the Ankhmahor's Tomb (Physician's Tomb) in Saqqara, Egypt, dating from 2,400 BC. One of the earliest surviving medical texts is the Ebers papyrus, a compendium dating from 1,550 BC. This 20 m long papyrus, found between the legs of a Mummy in Luxor and now in the University of Leipzig, describes, for the first time, the diagnosis and treatment of a number of urological conditions including retention, schistosomiasis and even bladder tumours.

Images of urological anatomy and our understanding of the subject was advanced by drawings from the fifteenth to sixteenth centuries, most notably by Leonardo da Vinci, Vesalius, Fallopius and Eustachius. They accurately demonstrated the structure of urological organs and their relations, based on cadaveric studies. However, it was not until 1895 that the first images were generated from a living person. Wilhelm Roentgen, who had discovered X-rays in November of that year, took the first X-ray of his wife Anna Bertha's hand. He was awarded the first Nobel Prize for Physics in 1901 'in recognition of the extraordinary services he has rendered by the discovery of the remarkable rays'.

Radiological imaging of the genitourinary system began the following year when John Macintyre set up the first radiology unit in the world at the Glasgow Royal Infirmary. He performed the first KUB X-ray in a patient with renal stones. This was followed by the first use of intravenous contrast by Dr. Leonard Rowntree of the Mayo Clinic in 1923. Using sodium iodide, he produced images of blood vessels and performed an intravenous urogram.

Over the last 40 years medical imaging has come on apace, particularly with the advent of cross-sectional imaging. Sir Godfrey Hounsfield, working for EMI in England, performed the first CT scan in 1972. Concurrently, a physicist, Dr. Allan Cormack, published work using a computer to reconstruct 3D images from X-ray data. Hounsfield and Cormack were subsequently awarded the Nobel Prize in Physiology or Medicine, in 1979, in recognition for their work.

MRI has its origins in scientific discoveries made in the 1930s when it was realised that the protons of water molecules align in a magnetic field. When the magnet is turned off the atoms revert to their steady state and in doing so emit photons which are detectable by a scanner. Raymond Damadian, a medical doctor and scientist in the United States, found that different tissues emit varying signals in a magnetic field, and in 1974 he filed for a patent for a diagnostic tool to identify cancer. This prompted Paul Lauterbur, Professor of Chemistry at State University New York, to use gradiants in the magnetic field to generate the first MRI images. Sir Peter Mansfield from the University of Nottingham then developed a mathematical technique that would allow scans to take seconds rather than hours and produce clearer images. He performed the first human cross-sectional MR scan in 1977. The importance of their discoveries was acknowledged when both men were awarded the Nobel Prize for Physiology or Medicine in 2003.

In medical practice today we rely heavily on images in the diagnosis and management of almost all our patients. For example, in diagnosis the majority of renal tumours are picked up incidentally on imaging prior to the patient developing symptoms, such that it is now rare to see people with any of the 'classic' triad of haematuria, a mass and loin pain. We use imaging to assess renal physiology, to assess disease extent and treatment response and as a permanent record for patient records, medico-legal and teaching purposes.

On her retirement Dr Parkinson made the collection of pathology images acquired throughout her distinguished career available to me for the purposes of continued education. At a similar time, sitting my exit exams, I was presented at each viva with an image to introduce a subject, in the same way that we are in everyday clinical practice. I had had the good fortune to be taught by Dr. Uday Patel, and reflecting on the advances in imaging and how medical practice had changed as a result, together we agreed to edit this book, collaborating with two outstanding teachers from the world urology stage, Prof. Bob Djavan and Prof. Peter Carroll.

This book is aimed primarily at trainee urologists, although radiology and histopathology trainees may also find it useful. Each chapter has been written as a series of 'cases' and edited by a radiologist, histopathologist and a urologist. The cases bring together a clinical scenario with the pathological process and relevant radiology and ask key questions about the scenario and imaging; below the images are the appropriate responses. The book is intended to cover the majority of urological conditions and the images that a practicing urologist will see. The text has been written to answer the questions posed about the images and does not pretend to cover comprehensively the whole of urology. However, we do hope the format acts as a more enjoyable way of learning, revising or just browsing the speciality of urology.

Simon Bott

Acknowledgements

Our very grateful thanks and appreciation to Dr. M. Connie Parkinson for providing the majority of the pathological specimen images and relevant text and for editing the whole manuscript on a number of occasions.

Most of the surgical specimens were photographed by members of the Department of Medical Art and Photography at The Institute of Urology during its years in Covent Garden. Subsequently their colleagues at The Middlesex Hospital and latterly in Media Resources at University College London continued this valuable service.

Tony Slade (Department of Photography, Illustration and Audio Visual Centre, University College, London) who gave us recurrent access to his knowledge and experience whilst allowing us to consume his time during the writing of the Introduction.

Dr. Ann Sandison, Consultant Histopathologist, Imperial College Healthcare NHS Trust for the illustrations for BXO, penile intra epithelial neoplasia, H&E and Immuno of the metastatic prostate cancer to bone.

Dr. Cathy Corbishley, Consultant Histopathologist, St George's Hospital, London for pathology images in the penile chapter.

Mr. Oliver Kayes SpR in Urology, for some penile cancer pathology images.

Mr. Paul Anderson for the hypospadias images.

Consultant Radiologists at Frimley Park Hospital who have offered help, advice and images: Drs Hywel Evans, Camilla Whitten, Jeremy Taylor and Rob Barker.

Contents

1 **Introduction: The Production of Radiological and Histopathological Images** ... 1
Uday Patel, M. Constance Parkinson, and Alex Freeman

2 **The Kidneys and Ureters** ... 21
Navin Ramachandran, Mark Ingram, and Uday Patel

3 **The Adrenal** ... 121
Anwen Newland, Dan Berney, and Andrea G. Rockall

4 **The Retroperitoneum** ... 147
Axel Martin and S. Aslam Sohaib

5 **The Bladder** ... 175
Dan Wood and Miles Walkden

6 **The Prostate** ... 231
Kevin Lessey and Susan Heenan

7 **The Testes and Their Adnexae** ... 295
Arjun Nair and James Pilcher

8 **The Penis** ... 347
Dan Magrill and Nick Watkin

9 **Urodynamics** ... 385
Manit Arya and Rizwan Hamid

Index ... 429

Contributors

Manit Arya, F.R.C.S. (Urol.) Department of Urology, University College Hospital, London, UK

Dan Berney, M.B., B.Chir., M.A., F.R.C. Path Department of Pathology, St Bartholomew's Hospital, London, UK

Alex Freeman, M.D., M.B.B.S., F.R.C. Path Department of Histopathology, University College Hospital, London, UK

Rizwan Hamid, F.R.C.S. (Urol.) Department of Urology, University College London Hospitals for Neurology & Neurosurgery, London, UK

Susan Heenan, M.A., M.Sc., F.R.C.P., F.R.C.R. Department of Radiology, St George's Hospital, London, UK

Mark Ingram, M.A., M.B.B.S., F.R.C.R. Department of Radiology, St George's Hospital, London, UK

Kevin Lessey, M.B.B.S. Department of Histopathology, St Thomas' Hospital, London, UK

Dan Magrill, M.R.C.S. Department of Urology, Frimley Park Hospital, Camberley, UK

Axel Martin, F.R.C.R. Department of Radiology, Royal Marsden Hospital, London, UK

Arjun Nair, M.B.Ch.B., M.R.C.P., F.R.C.R. Department of Radiology, St Georges Hospital, London, UK

Anwen Newland, M.B.Ch.B., M.R.C.P., F.R.C.R. Department of Radiology, Ealing Hospital NHS Trust, London, UK

M. Constance Parkinson, M.D., B.Sc., M.B.B.S., F.R.C. Path. Department of Histopathology, University College Hospital, London, UK

Uday Patel, M.B.Ch.B., M.R.C.P., F.R.C.R. Department of Radiology, St George's Hospital, London, UK

James Pilcher, M.B.B.S., M.Sc., M.R.C.P., F.R.C.P. Department of Radiology, St Georges Hospital, London, UK

Navin Ramachandran, M.B.B.S., B.Sc., M.R.C.P., F.R.C.R. Department of Radiology, University College Hospital, London, UK

Andrea G. Rockall, M.R.C.P., F.R.C.R. Department of Radiology, Imaging, Bart's Cancer Centre, St Bartholomew's Hospital, London, UK

S. Aslam Sohaib, M.R.C.P., F.R.C.R. Department of Diagnostic Imaging, Royal Marsden Hospital, London, UK

Miles Walkden, M.R.C.S., F.R.C.R. Department of Radiology, University College Hospital, London, UK

Nick Watkin, M.A., M.C.H.I.R., F.R.C.S. Deptartment of Urology, St George's Hospital, London, UK

Dan Wood, Ph.D., F.R.C.S. (Urol.) Department of Urology, University College Hospital, London, UK

Introduction: The Production of Radiological and Histopathological Images

1

Uday Patel, M. Constance Parkinson, and Alex Freeman

The urologist only ever sees the end product image, whether radiological or histological, but it is important to understand how these are produced. Only then can one fully appreciate their capabilities and limitations. Confident, informed interpretation directly follows from such basic knowledge. The following are brief explanations of how and why these images are created, their science and the practice. This chapter should be read before attempting the rest of this book, but equally the reader should periodically refer back to this section to ensure that his/her interpretative skills are based on a firm understanding of these essentials.

Production of Radiological Images

The common thread to the production of all radiological images is the detection of some form of tissue–energy interaction; broadly these can be subdivided as transmission radiology or emission radiology. With the former the energy source is external and passes through the body; examples are X-rays, ultrasound or magnetism, all being electromagnetic waves. Tissue–energy interactions alter the beam as it is transmitted through the body, and these are picked up by an external detector and converted into tissue-specific information. Emission radiology refers to nuclear medicine investigations, where the energy source is injected into the body, and the beam radiated out from inside the patient. Unlike tissue–energy interactions, nuclear medicine tests are used to study the handling of a given radioactive chemical by a particular tissue or organ. The emitted beam from the focus of concentration is detected by externally placed sources.

Urology is unique in that all these methods have their clinical place. The following is a brief explanation of how each of these work.

S. Bott et al. (eds.), *Images in Urology*,
DOI 10.1007/978-0-85729-769-3_1, © Springer-Verlag London Limited 2012

X-Rays and the Plain Radiograph

The X-ray was described by a German physicist – Wilhelm Röentgen – in December 1895. Its clinical value was immediately apparent and by 1896 a renal stone was diagnosed using this new ray (termed 'X' because its identity was initially unknown).

Although now very refined, the basics of X-ray production are not much changed from Röentgen's day. The ray is produced when electrons (the electrons are emitted by super-heating of a bare tungsten wire – the tungsten cathode) impact on to a separate tungsten plate (the anode) enclosed within a vacuumed tube. With the sudden deceleration of the electrons, and further interaction at an atomic level, energy is released in the form of an electromagnetic wave of a very short wavelength (approximately 10^{-10} m.) – an X-ray. When directed at the human body, this ray will travel through human tissues, but along the way it will be partly absorbed by these tissues, and this absorption (generally referred to as attenuation) is proportionate to the tissues' atomic number, density and thickness. Thus the exiting portion of the ray carries information about the consistency of the tissue that it has just traversed. In broad terms the density information prevails.

This information can be decoded either electronically or as hard copy. The traditional format is hard copy – the plain radiograph. This is formed when the X-ray falls on a conventional photographic film and converts invisible silver halide ions to stable and visible (dark) silver atoms. The amount converted is directly proportional to the strength of the X-ray (which, as explained above, is effected by the density of the tissue with which it has just interacted). Thus if the ray has traversed through a low-density substance such as air (e.g. the lungs), the ray is still powerful when it falls on the film and many silver atoms are formed. Thus the lungs are depicted as dark structures. In comparison, more of the ray will be absorbed when it encounters dense structures such as the bones (or renal stones), the beam is weakened and fewer silver ions are converted to atoms, and thus these structures are seen as relatively unexposed areas on the film, or white.

But silver is of course expensive, and also deteriorates over time, so the radiograph is now being gradually replaced by electronic image formats. These convert the information held by the X-ray into an arbitrary pixel-based electronic, or grey scale, that can be visualised on a computer screen. As the grey scale used is theoretically infinite, the contrast resolution of modern computer-based radiography (also called by an internationally recognised convention PACS – Picture Archiving and Communication Systems) is better than the traditional radiograph; however, its spatial resolution (i.e. the ability to resolve fine structures) is not as good. This relative deficiency is compensated by the superior storage capacity and general utility of PACS systems.

Computed Tomography (CT)

A major limitation of the radiograph (whether traditional or in the PACS format) is that it is limited to a two-dimensional image. There is no depth information. One can see the stone, but not how far it lies within the body. It could be in the kidney or in any other anatomical structure in front or behind, e.g. the gall bladder or back muscles. This limitation is overcome by computed tomography (CT). With CT the tube and mode of X-ray production is similar to that described above, except that the tube (and detector) rotates around the body, thus acquiring not only tissue-specific information but also spatial data (i.e. where in 3D space the tissue–energy interaction is located). Hence resulting detailed anatomical resolution of CT scanning. In modern scanners the anatomical information is sufficiently detailed to create accurate 3D anatomical maps.

Hounsfield or CT Units

As explained, CT also uses the (humble) X-ray and exploits similar density governed X-ray/tissue interactions as described before, except that the X-ray beam in the CT scanner is much narrower and this is detected by a diametrically opposite detector, to produce cross-sectional slices as fine as 0.6 mm thick in modern machines. The image itself is composed of individual picture elements, also called pixels. As there is no superimposition of images, contrast resolution is greater than the plain radiograph (a tenfold improvement). Each pixel is converted to a grey-scale value according to the sum attenuation of the tissue enclosed within the pixel, and the grey scale used to build a pixel-by-pixel image.

The attenuation is measured in CT or Hounsfield units (after the inventor of CT – Sir Godfrey Hounsfield). This is a subjective scale and water is assigned as the reference density (0 units) and all other values are measured relative to water. Air is −1000, fat −100 and bone >+200. The kidneys are in the soft tissue range of +40 to +60, rising to around 150 units after intravenous contrast. By common convention the image display parameters are set such that structures that have a high positive value are displayed as relatively white, e.g. bone/renal calculi and structures with a high negative value as relatively darker or black, e.g. air.

Window Levels and Width

The screen settings used to view CT images can be further focused onto the structure of interest. The window level signifies the Hounsfield unit that will be optimally seen and the window width is the range of Hounsfield units that will be best appreciated on the display monitor. For example, because the kidneys lie in the soft tissue range, the level is set at +40 and the window width is set at 200 Hounsfield units either side of +40. Any structure with a value inside the window width will be assigned a shade of grey and visible, but a structure >+200 will be white and those<–200 will appear black. Thus, when faced with a CT image the viewing settings have to be adjusted as described to optimise image evaluation. To an extent, this also applies when viewing other computer-based radiological images, e.g. PACS images, MR and US images.

Figure 1.1a–d shows examples of the various renal-specific protocols and CT techniques. Figure 1.1a is an axial CT image taken approximately 20 s after the start of the injection of intravenous iodinated contrast medium. Thus the arteries are seen to best advantage. Figure 1.1b is a 3D volumetric reconstruction of an arterial phase CT undertaken in a separate patient. There are two right and three left renal arteries. The highly detailed spatial information produced by modern CTs can be used to create anatomically faithful 3D images. Modern arterial CT has also virtually replaced traditional catheter angiography for the evaluation of the renal vasculature. Figure 1.1c and d are later phase CT scans, showing the nephrographic phase (approximately 60–90s post-injection) and the pyelographic phase (>4 min post-injection). These are optimised for evaluation of the renal parenchyma and collecting system respectively. Table 1.1 lists some of the common indications for CT in urological disorders.

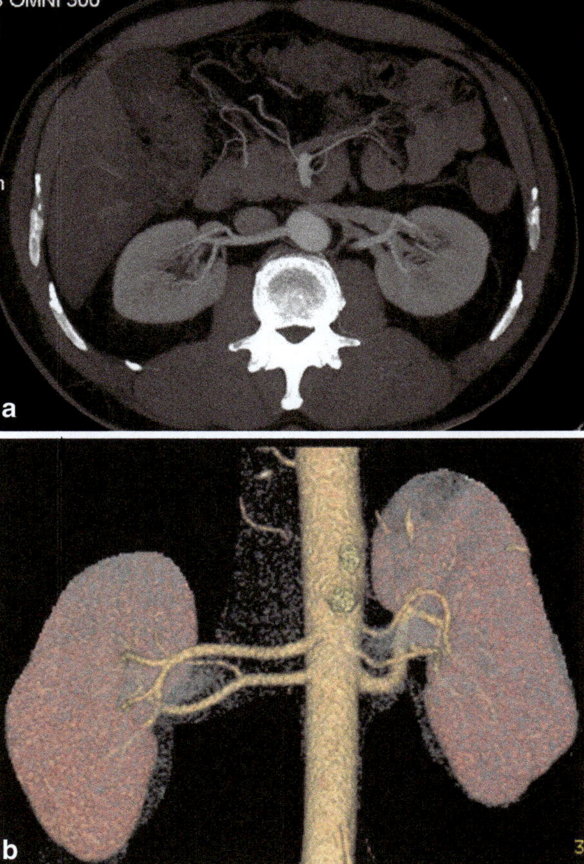

Fig. 1.1 (**a–d**) These are some examples of the various renal-specific CT protocols and techniques

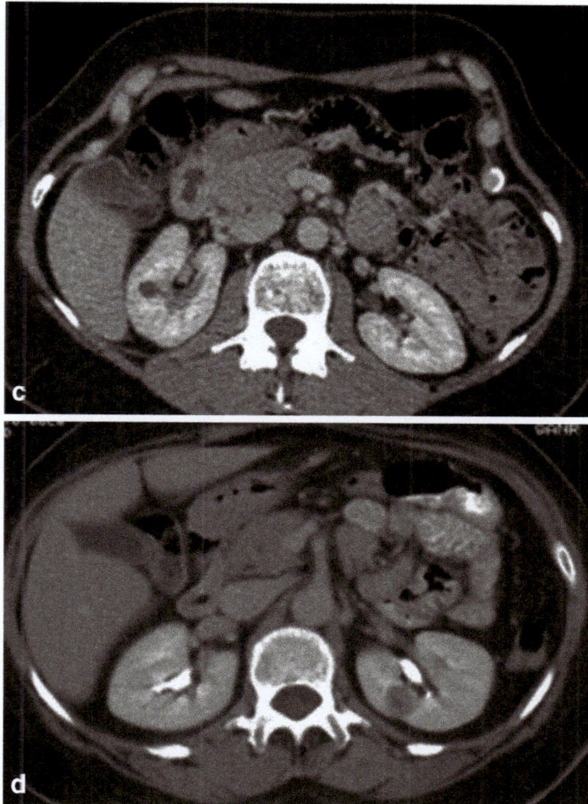

Fig. 1.1 (continued)

Table 1.1 CT in urological disorders

1. CT KUB – Accuracy almost a near perfect 100% (once interpretative error accounted for). Will also identify many of the renal colic mimics, such as appendicitis, diverticulitis etc.
2. CT of kidneys • Renal infections • Renal masses • Evaluation of renal anatomy, for surgical planning
3. CT angiography • Renal artery stenosis • Unexplained haematuria, for identification of arterio-venous disorders • Post-abdominal trauma
4. CT urography • Haematuria • Collecting system anatomy • Excluding synchronous lesions in high risk bladder cancer
5. Staging of urinary tract malignancy

Ultrasound (US)

Ultrasound employs sound waves beyond human hearing (>20 kHz), but which can easily penetrate human tissues. It is the most versatile of the imaging modalities (Table 1.2) as it is safe, patient friendly and a dynamic study. As a bedside imaging investigation it is unsurpassable. Furthermore, as sound waves are non-ionising, the technique is entirely safe and so far no serious tissue consequences have been proven.

The ultrasound probe acts as both an emitter and receiver of waves. An electric current applied to a piezoelectric disc results in alternating expansion and contraction of the crystal, which in turn emits a sound wave proportionate to the applied current (piezoelectric material = a material that generates an electric charge when mechanically deformed.). The emitted sound wave (in the range 3–20 MHz) will transmit through the body but, like all electromagnetic waves, it is also altered by intervening tissues and tissue–tissue interfaces. Of these, three interactions are exploited for sonography – the absorption of sound, the amount reflected or bounced back and a change in frequency induced by moving interfaces (the Doppler effect).

Table 1.2 US in urological disorders

1. Kidney • Haematuria • Loin pain • Suspected hydronephrosis • Renal impairment • Renal calculi
2. Bladder • Bladder outflow obstruction • Haematuria • Pelvic pain • Lower urinary tract symptoms
3. Scrotum • Testicular masses • Testicular pain • Suspected torsion • Infertility
4. Prostate • Lower urinary tract symptoms • Prostate size estimation • Suspected prostate cancer
5. Penis • Peyronie's disease • Erectile dysfunction

The first two are used to create the 'greyscale' ultrasound image, and the last for duplex/colour Doppler.

The strength of the returned sound (the 'echo') is detected by the probe and used to assign a grey-scale value. This strength is dependent on how much of the emitted ultrasound beam has been absorbed and/or reflected. Water hardly absorbs any sound and is also a poor reflector, while fat and air are good reflectors. Bone and calcium are highly sound attenuating and reflective, and demonstrate a sharp interface with a shadow beyond.

Doppler Ultrasound

As alluded to above, medical ultrasound is also subject to a frequency change when the beam encounters a moving interface, e.g. the surface of red blood cells. This frequency change can be back calculated to determine the velocity of the moving interface (see under further reading for the formula). Calculated velocities can be presented quantitatively as a waveform (duplex Doppler) or as a colour map of velocities (colour Doppler). The duplex Doppler waveform can be further converted into various Doppler indices, e.g. the resistive index, that reflect certain qualities of the supplied tissue, of which the principal one is the peripheral resistance offered by the tissue to blood flow. For example, neoplastic tissue offers little resistance because of tumour-induced neovascularity, necrosis etc., and will demonstrate lower resistive index values. In comparison, the acutely obstructed kidney will have a high resistive index, as the peripheral resistance is high. These semi-functional data can be used to further grey scale ultrasound evaluation.

The formula for resistive index (RI) is $RI = (PSV - EDV)/PSV$ (where PSV = peak systolic velocity, EDV = end diastolic velocity). RIs are measured on traces from segmental arteries throughout the kidney. The RI should be <0.70. Raised RI is a non-specific finding of an 'unwell' kidney. It does not indicate a particular pathology, other than increased peripheral resistance, but may be useful in monitoring the health of the kidney and response to treatment. It is also advocated by some as of value for the evaluation of acute renal obstruction. There are also some further Doppler ultrasound based semi-quantitative indices, all of some diagnostic value. These are not further covered here.

Magnetic Resonance Imaging (MRI)

The physics of MRI are complex but the essential is a powerful magnetic field (typically 1.5 T), which is capable of magnetising and re-aligning hydrogen nuclei in the body. By manipulating the external magnetic field, the alignment of the hydrogen nuclei can be further controlled to obtain weak radio signals, which can be amplified into the signal used to create the MRI (either MR image or MRI). The strength of the signal is used to create a grey-scale-based computer image. Spatial information can be obtained by the use of additional magnetic fields (or coils or gradients).

The acquired radio waves can be used to broadly quantify three signals – proton density, T1 recovery and T2 decay. Proton density reflects the number of protons per volume; T1 signal is caused by the nuclei giving up their recently acquired energy to the surrounding environment (also called spin–lattice relaxation). T2 signal occurs as the nuclei exchange energy between themselves (spin–spin relaxation).

An MRI contains information from all these processes but can focus on one or another by selectively manipulating the applied magnetic field. These are the basic parameters used to create an image, but there are many more allowing tissue contrast to be altered to detect different tissue features. Thus, unlike CT which is limited to X-ray attenuation (or tissue density) alone for creating an image, MRI allows for wider tissue characterisation. For example, T1 images show fluid as low signal (dark) and are generally good for anatomy. Blood products, e.g. haemorrhage such as that caused by prostate biopsy, are as a high T1 signal. Other causes of high T1 signal are colloid (e.g. some simple renal cysts, so-called hyperdense or Bosniak type 2 cysts) and melanin. T2 images show fluid as high signal (bright) and are useful for showing pathology which is usually associated with oedema (Fig. 1.2a), or for depicting fluid containing structures such as the urinary tract (Fig. 1.2b). Fat is usually bright on both sequences, but this can also be selectively suppressed.

MRI is generally used much less than CT for urological investigation (Table 1.3). Although it has many advantages, its greatest limitation in the urinary tract is its poorer precision for identifying calculi or calcification. Nevertheless, it performs better than CT for the local staging of prostate and bladder cancer and is equivalent for nodal staging and evaluation of renal masses. Further niche applications are for the evaluation of venous invasion by renal cancer (although modern multiplanar CT is making this application less necessary) and the evaluation of colic in pregnancy.

Radiographic Contrast Media (CM)

All contrast media (CM) have the common ability to improve the signal-noise ratio. The commonest agents used are radiographic contrast media, which are iodine (atomic number 127) containing agents. The iodine is bound to chemical compounds based on the benzene ring. Such compounds have a very short intravascular life and widely penetrate throughout the body tissues and extravascular space, transiently increasing the density of the soft tissues and hence improving the signal-noise ratio. The signal from the kidneys is especially increased because they are the principal source of excretion (99% being excreted by this route) with a half-life of 2 h. Renal excretion is by free glomerular filtration without tubular reabsorption, a fact that means CT contrast enhanced perfusion studies can be used to calculate glomerular filtration rate (GFR).

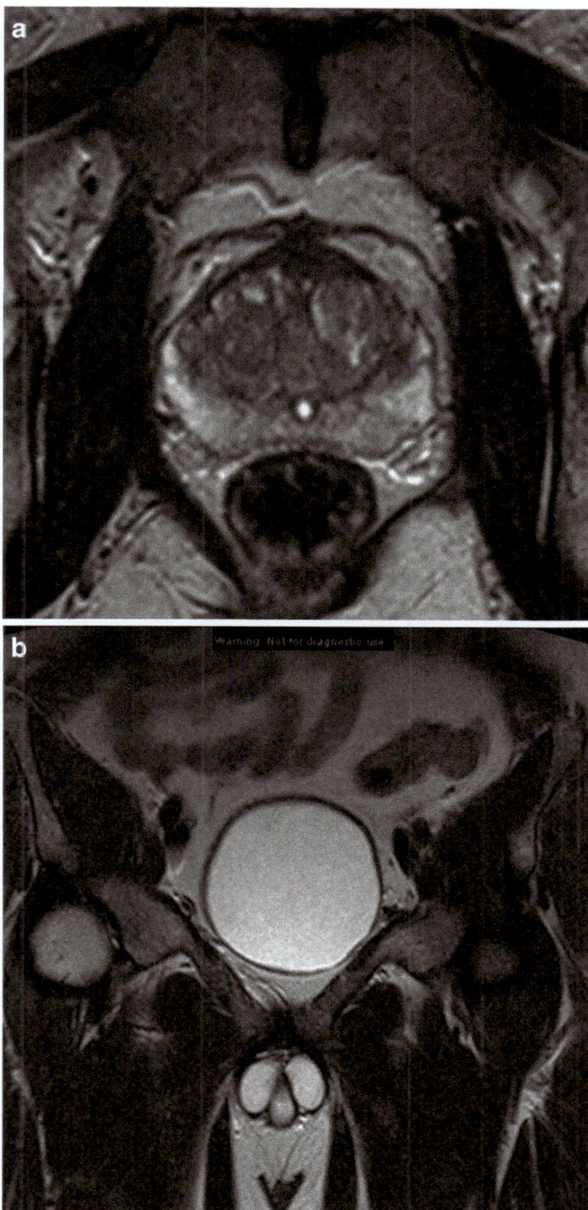

Fig. 1.2 (**a**, **b**) These are two T2 weighted MRI. The first shows a normal prostate gland with inner gland enlargement secondary to benign prostatic hyperplasia. Note the high T2 signal of the peripheral zone. The second image is a T2W tranverse study of the bladder. Urine is shown as high T2 signal

A limitation of current CM agents is their toxicity, either anaphylactoid or chemotoxicity. The exact mechanism of these is unclear and they can occur either early (within 1 h of administration) or be delayed (1 h to 1 week following administration). Anaphylactoid reactions occur independently of the dose or concentration of the agent. They are believed to be due to the ionic make up of the CM as earlier ionic agents caused severe anaphylactoid reactions. With the introduction of

Table 1.3 MRI and urological disorders

1. Staging prostate cancer
2. Renal imaging • Evaluation of indeterminate renal masses • Follow up of known renal masses • Staging of vascular invasion by known renal cancer
3. Staging of bladder cancer
4. MR urography • Especially in children with complicated urogenital anatomy
5. Penile imaging • Staging penile cancer • Priapism • Penile trauma
6. Pelvic floor imaging

non-ionic CM, the frequency of these reactions has reduced. Chemotoxic effects are related to the total dose, molecular toxicity and the physiological characteristics (such as osmolality) of each agent and thought to be responsible for nephrotoxicity. Modern CM, as well as being non-ionic, are also of low or iso-osmolality compared with plasma, and of lower chemotoxicity.

Contrast Nephropathy

Contrast media nephropathy is a diagnosis of exclusion, defined as an increase in serum creatinine by more than 25% or 44 μmol/l, occurring within 3 days of the use of iodine containing CM, with no alternative explanation. There is no characteristic or diagnostic biochemical or histological abnormality. Those with diabetes or pre-existing renal impairment, or other conventional risk factors for renal impairment, are at higher risk of CM-induced nephrotoxicity. The degree of pre-existing renal impairment also determines the severity of CM nephropathy. Its natural history is of slow natural recovery, and temporary dialysis may be necessary. Permanent renal damage is also possible.

Prevention of CM nephropathy is important. Since the causative mechanism is not known, specific therapeutic manoeuvres are not effective. Of all the prophylactic methods investigated, the evidence for simple hydration (commenced before and continued after contrast medium injection) is the most firm. See under further reading for a link to current recommendations regarding this subject.

Ultrasound CM

As with radiographic CM, certain injected agents can be used to enhance the sonographic signal/noise ratio. Essentially these agents are stabilised microbubbles (2–10 μ range), which are sono-visible. Only intravascular agents are available at the moment, with no soft tissue distribution but they are useful for vascular studies. They can improve the strength of the Doppler effect and allow more detailed vascular analysis. They can also, under some circumstances, return a signal of a specific frequency (or harmonic) which can be individually analysed. Such harmonic imaging is currently being evaluated and may expand the diagnostic range of grey-scale ultrasound.

MRI Contrast Media

MRI specific contrast media are also available. These are paramagnetic or superparamagnetic metal ions that affect the MR signal properties of surrounding tissues. Two main types are in use – non-specific extracellular agents (similar to radiographic and US contrast media) and organ-specific CM. The organ-specific contrast agents are mainly iron oxide based, used for liver imaging and therefore not that relevant to urological imaging.

Gadolinium chelates are the most widely used extracellular CM. They are strongly paramagnetic and shorten both T1 and T2 times of the hydrogen nuclei. Their pharmacokinetics are broadly similar to conventional iodinated CM, being short-lived intravascular, extracellular agents excreted by the kidneys. Their excretion is also by glomerular filtration without tubular secretion or reabsorption. Their safety profile is better than iodinated CM. Contrast-induced nephropathy is not a clinical concern but recently a causal link between certain gadolinium-based agents, renal failure and nephrogenic fibrosing dermopathy has been established (link below).

Nuclear Medicine

Nuclear medicine is emission-based imaging. It also uses electromagnetic waves, but in this case the commonest used is the short-lived gamma ray emitted by technetium-99. This is bonded to various organ- or physiology-specific chemicals. The radioactive chemical is injected intravenously and an external detector is used to measure the organ concentration or handling of the injected chemical. For the urinary tract, the agents in common use are DMSA (dimercaptosuccinic acid) and MAG3 (mercaptoacetyltriglycine) for the study of divided renal function and renal excretion respectively. Further agents used in urology are agents to measure glomerular filtration rate (glomerular filtration rate) and bone metabolism. For these, other chemicals are used, all still bonded with technetium.

Hazards of Radiological Imaging

As explained above the X-ray interacts at any atomic level within body tissues. This can damage the tissues, either at a cellular or genetic level. Ionisation of tissues by absorption of radiation energy is the cause, and the most vulnerable molecules are proteins and nucleic acid (DNA). Damage occurs either directly by rupture of the covalent bond or indirectly by free radical production. Terminologically, there are two broad groups of ionising hazards – stochastic effects and deterministic (non-stochastic).

Table 1.4 Effective radiation dose for patients undergoing radiological investigations

	Effective dose (mSv)	Approx of natural background radiation
Chest X-ray	0.02	3 days
Lumbar spine X-ray	1.3	7 months
IVU	2.5	14 months
Bone scan	4.0	1.8 years
CT		
Head	2.3	1 year
Abdomen (CT KUB)	10 (2–4)	4.5 years
Renal scan		
DTPA	1.0	6 months
Mag 3	1.0	6 months
Barium enema	7.0	3.2 years

Average effective dose in UK=2.2 mSv (87% Natural sources. 13% from artificial sources of which 11% is medical sources)

A stochastic effect means they arise by chance and have no threshold dose. The risk increases proportionately with the dose and an important example is cancer induction. Deterministic effects have a value below which they will not occur, i.e. there is a threshold dose, and include effects such as erythema and cataract formation. Once the threshold dose is exceeded, the likelihood increases rapidly until it becomes inevitable.

Doses in diagnostic radiology (measured in milli-Sieverts, or mSv) on the whole do not reach deterministic threshold levels, except in interventional radiology. Stochastic effects however are a risk with all X-ray imaging no matter how small the dose. It should be remembered that normal background radiation also has a risk of inducing a cancer. The quoted risk of inducing a cancer is 1:15,000 per mSv. Normal background radiation for a person in this country is approximately 2.2 mSv per year, unless you happen to live in Cornwall where radon gas increases this total to approximately 6 mSv per year. Imaging accounts for approximately 14% of this background radiation but is increasing. One of the main contributors to this increase is CT, which currently accounts for 10% of all radiological investigations and 40% of all radiation. Table 1.4 is a list of the typical doses seen in diagnostic radiology.

There are no described hazards of US imaging in routine clinical use, although experimentally there are concerns regarding local heating, especially with close contact scanning of the ovaries using the transvaginal route. MRI has also no reported hazards, although it is currently not approved for use in the first trimester of pregnancy.

Production of Histopathological Images

This is a brief guide outlining the production, utility, storage and governance of histopathological images with particular regard to Urological Pathology.

Aims and Uses

The primary aim of a histopathological image is to portray a clear and accurate representation of a surgical or biopsy specimen either macroscopically (as seen by the naked eye) or microscopically (as viewed using a light microscope), allowing important information to be conveyed visually. Furthermore, the image can either be printed or retained in a digital format and stored as a permanent record of the specimen.

Histopathological images have a clinical and educational value. An important use for these pictures is their correlation with preoperative images and intraoperative surgical findings, allowing constant audit of established and new techniques and providing information for research purposes. The value of such images is exemplified at multi-disciplinary team meetings where the extent of a surgical resection and the pathological process can be quickly visualised by colleagues from all disciplines. In addition, histopathological pictures can be used in undergraduate and postgraduate teaching, not only for medical students and trainee doctors, but also for those involved in related disciplines which include histopathology and anatomy.

In recent years, there has also been an increase in the use of histopathological images in medical consultations, often at the patient's request to facilitate their understanding. Occasionally, images are also used for medico-legal purposes.

As the endoscopic approach to urology increases, images of open surgical resections will allow urologists to see pathological processes in the context of adjacent anatomy.

Fixation and Photography of Operative Surgical Specimens

It is recommended that macroscopic photography be performed on completely fixed specimens. In unfixed specimens blood frequently obscures detail and produces reflections or specular highlights (making a smooth surface appear irregular). On and in fixed specimens blood solidifies and can be easily removed if necessary. The specimen pallor following fixation may be reversed prior to photography by immersing the specimen in absolute (100%) alcohol for a few hours.

The following sequential steps are important in ensuring the clarity and potential utility of macroscopic images:

Fresh surgical specimens for pathological examination are first immersed in a minimum of twice their volume of fixative for at least 24–48 h in a container of adequate size to limit distortion. Fixation inactivates enzyme activity, thereby preventing autolysis, preserves and hardens tissue to facilitate sectioning – the standard fixative is formalin. Complete bisection of a specimen is sometimes necessary to promote fixation but should be carried out in the laboratory. Incomplete incisions in non-anatomical planes or bivalving are to be avoided as they may produce anatomical distortion of the specimen and eversion of the internal tissue which may obliterate the boundaries of a tumour (Fig. 1.3). Complete fixation is necessary as partial penetration of fixative produces a variable colour change on the cut surface of the specimen which may confuse the non-pathologist (Fig. 1.4). The fixation process may be expedited in certain circumstances by microwave treatment to provide a pathological diagnosis the same day as the tissue is received in the laboratory.

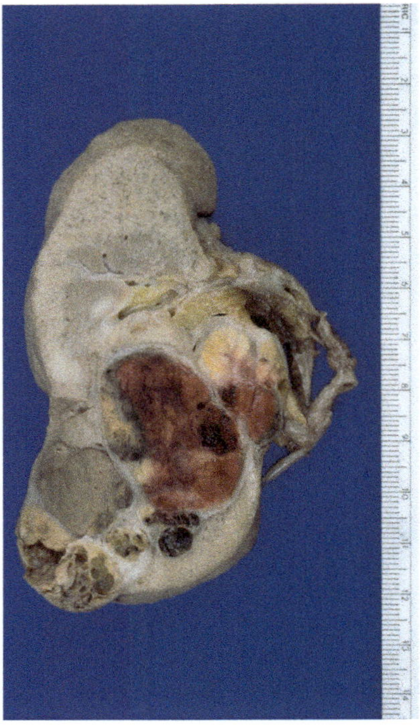

Fig. 1.3 Nephrectomy for carcinoma, the bright red area indicates failure of the fixative to penetrate to that site and not an inherent difference in the pathology

With respect to certain organs (especially kidney) removal of adventitial (adipose/connective) tissue and careful dissection may be necessary to give a clearer image of the lesion in relation to anatomical landmarks such as blood vessels, renal pelvis. During this process it is essential that subsequent tumour staging is not compromised. This may occur if peri-renal adipose tissue is entirely removed to obtain a clear external image with the loss of the precise tumour/adipose tissue interface necessary for staging. Thus photography and tissue sampling may have to be synchronised.

After fixation the specimen is sliced considering national and local protocols with an awareness of the plane of section seen in preoperative imaging, using a long sharp knife to reduce artefactual irregularities in the surface or 'hesitant' cuts.

Low-magnification photographs are then taken of the external and internal (cut) aspects of the specimen, filling the entire frame but including a scale (ruler or digital), not obscuring the relevant surface of the specimen. For certain large specimens a photograph following tissue sampling may also be valuable to allow correlation with microscopic findings, e.g. the site and depth of tumour invasion or the tumour types equating to the different macroscopic appearances within a mixed germ cell testicular tumour.

High-magnification views of areas of interest, if possible including a recognisable landmark to indicate the anatomical relationships of the lesion and to orientate the viewer. For demonstration purposes it may be worth combining the images derived from the last two steps (Fig. 1.5).

When all or most of the above guidelines have not been followed, it is occasionally possible with ingenuity and patience to obtain a contributory image (Figs. 1.6 and 1.7).

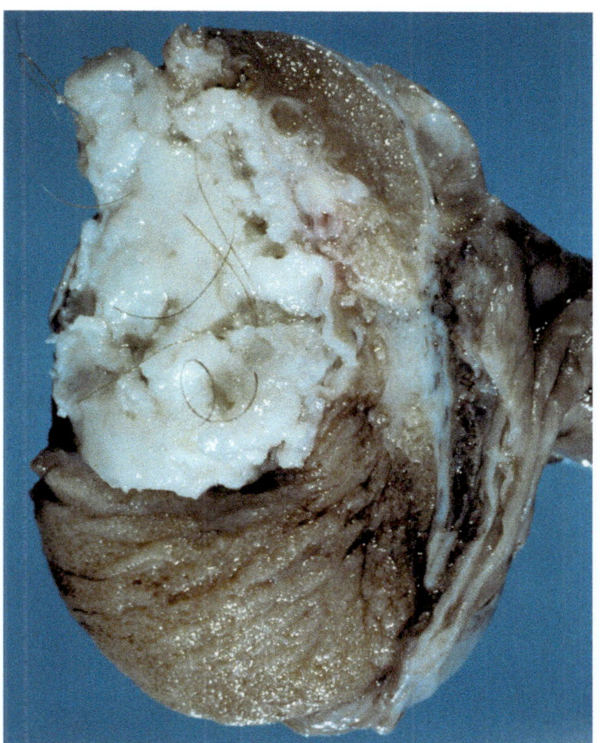

Fig. 1.4 Bivalved orchidectomy for differentiated Teratoma in which the tumour has everted obscuring the tunical limit

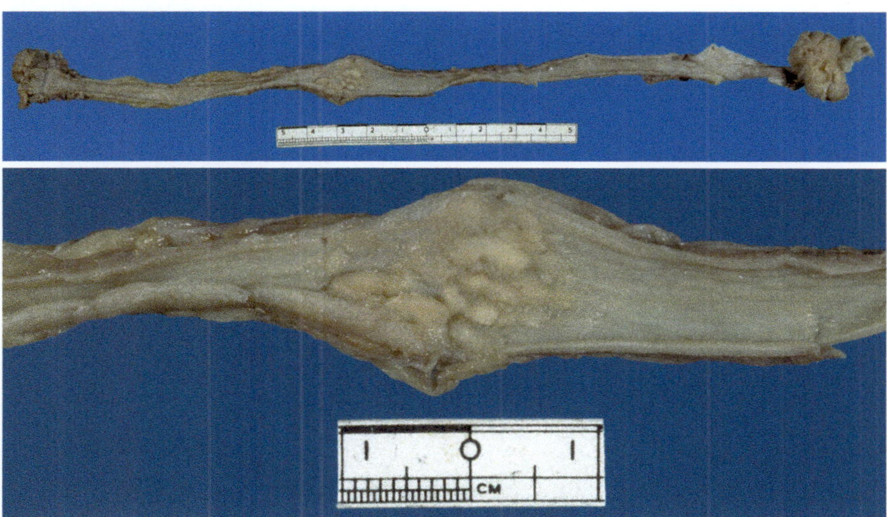

Fig. 1.5 Ureterectomy for carcinoma demonstrating the value of different magnifications within the same image

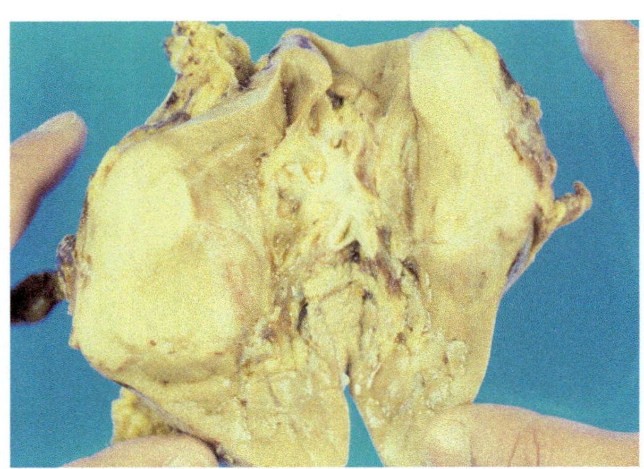

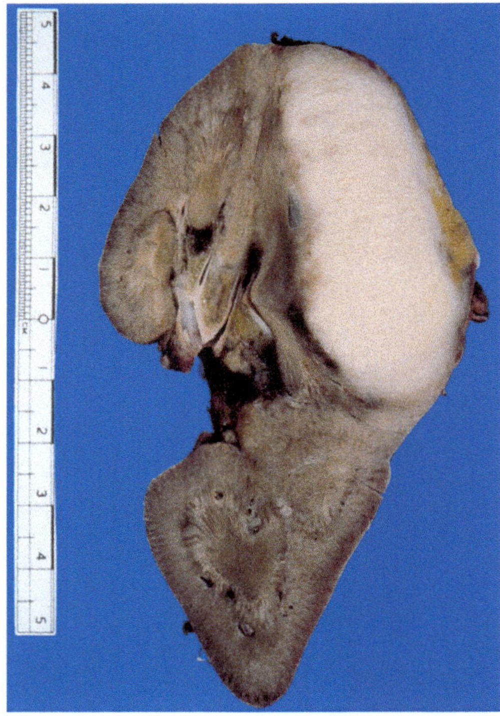

Fig. 1.6 and 1.7
A nephrectomy was said 'to have been photographed' (Fig. 1.6) but both specimen presentation and photography limited image clarity. Microscopy revealed the rare diagnosis of Wegener's Granulomatosis presenting as a solid mass. Further dissection, recolourisation, transection in a recognisable plane and professional photography produced a contributory image (Fig. 1.7)

Photography Technique and Related Issues

When purchasing a digital single lens reflex (DSLR) camera it is advisable to buy the best quality lens possible and a camera body of at least 8 megapixels. All DSLRs produce very acceptable images whichever manufacturer is selected. Buying the best quality macro lens will improve image quality.

A rigid system is essential to hold the camera, thereby leaving the hands free and avoiding camera shake at slow shutter speeds. Lights or flash should be used, the aim being to give a balanced, clean, crisp effect to minimise harsh shadows and reflections or specular highlights. A lightbox as a background and two lamps angled at 45° for foreground give optimum results.

It is useful to establish the correct positioning of the specimen against a clean, smooth background which must be spongeable (glass or Perspex) and of suitable colour or white/translucent. (It is possible to 'clean-up' and change background colour subsequently but requires a high level of skill and is time consuming.)

Processing of Tissue and Photography of Microscopic Sections

The factors required for good microscopic images include the following.

Selection of the appropriate tissue samples, limited by the size of the cassettes (perforated plastic containers) but not exceeding 4 mm in thickness. The cassetted tissue samples are dehydrated and infiltrated with paraffin wax in an automated process to produce rigid wax blocks. From these blocks uniform sections 3–5 μm in thickness can be cut, placed on glass slides and in a second automated process cleared of wax, subjected to various solvents and alcohols and stained, usually with haematoxylin and eosin (H and E).

Haematoxylin binds to acidic components including DNA, RNA and certain mucins, all referred to as basophilic. Thus nuclei appear deep blue/purple and cytoplasm if rich in ribosomes may have a blue tinge. Eosin predominantly stains intra and extracellular proteins, thus cell cytoplasm and collagen fibres appear pink or eosinophilic.

Various cellular and extracellular components, e.g. glycogen, fat or mucin, can be demonstrated by histochemical stains, but identification of cellular and extracellular constituents is commonly the province of immunohistochemistry (I.H.). In this automated technique a section is exposed to a monoclonal (primary) antibody raised against an antigen in the specific tissue component to be demonstrated. The site of the antigen/antibody binding is localised by a second monoclonal antibody (raised against the primary antibody) to which a coloured tracer is attached. Immunohistochemistry is commonly used in the demonstration of prostate-specific antigen in tumours of possible prostatic origin.

The wax blocks and sections on glass slides (both H and Es and I.H. preparations) are then stored in the histopathology tissue bank. Further sections can be cut from the blocks as required. It is important to appreciate that sections adequate for diagnosis may be suboptimal for an educational image. Although the H and E stain is regarded as permanent, it may fade over time and the original sections used for diagnosis may include artefacts, such as thickness irregularity and tears which diminish the clarity or obscure the image of the required field. Thus having selected fields for photography, if any of the above problems are present it is important to obtain a newly cut and stained section. Although image manipulation software may be helpful, they are limited to enhancing colour or contrast and take time and skill.

A low-magnification image enables an overview of the areas of interest. Scanning equipment has and is being developed to process large amounts of standard image data. The high resolution of these scans will allow for zooming on a computer monitor, but problems arising from the non-standard nature of microscopic images will have to be overcome. Higher magnification images allow pathological processes such as an invasive edge, vascular and perineural infiltration and specific cellular or nuclear features including nucleoli, chromatin pattern, mitotic figures, some cytoplasmic detail and cell walls to be visualised.

Microscopic photographs may include a range of low- and high-power magnification views to allow correlation of areas of the specimen marked on the original macroscopic picture with their microscopic and cellular appearances. (See Fixation and Photography, above.)

From the above guidelines it is apparent that histopathologists must either perform or be closely involved in all the practical aspects of specimen photography/scanning techniques.

Governance and Storage of Histopathological Images

The production of these images results in a valuable and potentially retrievable record of pathology specimens at both a macroscopic and microscopic level. This could be viewed as part of the clinical patient record and thus requires consideration of issues regarding confidentiality and freedom of information. It is important to be aware of legislation and advice surrounding these areas including the Data Protection Act (1998), the Caldicott Principles (1997) and the Freedom of Information Act (2000).

The Human Tissue Act (2004, England and Wales) whilst regarding the making and displaying of images as outside its scope endorses the guidance given on this topic by the General Medical Council (which effectively states that anonymised images may be used for educational purposes without patient consent).

Under the Copyright Act (1998), ownership of specimen images taken by an employee of a hospital or university (photographer or doctor) lies with the employer and not the individual creating the images. However, local agreements commonly allow such images to be retained and used for educational and examination purposes by the histopathology and photographic departments. In the case of a freelance photographer working within an institution or a doctor taking photographs within private practice, copyright is held by these individuals unless they have a contractual agreement to the contrary. Copyright is for a fixed term, currently 70 years following European harmonisation. All images that are published commercially or shown in public should be credited either by using the universal copyright convention symbol © followed by the name of the copyright owner and date, or in the text. Doctors are most likely to infringe copyright when digital images are sent electronically to colleagues and subsequently shared with others, such that knowledge of their origin is lost and a credit not applied. Departmental policies should be developed to cover the exchange of digital images and the use of images as doctors relocate to new posts in different institutions.

Recently, options for scanning microscopic slides with high-resolution scanners have been promoted and it is possible to archive the electronic information in a specialised database, ensuring it is anonymised and password-protected, either held on a local computer or on a remote server.

It is worth investigating the options available for long-term storage of histopathological images with close interaction with the local Information Technology and Clinical Governance teams as the rules may vary between regions and NHS Trusts, but will generally follow the standards followed by the Institute of Medical Illustrators.

Further Reading

Caldicott principles 1997. www.dh.gov.uk
Copyright Act 1998. www.copyrightservice.co.uk
Data protection Act 1999. www.hmso.gov.uk
ESUR Guidelines on Contrast Media. www.esur.org
Freedom of Information Act 2000. www.foi.gov.uk
Human Tissue Act 2004. www.hta.gov.uk
Making the best use of clinical radiology services (MBUR), 6th edition (2007). www.rcr.ac.uk
Patel U, Walkden M. Principles of radiological imaging. In: Mundy AR, Fitzpatrick J, Neal DE, George NJR, eds. *The Scientific Basis of Urology*. 3rd ed. London: Informa; 2010.

The Kidneys and Ureters

2

Navin Ramachandran, Mark Ingram, and Uday Patel

Case 2.1

1. Describe the images shown and their orientation.
2. What are the normal greyscale (i.e. not Doppler) ultrasound appearances of the kidneys and ureters?
3. Image 2.1.2 is the cut surface of a normal kidney, label 1–7.

S. Bott et al. (eds.), *Images in Urology*,
DOI 10.1007/978-0-85729-769-3_2,

Fig. 2.1.1

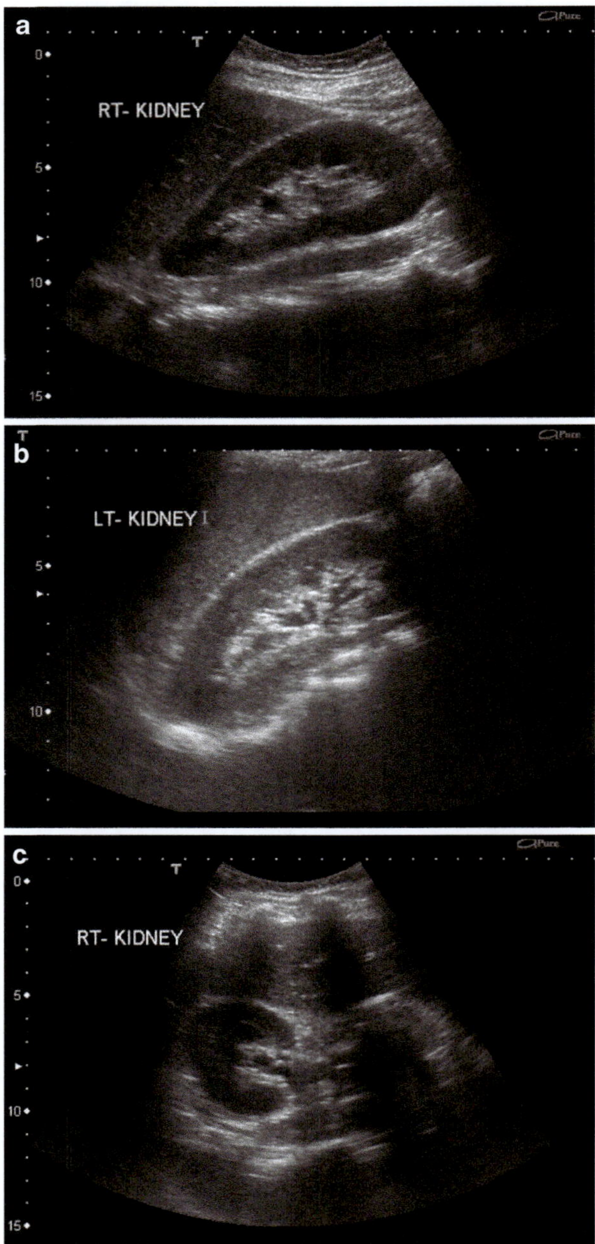

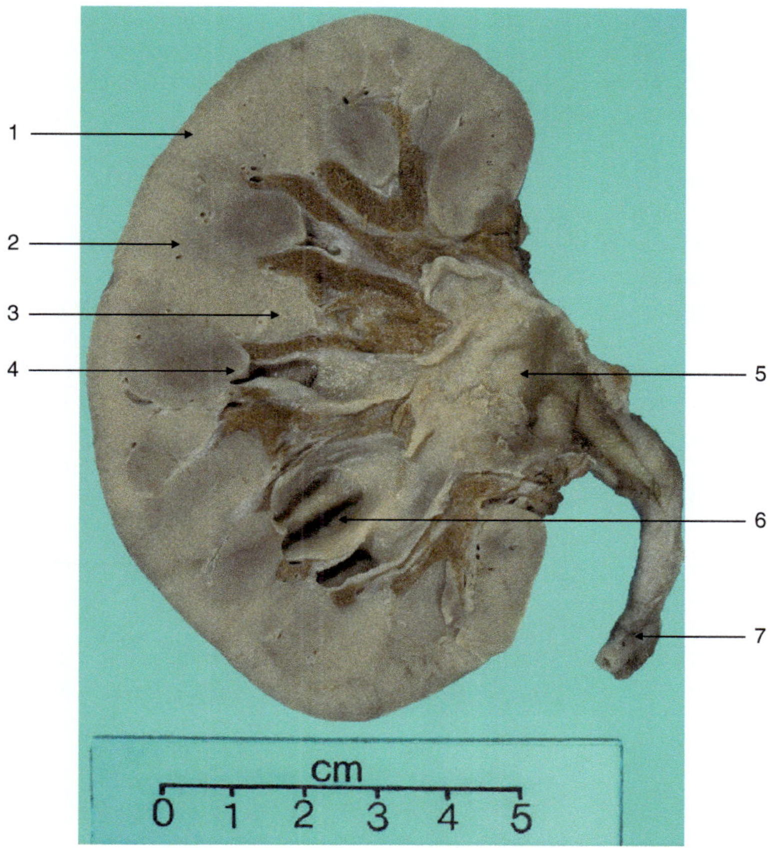

Fig. 2.1.2

Answers to Case 2.1

1. Figure 2.1.1a-c are longitudinal ultrasound images through a normal right (a) and left (b) kidney, and transverse image through the right kidney (c). The left side of the image corresponds to the cranial or right side of the patient, depending on whether the probe is orientated longitudinally or transversely. Lying immediately above/adjacent to the kidney on the right is the liver, and on the left the spleen.
2. The kidneys have a hypoechoic (i.e. darker) outer cortex which should be iso- or hypoechoic compared to the adjacent liver or spleen. If the cortex is hyperechoic, this is a non-specific sign of renal parenchymal disease. In thinner patients the medullary pyramids may be distinguished from the renal cortex, lying more centrally adjacent to the renal sinus. These are normally hypoechoic compared to the cortex. The renal sinus, seen centrally/medially, is hyperechoic due to its high fat content. The renal vessels and pelvicalyceal system may be seen within this region. Non-dilated ureters are not usually well seen on ultrasound except at the vesicoureteric junction.
3. Cut surface of a normal kidney showing (1) renal cortex (2) medullary ray (3) column of Bertin (4) renal papilla (5) renal pelvis (6) calyx (7) ureter.

Further Reading

Hangiandreou NJ. AAPM/RSNA physics tutorial for residents: topics in US. B-mode US: basic concepts and new technology. *Radiographics*. 2003;23: 1019–1033.

Case 2.2

1. Describe the images shown. What accounts for their different appearances and why?
2. What are the various urinary system focused CT protocols and their indications.
3. What is the imaging modality used in Fig. 2.2.2a,b. Explain the differences between these two studies.

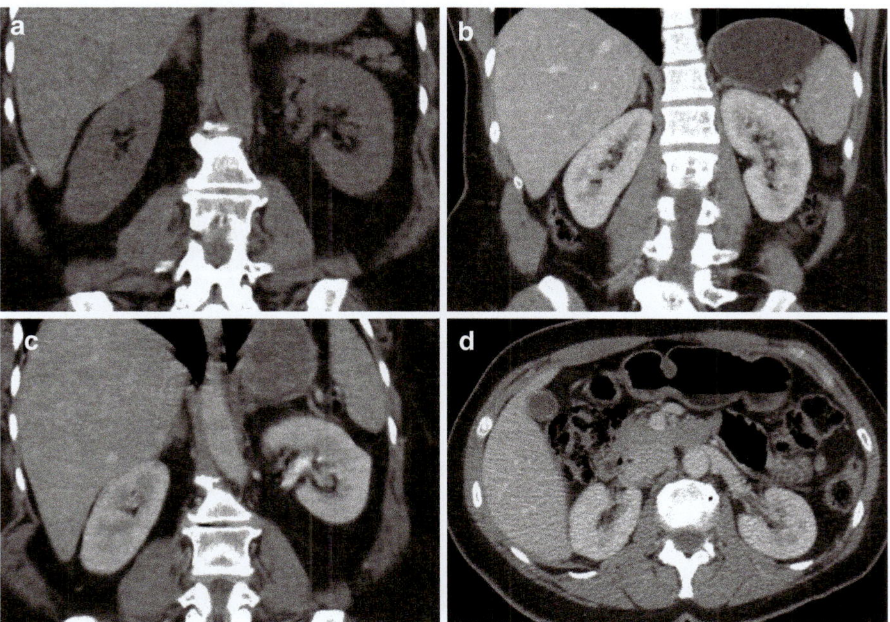

Fig. 2.2.1

Fig. 2.2.2

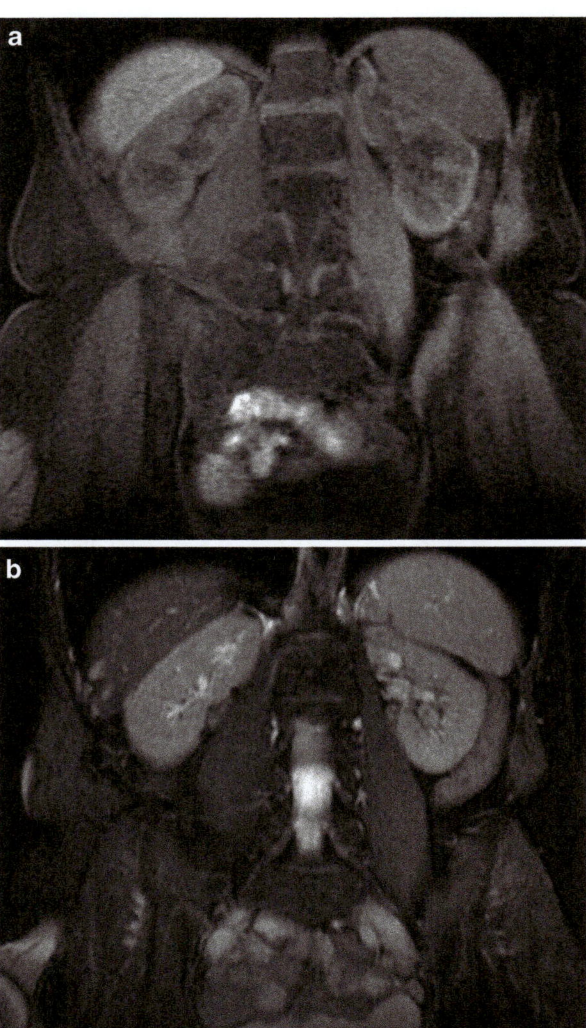

Answers to Case 2.2

1. Figure 2.2.1a–d are coronal and axial images through the kidneys acquired at different times before and following intravenous contrast administration.
   a. Pre-contrast studies (Fig. 2.2.1a).
   b. Cortico-medullary phase, 30–60 s following contrast. The cortex and medulla can be differentiated (Fig. 2.2.1b).
   c. In Image 2.2.1c two boluses of contrast have been administered, 4–10 min prior to the scan and again at 60–90 s before the scan. The early contrast has been excreted and outlines the collecting system i.e. produces a urogram. The later bolus gives good enhancement of the kidney (as in Fig. 2.2.1b). This is an example of a split bolus technique to optimally demonstrate both the renal parenchyma and collecting system on a single study. This technique is used for CT Urography.
   d. Nephrographic phase axial image through the kidneys at 60–90 s post contrast (Fig. 2.2.1d).

   When looking at a CT scan, compare the kidney to adjacent muscle such as the psoas. If contrast was given immediately prior to the scan, the kidney will have enhanced much more than the muscle. If the pelvicalyceal system is outlined, contrast was administered at least a few minutes prior to the scan.
2. The specific protocols vary between centres, but the reasoning remains the same.
   - A CT KUB. No intravenous contrast and low radiation dose. Used to investigate renal colic.
   - 'Renal mass' protocol CT involves pre- and post-contrast scans, looking at the enhancement of the kidney and renal masses and cysts to assess their malignant potential.
   - CT urogram evaluates the renal parenchyma, the pelvicalyceal system, ureters and bladder as a global investigation for haematuria. The simplest version of this protocol involves a precontrast scan to look for calcification, a 60–90 s scan to look for abnormal enhancement of the urothelium, and a delayed scan at around 15 min (when contrast has been excreted) to look for filling defects. This is effectively three separate CT scans, and comes with a high radiation burden, and there are many variations designed to reduce this (e.g. the split bolus technique discussed under answer 1 above).
3. T1 (Fig. 2.2.2a) and T2 (Fig. 2.2.2b) weighted coronal MRI images of the abdomen. T1 images are distinguished from T2 studies by the appearances of fluid (e.g. in the collecting systems, the bladder or the cerebro-spinal fluid) which is bright white on T2 images and dark on T1. Fat is usually bright on both sequences, but fat signal can be selectively suppressed as in the images above – note the low signal within the subcutaneous fat. Corticomedullary differentiation is best appreciated on T1 images, and this can be further enhanced by the use of gadolinium based MR contrast agents.

Further Reading

Patel U. Principles of radiological imaging of the urinary tract. In: Mundy AR, Neal D, George NJR, Fitzpatrick J, eds. *Scientific Basis of Urology*. 2nd Ed. London: Taylor and Francis; 2004.

Case 2.3

1. Figure 2.3.1a,b shows the CT scans of a 25-year-old male who was involved in a road traffic accident (RTA). Describe the findings. Compare these with the CT images in Fig. 2.3.2a,b from another patient involved in an RTA.
2. What is the grading system most commonly used in renal trauma and how is each grade managed?
3. What does Fig. 2.3.3 show and what investigation should the patient undergo prior to nephrectomy?

Fig. 2.3.1

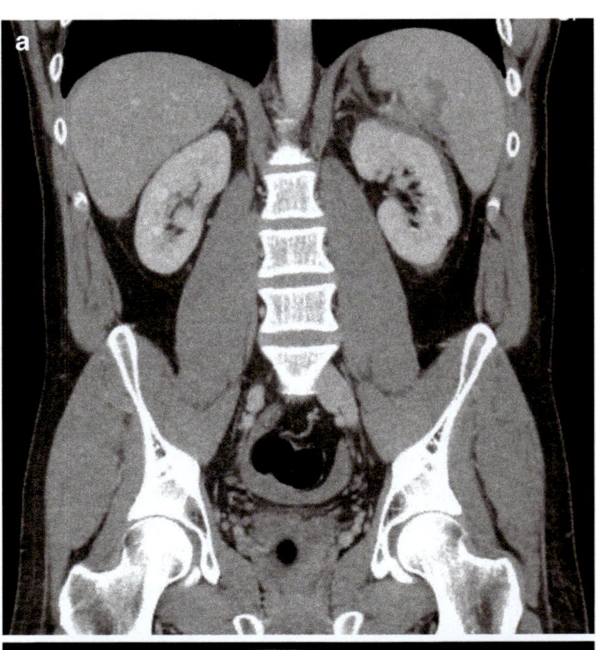

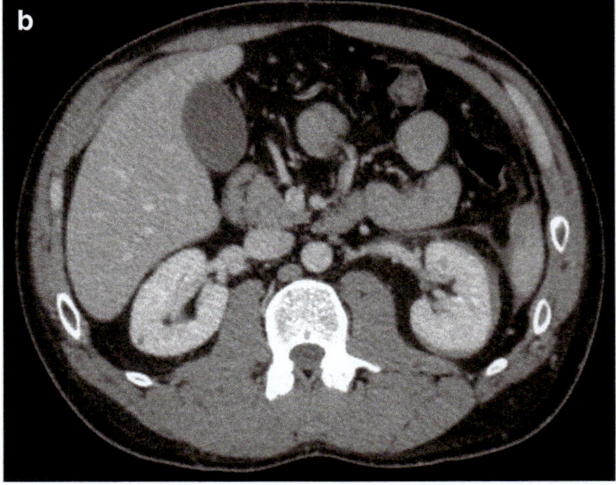

Fig. 2.3.2

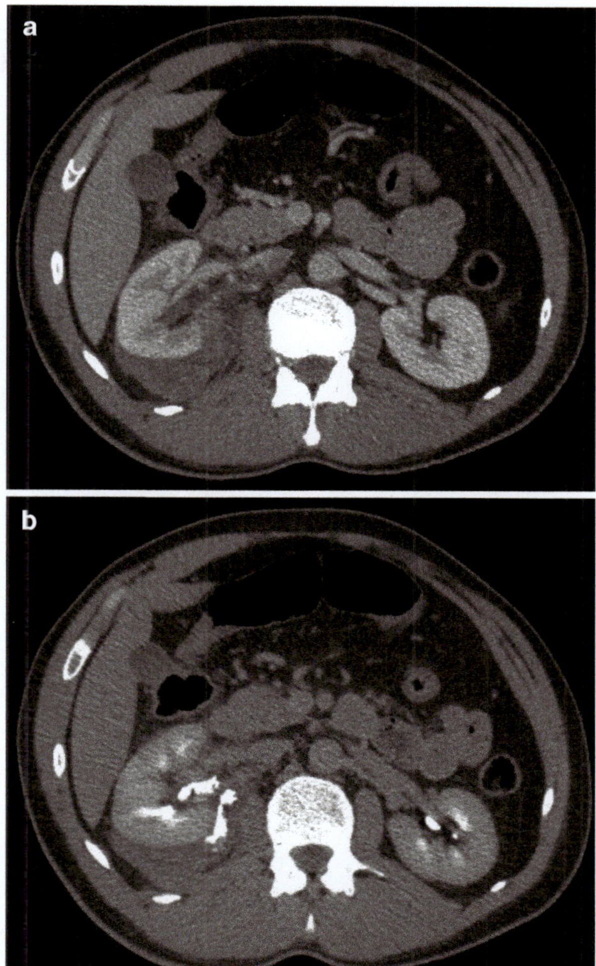

Fig. 2.3.3

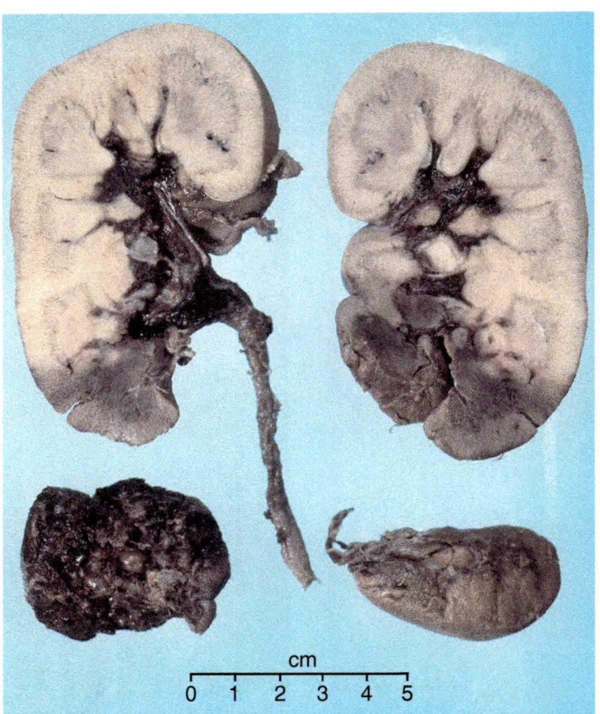

Answers to Case 2.3

1. Figure 2.3.1a,b are postcontrast coronal and axial CT images through the abdomen. There is a crescentic low attenuation region following the convexity of the left renal cortex, compatible with subcapsular haematoma. The left kidney is normal. There is also linear low attenuation within the spleen, consistent with a laceration and a small amount of free fluid tracking medially from the spleen. This is a Grade I renal injury.

   Figure 2.3.2a,b are post-contrast axial images through the kidneys showing a low attenuation region posteromedially in the right kidney, extending into the renal pelvis. In the context of recent trauma this represents a laceration. This extends outside the kidney resulting in a perinephric haematoma or collection. On the delayed phase image (Fig. 2.3.2b) contrast excreted into the collecting system has also leaked into the collection confirming damage to the collecting system i.e. grade IV injury.
2. The American Association for the Surgery of Trauma (AAST) classification is most commonly used:

   Grade I – Renal contusion or small non-expanding subcapsular haematoma associated with microscopic or rarely macroscopic haematuria.

   Grade II – Parenchymal laceration (<1 cm) in renal cortex only. May be associated with minor perinephric haematoma.

   Grade III – Laceration (>1 cm) extending from cortex into medulla, but sparing the collecting system. May be associated with significant retroperitoneal haematoma.

   Grade IV – Laceration (>1 cm) associated with collecting system or segmental renal vessel damage with contained haemorrhage or thrombosis within vessel.

   Grade V – Shattered kidney or renal vessel avulsion.

   Blunt trauma causing grades I–IV trauma can usually be treated conservatively. Life-threatening haemodynamic instability, due to renal haemorrhage, is an absolute indication for renal exploration, as is an expanding or pulsatile perirenal haematoma identified at laparotomy performed for associated injuries. Grade 5 vascular renal injuries are, by definition, regarded as an absolute indication for exploration, though there have been reports of shattered kidneys being managed conservatively. Penetrating injuries are frequently explored to exclude abdominal visceral injuries. Renal injuries with urinary extravasation and devitalised fragments may be managed conservatively or endoscopically if the patient is haemodynamically stable. These injuries are, however, associated with an increased rate of complications.
3. Figure 2.3.3 is a nephrectomy specimen following a road traffic accident, the lower pole was avulsed. This patient was haemodynamically unstable as a result of a ruptured spleen and an expanding retroperitoneal haematoma was found at laparotomy. A one-shot intra-operative IVU should be performed on the operating table prior to nephrectomy if a normal contra-lateral kidney has not been demonstrated on preoperative imaging.

Further Reading

Djakovic N, Plas E, Martínez-Piñeiro L, Lynch Th, Mor Y, Santucci RA, Serafetinidis E, Turkeri LN, Hohenfellner M. EAU guidelines on urological trauma. *Eur Urol.* 2010;57(5):791–803.

Santucci RA, Wessells H, Bartsch G, Descotes J, Heyns CF, McAninch JW, Nash P, Schmidlin F. Evaluation and management of renal injuries: consensus statement of the renal trauma subcommittee. *BJU Int.* 2004;93:937–954.

Case 2.4

1. What is this study? What does it show in this man with a long history of ankylosing spondylitis and recurrent bilateral loin pain?
2. How do appearances vary according to disease stage?
3. Describe the appearance of the specimen from an autopsy of an elderly man in image 2.4.2.
4. What are the causes of this condition?

Fig. 2.4.1

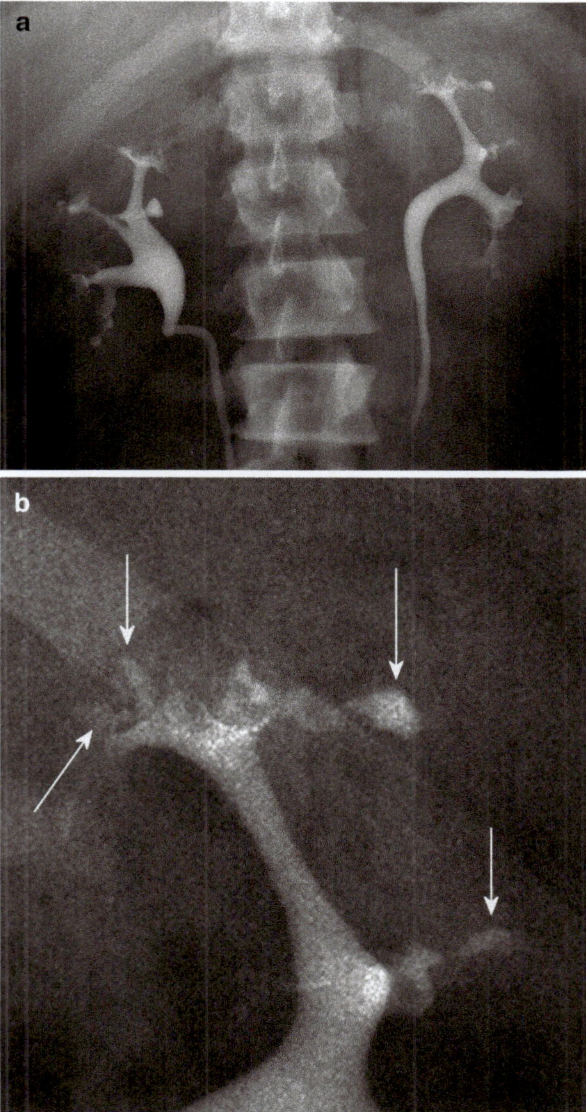

Fig. 2.4.2

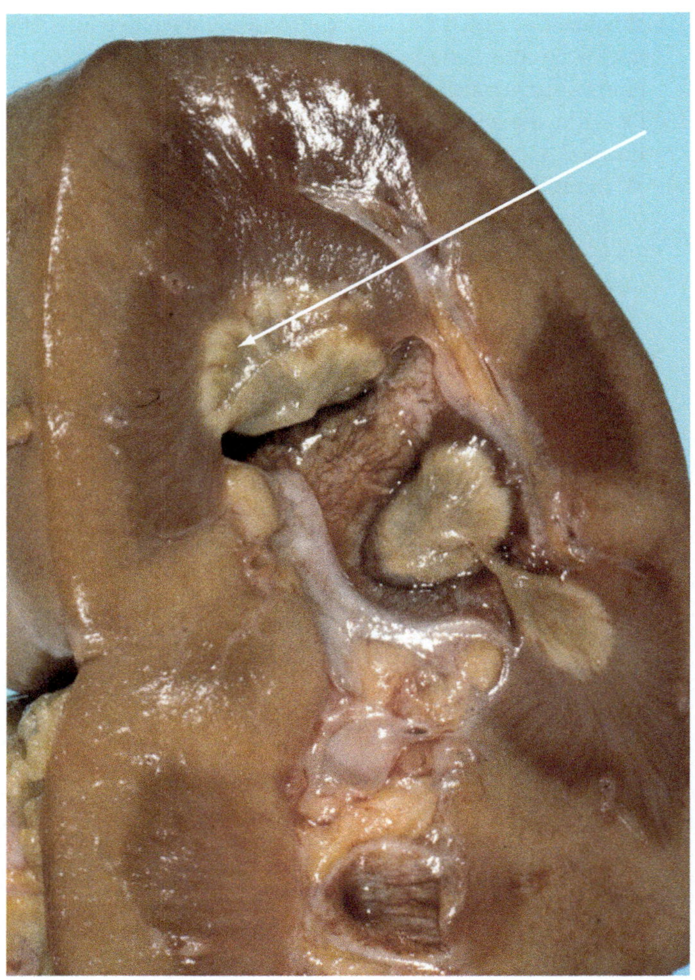

Answers to Case 2.4

1. Figure 2.4.1a is a 5-min post-contrast image from an IVU showing irregular calyces with contrast tracking out from the fornices into the papillae, producing an 'egg in cup' appearance. Figure 2.4.1b is a close-up image of the left upper pole with the tracking contrast arrowed. Appearances are consistent with papillary necrosis, and in this case it was secondary to analgesic use.
2. Early on, normal appearances or subtle papillary swelling. Later, contrast tracks into the papillae as shown above. The necrotic papillae then cavitate and slough off from the medulla. If they remain in the calyx they give a 'egg in cup' appearance on IVU. Detached papillae may cause filling defects within the pelvis or ureteric obstruction. Subsequently necrotic papillae may calcify. In the sites from which papillae have been lost calyces appear clubbed and the medulla overlying the damaged papillae becomes scarred causing an irregular cortical outline.
3. Figure 2.4.2 shows the upper pole of a bisected kidney removed from an elderly man who had untreated bilateral urinary tract obstruction and pyelonephritis. The papillae are yellow and necrotic and show early central cavitation. The sloughed papillae may also calcify due to Proteus colonisation. The renal outline may become wavy due to focal atrophy.
4. A mnemonic for the causes of papillary necrosis: POSTCARDS
   P – pyelonephritis
   O – obstruction
   S – sickle cell
   T – TB
   C – cirrhosis
   A – analgesic abuse
   R – renal vein thrombosis
   D – diabetes mellitus
   S – systemic vasculitis

Of all these, sickle cell disease and diabetes mellitus are the most common causes in contemporary practice.

Further Reading

Jung DC, Kim SH, Jung SI, Hwang SI, Kim SH. Renal papillary necrosis: review and comparison of findings at multi-detector row CT and intravenous urography. *Radiographics*. 2006;26(6):1827–1836.

Case 2.5

1. What do these images show and what is the diagnosis in this middle aged female with recurrent loin pain resistant to antibiotics?
2. What is the treatment for this condition?

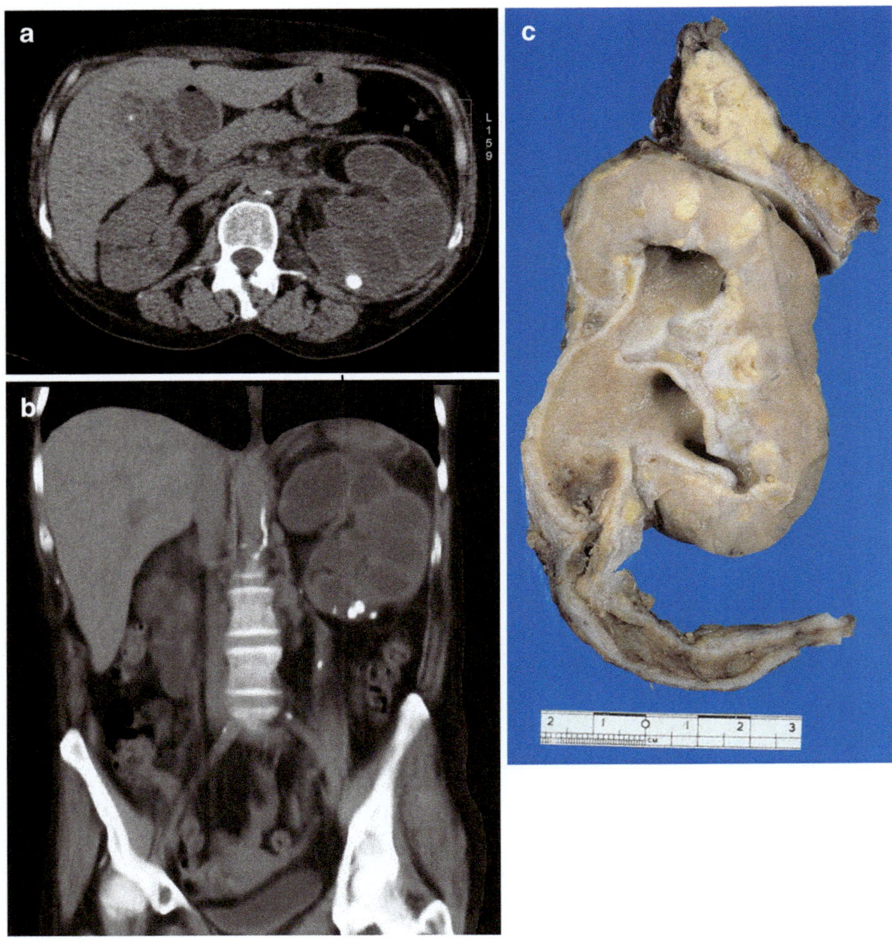

Fig. 2.5.1

Answers to Case 2.5

1. Axial (Fig. 2.5.1a) and coronal MPR* (Fig. 2.5.1b) images through the left kidney. The left kidney is enlarged and contains multiple large, round, low attenuation (−10–30 Hounsfield units) lesions, but maintains a normal shape. The low attenuation lesions represent enlarged calyces, abscesses or granulomas. This is sometimes called the bear paw sign. A few calculi are seen within the kidney (but not obstructing the renal pelvis – obstructing calculi are seen in 75% of cases with this condition). There is perinephric stranding and thickening of Gerota's fascia. Appearances are of Xanthogranulomatous pyelonephritis (XGP).

   Figure 2.5.1c is a nephrectomy specimen with thickened and dilated upper ureter and pelvis. Yellow deposits produce space occupying lesions throughout the kidney and extend into adipose tissue adjacent to the upper pole. Microscopically the yellow deposits are a xanthogranulamatous inflammatory reaction. This is a chronic inflammatory process in which lipid-laden histiocytes destroy the renal parenchyma with potential extension of an inflammatory mass into the perinephric space adjacent psoas muscle and posterior abdominal wall. Squamous cell carcinoma is a rare complication.

   When it extends outside the kidney, XGP may mimic tumour. No radiological features are definitive of XGP, but the low density lesions in the presence of an obstructive calculus, which is often a staghorn, are highly suggestive. Diagnosis is made histologically by the presence of foamy lipid-rich macrophages accompanied by acute- and chronic-phase inflammatory cells.
2. Antibiotics and conservative therapy do not tend to be successful. Nephrectomy is the treatment of choice, with the removal of all the granulomatous tissue to prevent ongoing inflammation leading to fistula formation. Partial nephrectomy may be appropriate if only a part of the kidney is involved.

Further Reading

Craig WD, Wagner BJ, Travis MD. Pyelonephritis: radiologic-pathologic review. *Radiographics*. 2008;28(1):255–277.

Korkes F, Favoretto RL, Bróglio M, Silva CA, Castro MG, Perez MD. Xanthogranulomatous pyelonephritis: clinical experience with 41 cases. *Urology*. 2008;71(2):178–180.

* MPR = multiplanar reformat. This method uses the three-dimensional data acquired by the CT scanner to reconstruct images in any plane. For example the coronal plane of the kidney, rather than the coronal plane of the whole body has been chosen in this case.

Case 2.6

This woman presented with a history of recurrent urinary tract infections.

1. Describe the study and findings in the path specimen.
2. What is the differential diagnosis in the radiological study?
3. What is the most likely diagnosis?

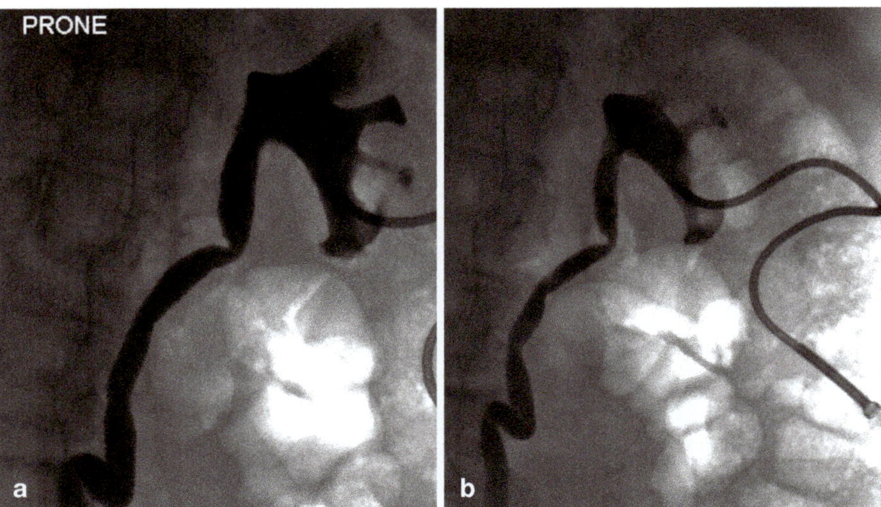

Fig. 2.6.1

Fig. 2.6.2

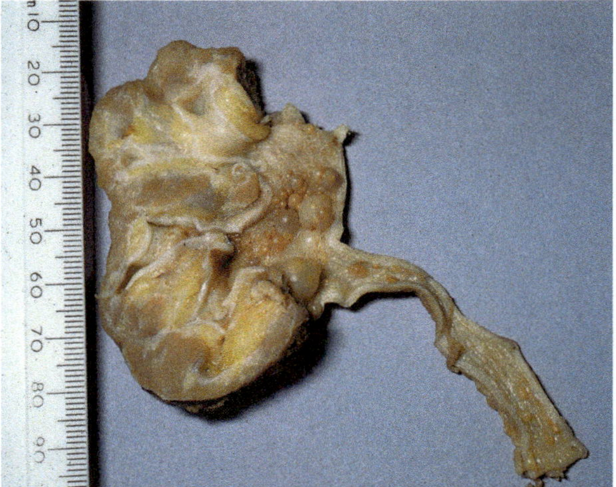

Answers to Case 2.6

1. Figures 2.6.1a,b are from a nephrostogram study of the left urinary tract, showing multiple subtle but persistent filling defects in the left upper ureter, just beyond the pelviureteric junction. These filling defects appear to be mucosal in location, and extend into the lumen from the ureteric wall (note the irregularity of the mucosal outline). The nephrectomy specimen (Figure 2.6.2) shows the cut surface of the kidney and upper ureter demonstrating pyelonephritic scarring and numerous subepithelial cysts of varying size in the pelvis and ureter with microscopic features of pyeloureteritis cystica.
2. The differential for these radiographic appearances is wide:
   - Pyeloureteritis cystica
   - Multifocal TCC
   - Adherent thrombus
   - Vascular impressions
   - Metastases e.g. from prostate, stomach, breast (rare)
   - TB
   - Schistosomiasis
3. In this case the diagnosis was pyeloureteritis cystica, given the history of chronic infections. However, malignancy must be excluded by endoscopic evaluation or cytology as appropriate. Pyeloureteritis cystica is thought to occur due to proliferation of epithelial cells secondary to chronic obstruction/infection, resulting in multiple subepithelial cysts measuring 1–4 mm. On IVU/retrograde ureterography/nephrostogram, this causes multiple well-defined filling defects and ureteric scalloping as seen in this example. The cysts slowly resolve over months to years following treatment of the underlying condition. They are not premalignant and do not cause obstruction.

Further Reading

Menéndez V, Sala X, Alvarez-Vijande R, Solé M, Rodriguez A, Carretero P. Cystic pyeloureteritis: review of 34 cases. Radiologic aspects and differential diagnosis. *Urology*. 1997;50(1):31–37.

Case 2.7

A 45-year-old man presents with dysuria and urinary frequency. Initial urinary tests reveal microscopic haematuria and sterile pyuria. A second 84-year-old man presents with night sweats and a swelling in his loin.

1. Describe the images shown and the likely diagnosis.
2. What are the macroscopic changes seen in the kidney and ureter in this condition?
3. What other findings may be present on plain film and intravenous urography in this condition?
4. Describe the appearances seen in the kidney in Fig. 2.7.3 and the likely diagnosis.

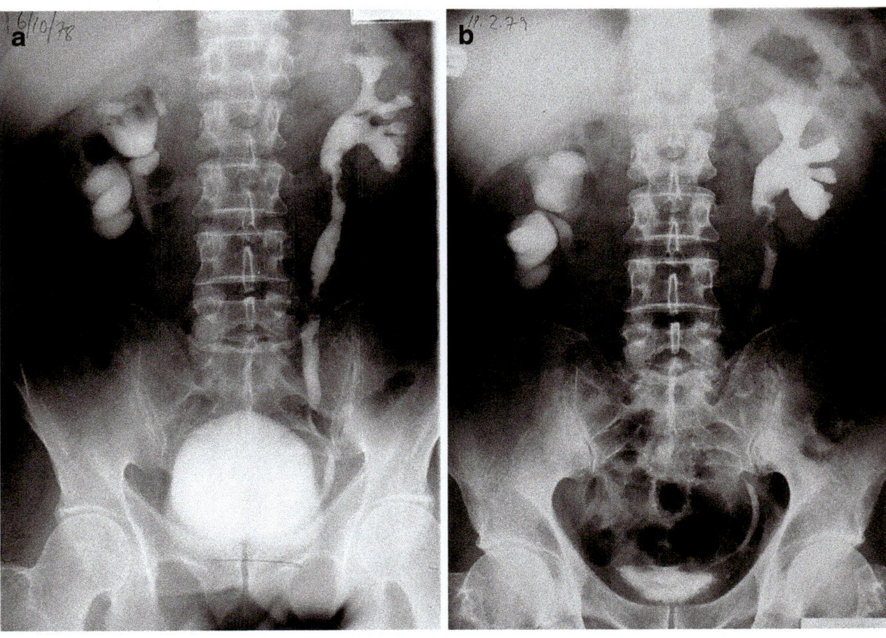

Fig. 2.7.1

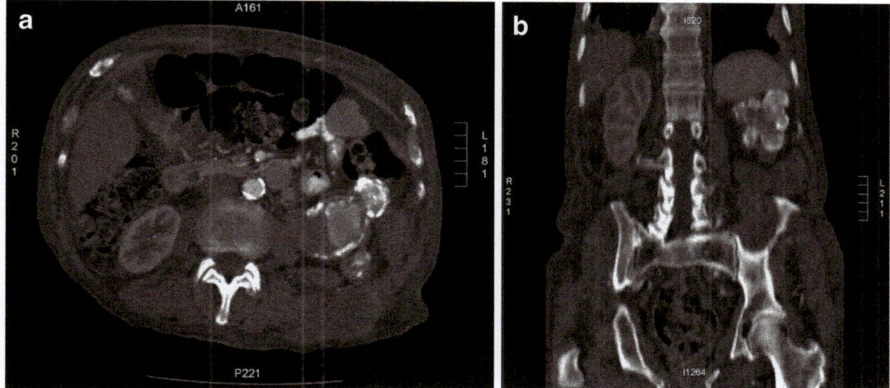

Fig. 2.7.2

Fig. 2.7.3

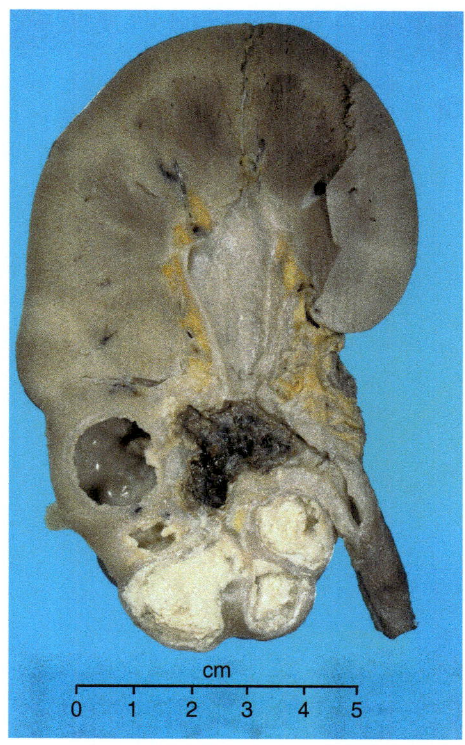

Answers to Case 2.7

1. Figure 2.7.1a,b are two IVU films taken 4 months apart and show marked abnormality of both renal collecting systems and left ureter. The left kidney shows blunted, dilated calyces and the left ureter demonstrates an irregular 'jagged' contour with alternating strictures and dilatations. The right kidney shows dilated calyces secondary to infundibular strictures, and cephalic retraction of an atrophic renal pelvis. The appearances are highly suspicious for renal and ureteric tuberculosis. Figure 2.7.2a is an axial and Fig. 2.7.2b a coronal contrast enhanced CT of the older man showing a calcified and atropic right renal parenchyma with an associated fluid collection involving the posterior abdominal wall. Aspiration of the fluid collection and culture revealed mycobacterium bovis.
2. The classic findings of renal tuberculosis include parenchymal destruction and scarring with associated cavity formation. Granuloma formation leads to parenchymal masses and fibrosis with secondary strictures of the ureters and collecting systems. The organisms reach the kidney through haematogenous spread, and then propagate distally down the ureters to the bladder.
3. Plain abdominal radiographs demonstrate a wide variety of calcification ranging from amorphous granular calcification to dense punctuate calcification. In end-stage renal TB, intravenous urography often shows a shrunken hydronephrotic kidney or complete absence of function (autonephrectomy). Chest radiographs show evidence of active or healed tuberculosis in only 30%.
4. In Fig. 2.7.3 the kidney shows loss of parenchyma at the lower pole and replacement by caseous tissue. Microscopy revealed caseous granuloma and acid fast bacilli on Zeihl-Neelsen staining.

Further Reading

Gibson MS, Puckett ML, Shelly ME. Renal tuberculosis. *Radiographics.* 2004;24:251–256.

Case 2.8

A 75-year-old diabetic woman presented with fever and flank pain.

1. Describe the images and the most likely diagnosis?
2. What is the aetiology?
3. What is the radiographic differential diagnosis?

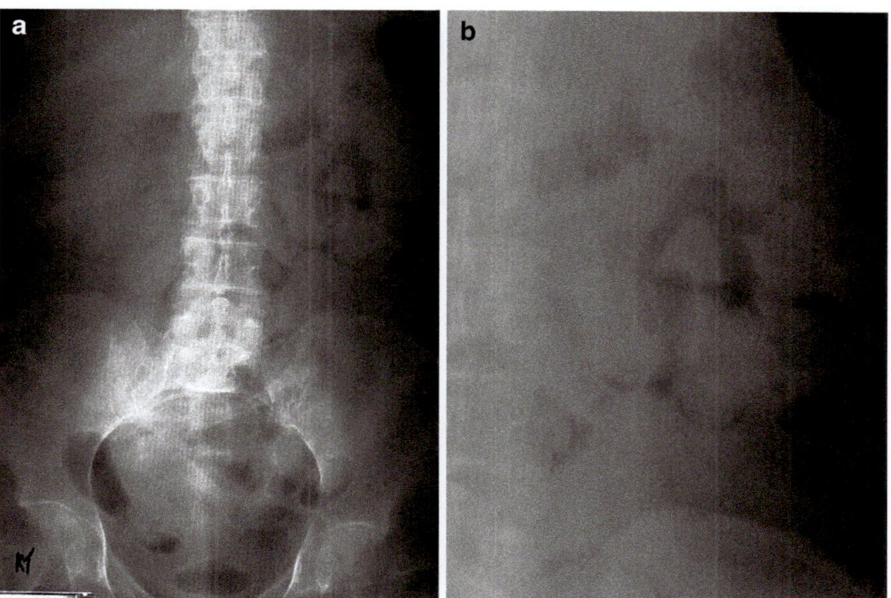

Fig. 2.8.1

Answers to Case 2.8

1. Plain film of the abdomen (Fig. 2.8.1a) with a magnified image of the left upper quadrant (Fig. 2.8.1b). There is an abnormal gas shadow outlining the left pelvi-calyceal system and a further gas shadow centrally in the pelvis which outlines the bladder. Appearances are highly suggestive of emphysematous pyelonephritis.
2. This is an acute, life-threatening infection of the kidney with gas formation. It is associated with diabetes most commonly, but also immunocompromise or ureteric obstruction. The usual organisms are *E. coli, Klebsiella or Proteus*.
3. Similar radiographic appearances may be seen with enterovesical fistula (iatrogenic, tumour, Crohn's disease), a psoas abscess fistulating into the renal collecting system or after recent endourological intervention.

Further Reading

Craig WD, Wagner BJ, Travis MD. Pyelonephritis: radiologic-pathologic review. *Radiographics*. 2008;28(1):255–277.

Case 2.9

These studies are from a 20-year-old man with vague back pain.

1. Describe these images and what is the likely diagnosis.
2. What is the differential diagnosis?
3. The patient reports that his father passed away from a sudden 'bleed in the brain'. What is the most likely diagnosis?
4. Name some associations/complications of this condition
5. What does the surgical specimen (Fig. 2.9.2) show?

Fig. 2.9.1

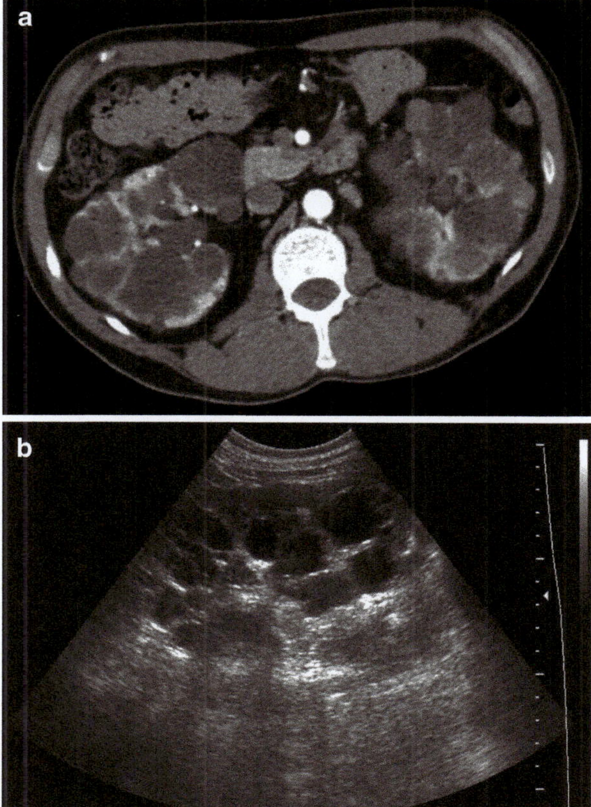

Fig. 2.9.2

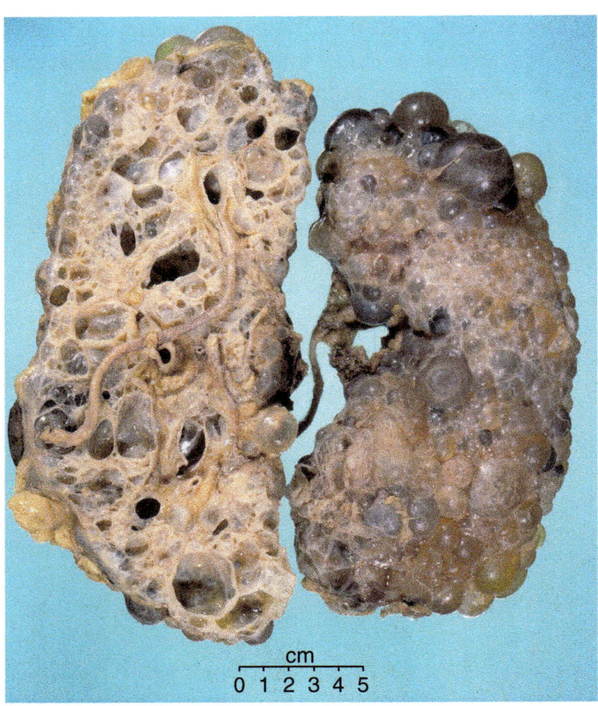

Answers to Case 2.9

1. Both the CT (Fig. 2.9.1a) and USS (Fig. 2.9.1b) images show multiple bilateral renal cysts. Although no pre contrast CT is available to fully characterise the cysts, the overall appearances are of numerous bilateral simple (or Bosniak type 1 cysts). One to three simple cysts in this age group would be consistent with normal age related simple cysts, but the numerous bilateral cysts as seen in this case, is in keeping with an underlying renal cystic syndrome.
2. In an adult, the most common renal cystic syndromes are autosomal dominant polycystic kidney disease (ADPKD), von Hippel Lindau (VHL) disease, tuberous sclerosis (TS).
3. The family history of possible subarachnoid haemorrhage makes ADPKD most likely, as this is associated with intra-cerebral aneurysms. This condition is associated with at least two different genetic mutations: ADPKD1 on chromosome 16p in 85–90% of patients, ADPKD2 on chromosome 4q in 5–15%.
4. Associations and complications are listed below:
   - Renal: Large kidneys with multiple renal cysts which can become infected or haemorrhage. Pain and haematuria. Progressive renal failure – 50% develop end stage renal failure. Calculi and renal cyst calcification
   - Other cysts: liver, pancreas, seminal vesicles, testis, ovary
   - Cardiovascular: hypertension, thoracic aortic aneurysm
   - Neurological: Berry aneurysm causing subarachnoid haemorrhage.
5. Figure 2.9.2 shows bilateral nephrectomy specimens for ADPK prior to transplantation showing cut and outer surfaces. The kidney parenchyma is replaced by cysts of varying size with focal haemorrhage. Nephrectomy is performed in these cases in the event of pain, due to size, bleeding, cystic infection or malignant transformation.

Further Reading

Wilson PD. Polycystic kidney disease. *N Engl J Med.* 2004;350(2):151–164.

Case 2.10

1. Describe the CT findings in Figs. 2.10.1a,b and 2.10.2a,b and the abnormality seen in the kidney specimens Figs 2.10.1c and 2.10.2c and d.
2. What is the Bosniak classification for these lesions? What are the CT features of lesions with this Bosniak classification?
3. What is the likelihood of malignancy?
4. What is meant by a renal protocol CT?

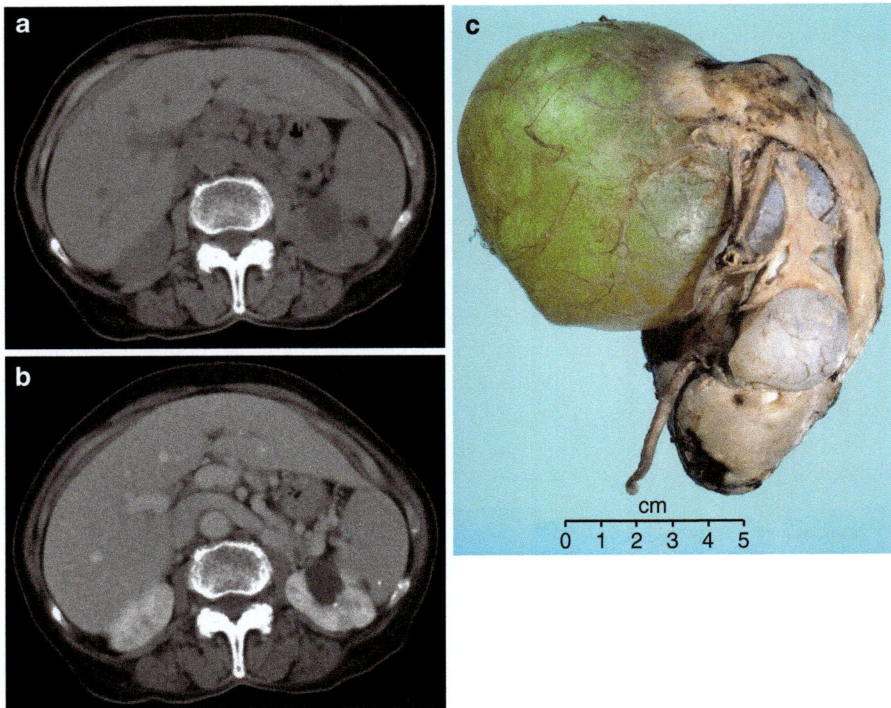

Fig. 2.10.1

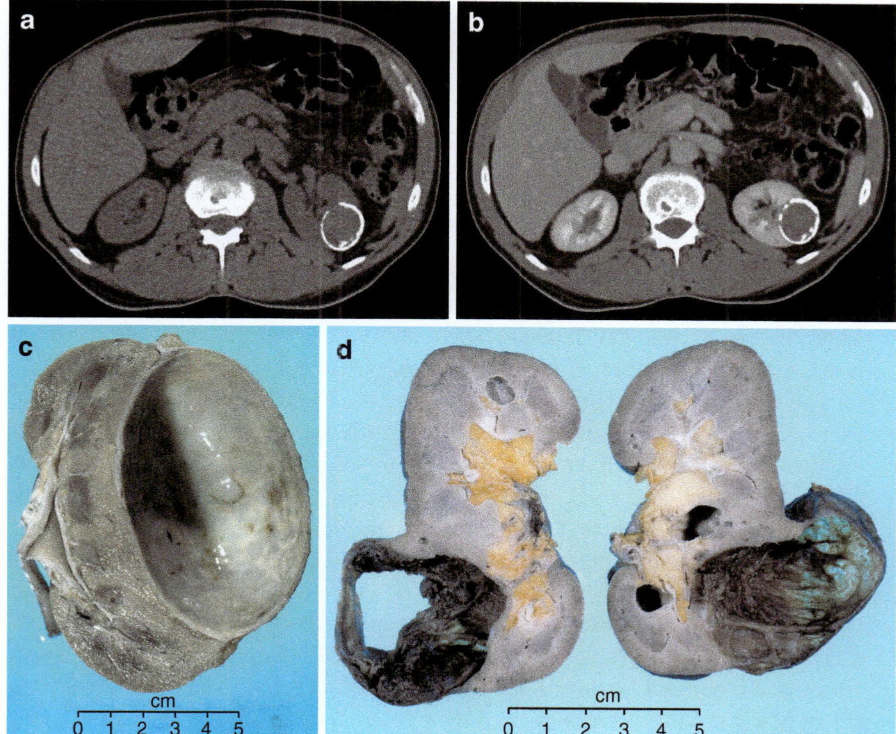

Fig. 2.10.2

Answers to Case 2.10

1. Figure 2.10.1a,b are pre- and post-contrast axial CT images through the upper abdomen showing a simple cyst in the upper pole of the left kidney. There is no evidence of wall-thickening, septations, enhancement or calcification. Figure 2.10.2a,b pre- and postcontrast axial CT images through the upper abdomen showing a cystic left renal lesion with thick peripheral calcification. There is no evidence of septation, enhancement or solid elements. Figure 2.10.1c is a nephrectomy specimen including a large simple upper pole cyst. Its straw coloured fluid content is visible through its very thin wall.
2. Figure 2.10.1a,b show a Bosniak type I cyst. As it is a single cyst it is a simple age related renal cyst. A Bosniak I cyst is a simple benign cyst with a hairline-thin wall that does not contain septa, calcification or solid components. It has the same density as water (CT density < 20 units), does not enhance with contrast and has a sharp interface with adjacent renal parenchyma.

   The CT features of typical type II cysts may include a few hairline-thin septa, thin calcification in the wall or septa. Hyperdense cysts are uniformly high-attenuation lesions of <3 cm. Type II cysts do not enhance. The cyst shown here (Figure 2.10.2a,b) has thick peripheral calcification and is classified as Bosniak IIF (Follow-up). These cysts might contain more hairline-thin septa, minimal enhancement of a hairline-thin septum or wall may be seen and there may be minimal thickening of the septa or wall. The cyst may contain calcification that might be nodular and thick, as here, but there is no contrast enhancement and there are no enhancing soft-tissue elements. The follow-up protocols for Bosniak IIF cysts are currently not well defined, one protocol is to repeat the study (either CT or MRI) at 6 and 12 months, and then yearly for 3 years.

   Figure 2.10.2c is the cut surface of a kidney including a large unilocular cyst with fibrous wall and areas of calcification, this would appear as a Bosniak II cyst on CT imaging. Figure 2.10.2d is a bisected kidney including cysts of various size. The lower pole cyst shows evidence of previous haemorrhage and is transected by septa.
3. There is no chance of malignancy with Type I cysts, except in von Hippel Lindau disease when any renal cyst can undergo malignant transformation. The majority of Bosniak II cysts are benign, less than 15% Bosniak IIF cysts are malignant.
4. The renal mass protocol CT includes a pre and post contrast fine cut CT focused on the kidneys. The timings of the post contrast study may vary from 45–120 s, but most favour 60–90 s. With the benefit of a pre and post contrast study enhancement can be objectively evaluated – a >20 unit density change after contrast implies vascularised tissue, and this is a key evaluation when searching for neo-vascularity. But benign pathology, such as inflammation, can also show enhancement in the same manner, thus a renal mass should always be evaluated in the context of the clinical setting.

Further Reading

Israel GM, Bosniak MA. How I do it: evaluating renal masses. *Radiology*. 2005;236(2):441–450.

Case 2.11

A 55-year-old man presented with macroscopic haematuria.

1. What are the findings on CT?
2. What is the Bosniak classification for this lesion? What are the other CT features of lesions with this Bosniak classification?
3. What is the likelihood of malignancy? Describe the management options.

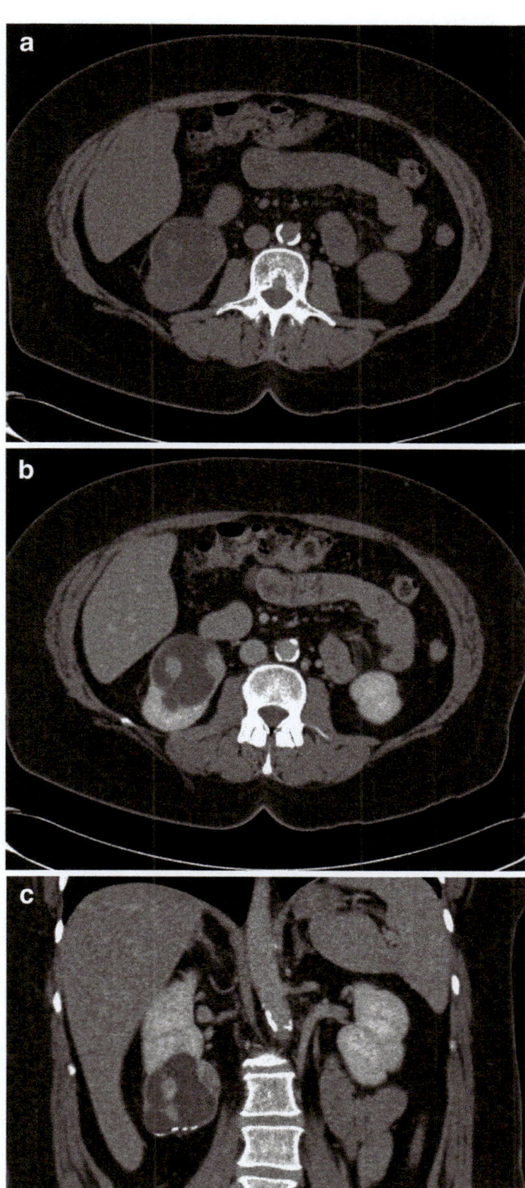

Fig. 2.11.1

Answers to Case 2.11

1. Figure 2.11.1a,b,c are CT images through the upper abdomen. There is an exophytic multilocular cystic lesion arising from the anterior aspect of the lower pole of the right kidney. This demonstrates nodular wall thickening and multiple enhancing nodular septations within it.
2. This is a Bosniak type 3 cyst. Other CT features that may be seen with a type 3 cyst are thick or irregular calcification, irregular margin or nodularity or a non-enhancing nodular cyst.
3. With a type 3 cyst the likelihood of malignancy is 50% (ranging from 30 to 60%), and surgery (partial or total nephrectomy) is indicated in many of these patients. Patients who are not suitable for surgery due to co-morbidity may be considered for minimally invasive treatment such as cryotherapy or radiofrequency ablation. Where the history or clinical findings strongly suggest an alternative diagnosis (such as infection) interval follow-up or biopsy of the lesion may be indicated.

Further Reading

Israel GM, Bosniak MA. How I do it: evaluating renal masses. *Radiology*. 2005; 236(2):441–450.

Case 2.12

This abnormality was an incidental finding on ultrasound examination for suspected abdominal aortic aneurysm, and a renal protocol CT was later undertaken.

1. Describe the USS and CT findings. What is the Bosniak classification for this lesion? What are the CT features of lesions with this Bosniak classification?
2. What is the differential diagnosis?
3. What is the likelihood of malignancy?
4. Describe the nephrectomy specimen Fig. 2.12.2.

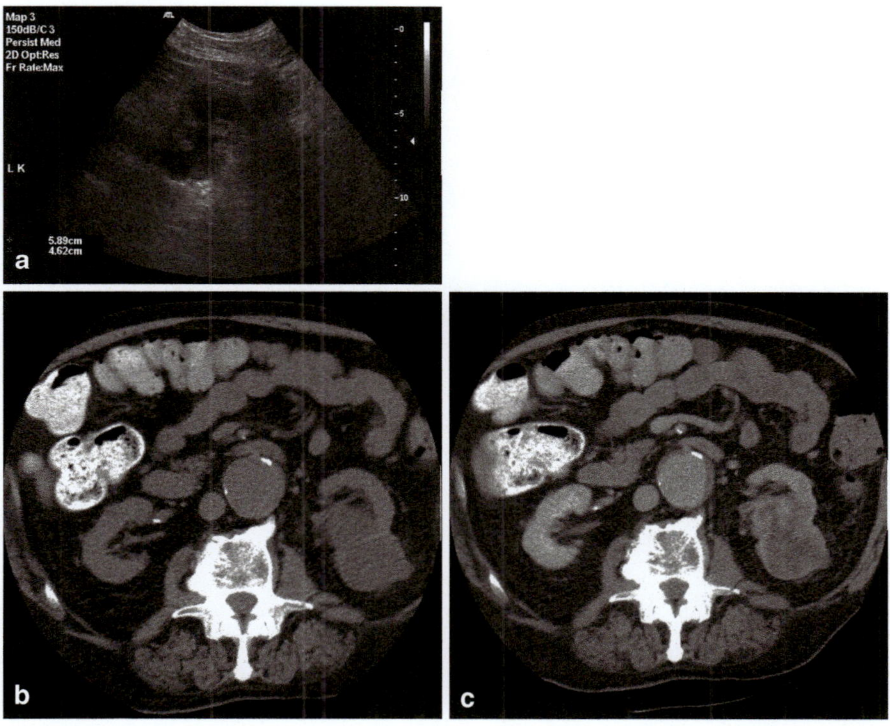

Fig. 2.12.1

Fig. 2.12.2

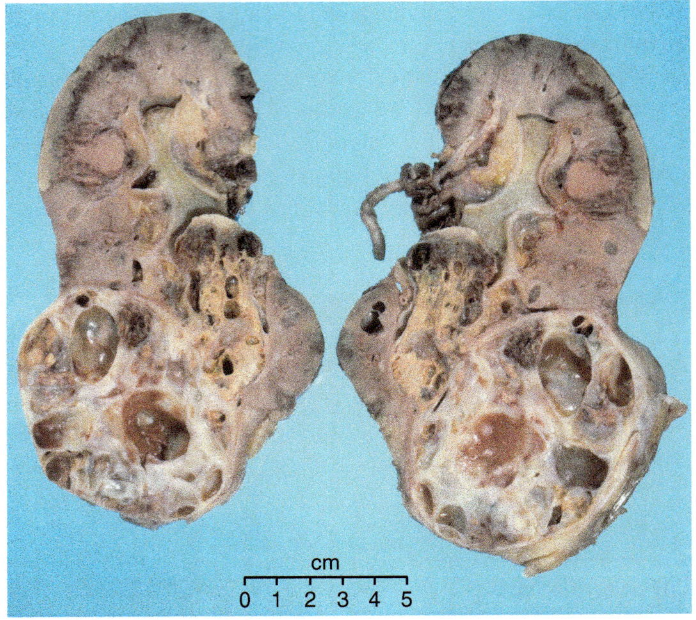

Answers to Case 2.12

1. Figure 2.12.1a is an ultrasound, and Fig. 2.12.1b, c are pre- and postcontrast axial CT images, respectively, through the upper abdomen showing a partially enhancing, cystic left renal mass. On CT it has a low density centre, which on US is seen to be cystic (note the posterior acoustic enhancement on ultrasound – posterior enhancement implies a water like density). Thus this is a complex cyst, or possibly a solid mass that has undergone central liquefaction or necrosis – either way it is a Bosniak IV cyst.
2. An abscess is unlikely in an asymptomatic patient, especially as there are no surrounding perinephric changes that would be expected with an inflammatory mass. In an asymptomatic patient, this is most likely a malignant cystic mass. Metastasis is also unlikely, unless the patient has a history of concurrent active non-renal malignancy.
3. The likelihood of malignancy is nearly 100% with a Bosniak type IV cyst.
4. Figure 2.12.2 is the cut surface of a nephrectomy specimen showing a cystic renal mass with adjacent solid yellow areas replacing the lower pole and bulging into the renal pelvis. These appearances would be consistent with a Bosniak type IV cyst on CT. Microscopy revealed a clear cell renal call carcinoma (RCC).

Further Reading

Israel GM, Bosniak MA. How I do it: evaluating renal masses. *Radiology*. 2005;236(2):441–450.

Case 2.13

A 30-year-old women presents with non-specific chronic back pain.

1. Describe images 2.13.1a–c. What is the diagnosis?
2. What is the aetiology of the mass?
3. What are the potential complications of this condition?
4. What procedure has been performed in Fig. 2.13.2?
5. What is shown in the nephrectomy specimen Fig. 2.13.3

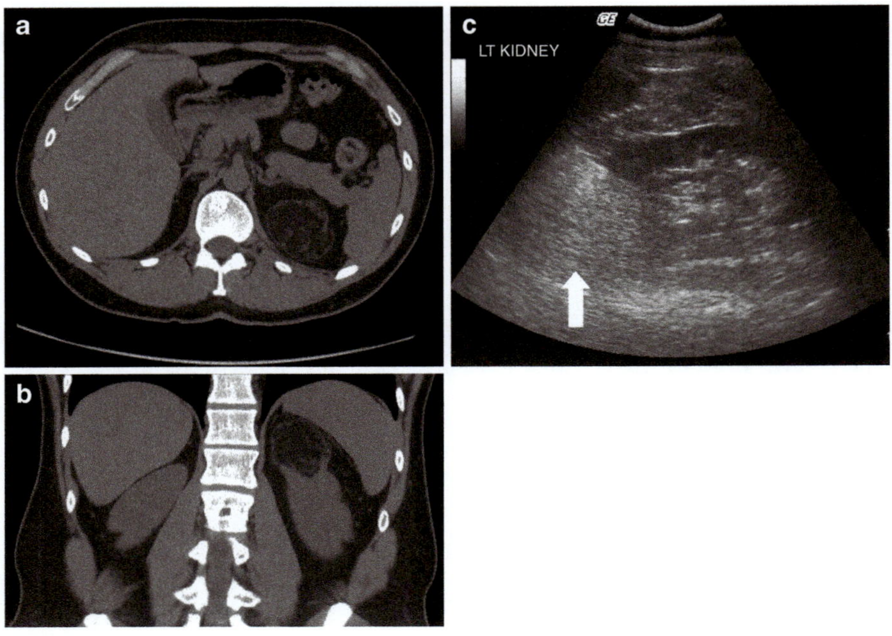

Fig. 2.13.1

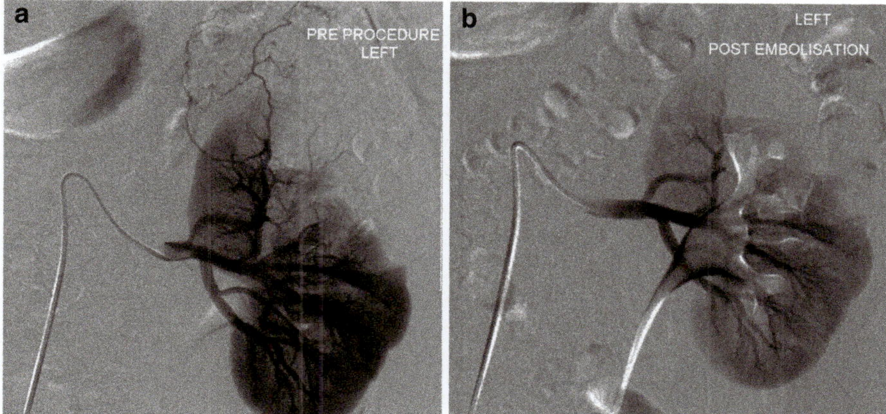

Fig. 2.13.2

Fig. 2.13.3

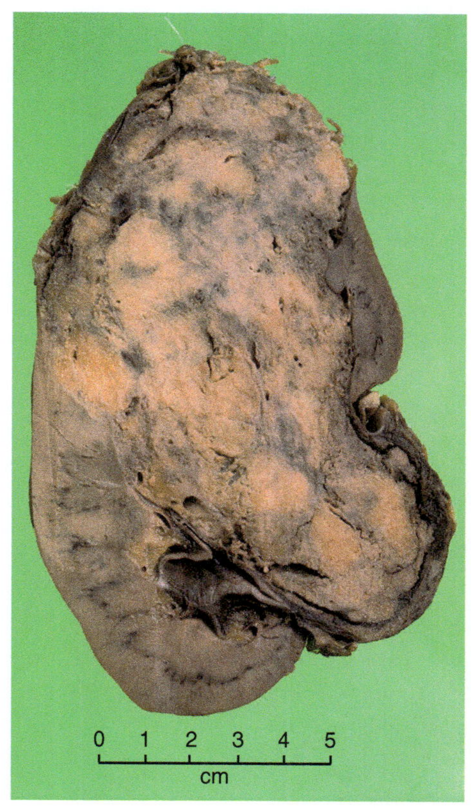

Answers to Case 2.13

1. Axial (Fig. 2.13.1a) and coronal (Fig. 2.13.1b) non-contrast CT images of the upper abdomen, and an ultrasound image (Fig. 2.13.1c) of the left kidney showing an exophytic mass in the upper pole of the left kidney. This mass has similar density to the subcutaneous and retroperitoneal fat on both CT and USS. The diagnosis is angiomyolipoma (AML). Diagnosis can be made on CT (or MRI) if the mass has a density of <0 HU (or is fatty on T1 MRI), but some atypical fat-poor AMLs have a higher density.
2. AML is a hamartoma including various proportions of adipose tissue, spindle and epithelioid smooth muscle and abnormal blood vessels. Approximately 80% are solitary and sporadic, 20% are multifocal and associated with tuberous sclerosis. Tuberose Sclerosis (TS), an inherited autosomal dominant syndrome, is caused by mutation of either of two genes, TSC1 and TSC2 located on chromosomes 9q34 and 16p13, respectively. The vast majority of AMLs are benign, but rare malignant variants have been described. Sporadic cases are more common in females (4:1); there is no apparent sex predilection in TS patients. The increased incidence of sporadic AML in females and their increased growth rate in pregnancy, the onset of AML after puberty and progesterone immunoreactivity support a hormonal influence.
3. The majority of tumours are asymptomatic, but symptoms include abdominal/flank pain, hypertension, weight loss and nausea. Tumours >4 cm have an increased risk of spontaneous haemorrhage (Wunderlich syndrome), which may be catastrophic, and therefore this is usually deemed as the threshold for prophylactic treatment – ideally with a nephron preserving procedure such as embolisation or partial nephrectomy.
4. Figure 2.13.2a,b are arteriograms of the left renal artery before and after selective embolisation of the branch feeding the AML. No residual flow is seen within the vessel following embolisation, but the tumour can recur in the long term, especially in patients with TS.
5. Figure 2.13.3 is the cut surface of a nephrectomy specimen showing a heterogeneous mass expanding the upper pole and bulging into the hilum. The macroscopic predominance of fat and the presence of obvious transected vascular lumena is typical of AML. This diagnosis was confirmed by the microscopic identification of all the tissues described in answer 2.

Further Reading

Sooriakumaran P, Gibbs P, Coughlin G, Attard V, Elmslie F, Kingswood C, Taylor J, Corbishley C, Patel U, Anderson C. Angiomyolipomata: challenges, solutions, and future prospects based on over 100 cases treated. *BJU Int.* 2010;105(1):101–106.

Case 2.14

A 65-year-old gentleman complained of intermittent flank pain and underwent a CT scan.

1. Describe the findings and differential diagnosis. What is the likely diagnosis here?
2. Are there any CT features which are specific to this condition?
3. Which other radiological investigation may be useful?
4. The nephrectomy specimen shows a solitary lesion with the same pathological diagnosis, describe what you see.

Fig. 2.14.1

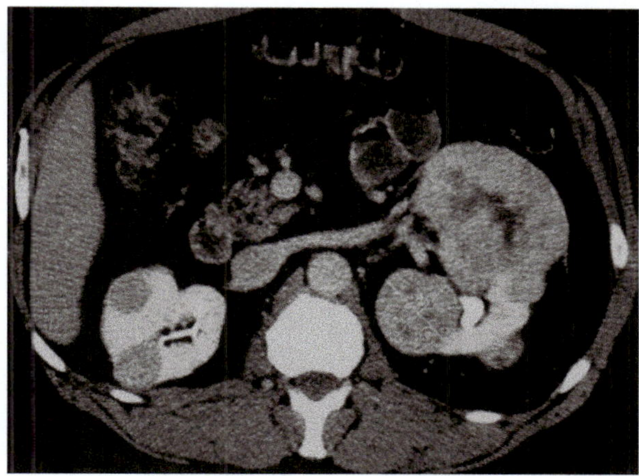

Fig. 2.14.2

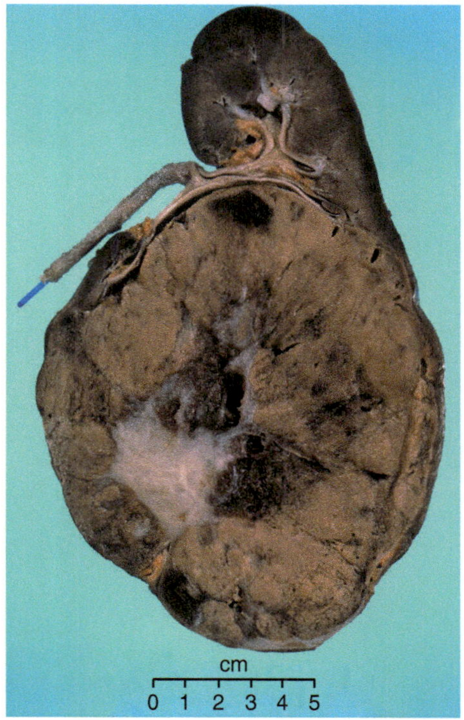

Answers to Case 2.14

1. Figure 2.14.1 is an axial CT showing multiple well-demarcated solid enhancing masses in both kidneys. The largest in the left kidney contains a central low attenuation scar. The appearances are non-specific and the differential diagnosis includes multiple renal cell carcinomas, renal metastasis, renal lymphoma and multiple oncocytomas. Multiple angiomyolipoma are unlikely because of the absence of fat. Bilateral pyelonephritis can rarely present with multiple focal areas of altered enhancement, but there would be a history of infection. The central stellate scar within the largest mass suggests oncocytoma but this is not diagnostic.
2. There are no firm diagnostic features of oncocytoma. Oncocytomas are benign tumours in which the predominant cell, the 'oncocyte' has deeply eosinophilic, copious glassy cytoplasm containing numerous mitochondria with a dearth of other organelles. Pre operative biopsy may not aid the diagnosis because well-differentiated renal carcinomas may contain eosinophilic cells, and up to 30% of tumours that are predominantly oncocytomas contain foci of clear cells, typical of some renal carcinomas.
3. Angiography typically demonstrates a 'spoke-wheel' configuration of radiating vessels, but is now rarely used. MRI does not provide any additional information.
4. Figure 2.14.2 is the cut surface of a nephrectomy specimen containing a well circumscribed brown tumour with a central scar expanding the lower pole. Light and electron microscopy showed the typical features of oncocytoma, as described in answer 2.

Further Reading

Gudbjartsson T, Hardarson S, Petursdottir V, Thoroddsen A, Magnusson J, Einarsson GV. Renal oncocytoma: a clinicopathological analysis of 45 consecutive cases. *BJU Int.* 2005;96:1275–1279.

Tickoo SK. Pathologic features of renal cortical tumors. *Urol Clin N Am.* 2008;35:551–561.

Case 2.15

These are the radiological images of a 58-year-old woman, who presented with haematuria and flank discomfort.

1. Describe what you see on her CT and US scans?
2. What is the differential diagnosis, and what findings would favour each?
3. What does the nephrectomy specimen (Fig. 2.15.2) show?
4. Describe the management options?

Fig. 2.15.1

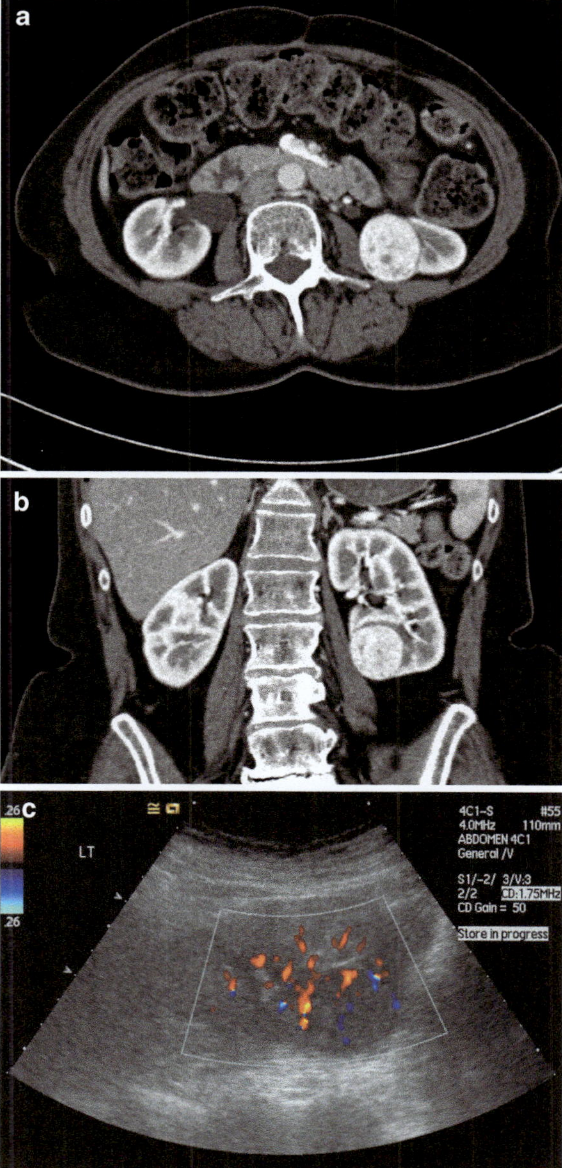

Fig. 2.15.2

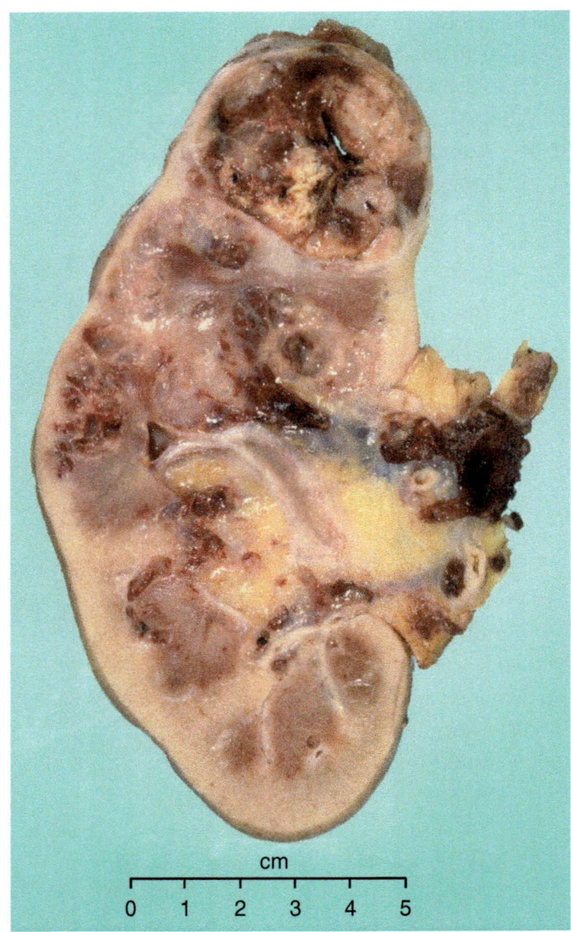

Answers to Case 2.15

1. Figure 2.15.1a axial and Fig. 2.15.1b coronal postcontrast CT images through the upper abdomen showing an enhancing exophytic mass in the lower pole of the right kidney. This lesion is hypoechoic and vascular on ultrasound (as seen in Fig. 2.15.1c).
2. The differential diagnosis includes:
   - Renal cell cancer (RCC) – more likely if there is renal vein involvement.
   - Transitional cell cancer (TCC) – more likely if there is renal pelvic / ureteric involvement or a synchronous urothelial lesion elsewhere.
   - Oncocytoma – a central scar may be present , but as discussed in Case 2.14 this is not always seen.
   - Fat-poor angiomyolipoma (AML) a rare variant of AML, more likely if the patient has tuberous sclerosis.
   - Lymphoma – consider if there is lymphoma elsewhere.
   - Metastasis from another primary – probable if the renal mass follows the course of the disease elsewhere.

   This proved to be a renal cell cancer. Most large renal masses are likely to be RCCs, but a large minority (up to 30% in some series) of small (<3 cm) incidental renal masses are proving to be non-RCCs in contemporary series, either oncocytomas or angiomyolipomas.
3. Figure 2.15.2 is the cut surface of a kidney showing a yellow, haemorrhagic tumour replacing the upper pole, invading veins and distorting the hilum. Microscopy showed clear cell RCC.
4. Management has to be tailored to the patient, taking account of their age and co-morbidity, and also the likely tumour type.
   - Small masses may be monitored – there is a negligible metastatic risk if the tumour is <3 cm.
   - Excision via (radical or partial) nephrectomy.
   - Ablative therapy – either cryotherapy or radiofrequency ablation.
   - Percutaneous biopsy under CT or ultrasound guidance may help determine the cell type and help the most appropriate therapy to be chosen. As discussed above, not all small, incidental renal masses are malignant.

Further Reading

Russo P. Partial nephrectomy for renal cancer: part I. *BJU Int.* 2010;105(9): 1206–1220.

Case 2.16

1. A 28-year-old female patient with pancreatic insufficiency was found to have multiple renal cysts on routine imaging. Describe the findings on her CT scan.
2. What is the likely unifying diagnosis?
3. What are the non-renal manifestations of this condition?
4. What is the risk of renal malignancy in this patient and how should she be followed-up?
5. Describe what you see in the nephrectomy specimen (Fig. 2.16.2), what tumour subtype are these likely to be.

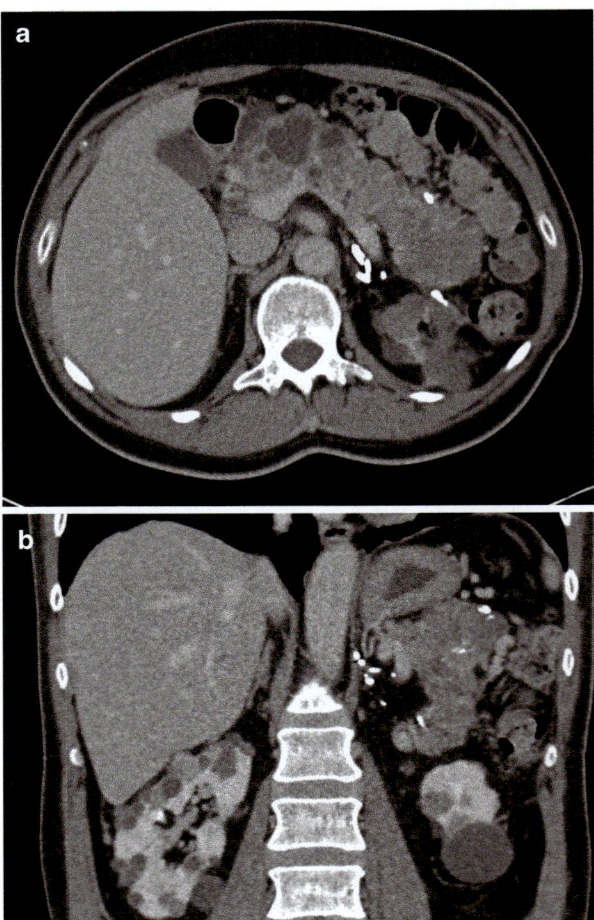

Fig. 2.16.1

Fig. 2.16.2

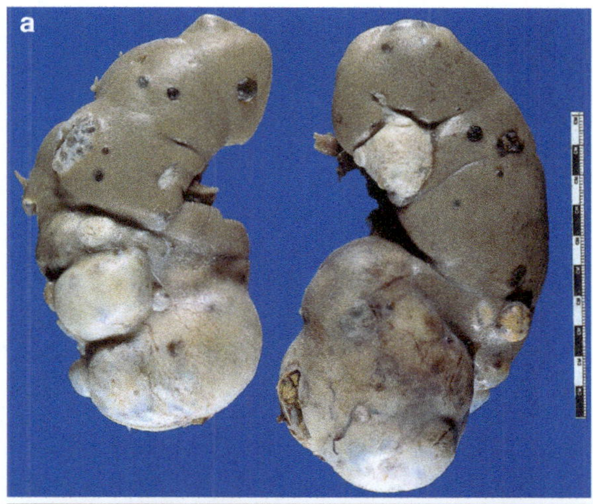

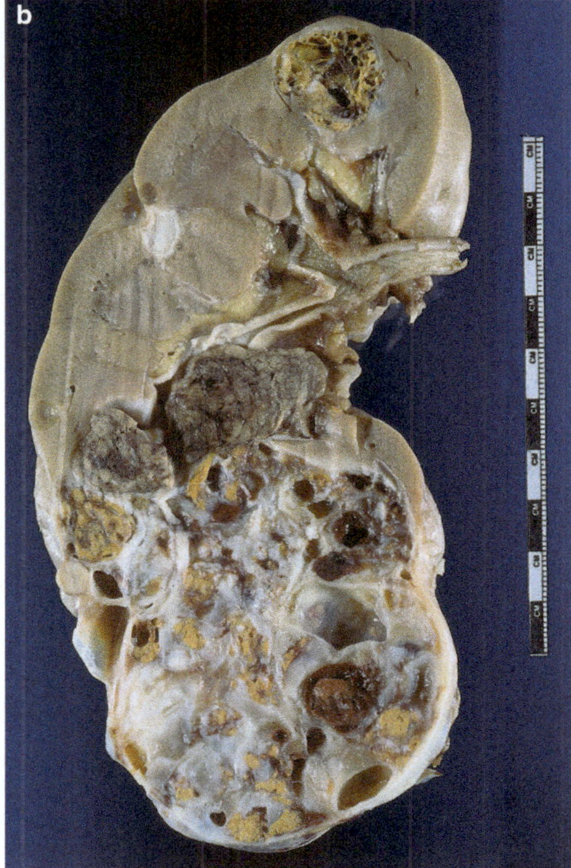

Answers to Case 2.16

1. Axial (Fig. 2.16.1a) and coronal (Fig. 2.16.1b) post-contrast CT images through the upper abdomen. There are multiple cysts within the pancreas and kidneys. The renal cysts are seen to be of a variety of types, from simple cysts to some more complex ones with thick walls and at least one appears virtually solid. Multiple pancreatic and renal cysts of a variety of types are characteristic of von Hippel Lindau (VHL) disease.
2. von-Hippel Lindau disease is an autosomal dominant condition. The von Hippel-Lindau gene is located on the short arm of chromosome 3 (3p26–p25), only 20% are familial, the rest are sporadic mutations.
3. The non-renal manifestations of this condition are capillary haemangioblastomas of the CNS and retina, phaeochromocytomas, pancreatic cysts and tumours, neuroendocrine tumours, endolymphatic sac tumours of the inner ear and cystadenomas of the epididymis and broad ligament.
4. There is a high risk of renal malignancy with this condition and 20–45% of patients with VHL will develop renal cell carcinoma and up to 70% of patients if they reach the age of 60 years. Renal carcinoma is the leading cause of death in these patients, followed by CNS haemangioblastomas (most commonly in the cerebellum or spinal cord). In the images shown one or two of the masses are malignant on conventional CT criteria (those with thick, nodular enhancing walls).

   Renal cysts form a histopathological continuum ranging from benign cysts (with one to two cell layers of bland epithelium), atypical cysts (demonstrating epithelial hyperplasia with or without mild cytologic atypia), to malignant cysts harbouring RCC. The presence of atypia or foci of carcinoma does not correlate with cyst size. Furthermore, lesions that appear radiologically or grossly solid range from conventional solid RCC, to predominantly hyalinized, fibrotic nodules.

   In contrast to simple cysts occurring in the general population, which are virtually always benign, renal cysts in patients with von Hippel-Lindau disease may contain occult carcinoma. Radiologic evaluation, visual inspection at surgery and even frozen section analysis of cystic lesions cannot be relied on to detect small foci of carcinoma. Close surveillance is therefore mandatory. Repeated nephron sparing procedures (ablation or partial nephrectomy) is the treatment of choice, but the decision regarding when to intervene is often difficult to reach in the presence of so many renal masses.
5. A large lower pole yellow cystic tumour is seen in addition to several smaller tumours and cysts of varying size, scattered throughout the parenchyma. Microscopy confirmed that all the tumours were of clear cell type.

Further Reading

Coleman JA. Familial and hereditary renal cancer syndromes. *Urol Clin N Am.* 2008;35:563–572.

Meister M, Choyke P, Anderson C, Patel U. Radiological evaluation, management, and surveillance of renal masses in Von Hippel-Lindau disease. *Clin Radiol.* 2009;64(6):589–600.

Solomon D, Schwartz A. Renal pathology in von Hippel-Lindau disease. *Hum Pathol.* 1988;19(9):1072–1079.

Case 2.17

A 67-year-old man presented with macroscopic haematuria. Cystoscopy was normal.

1. Describe the findings and likely diagnosis.
2. What is the differential diagnosis?
3. How would you manage this patient?
4. Describe what you see in the nephrectomy specimen (Fig. 2.17.2).

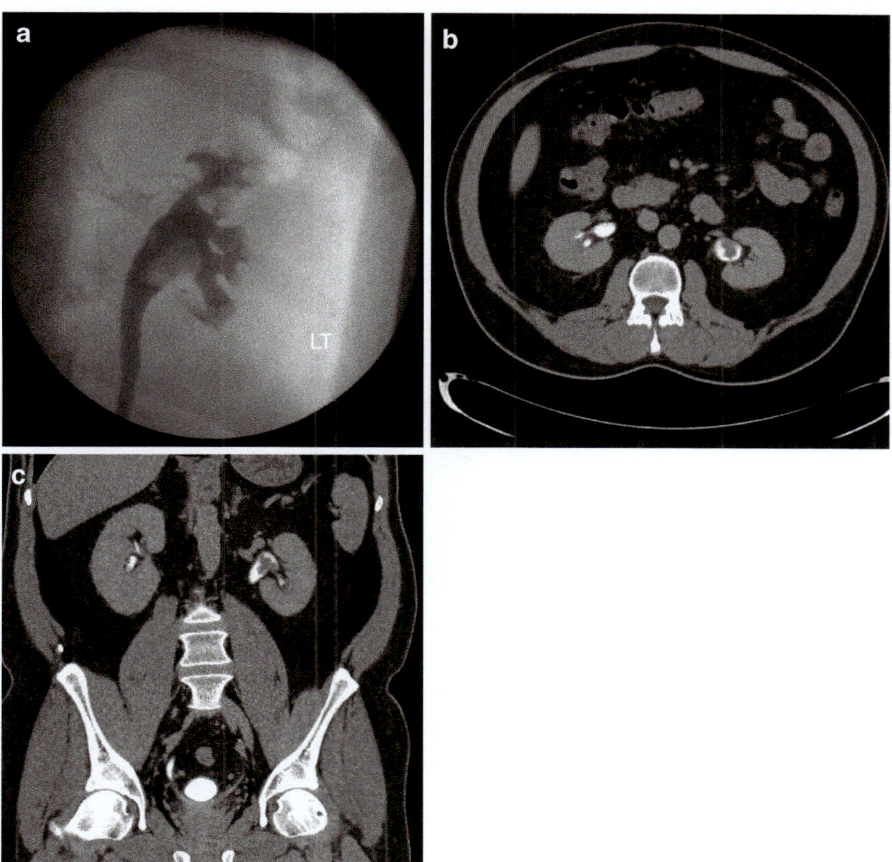

Fig. 2.17.1

Fig. 2.17.2

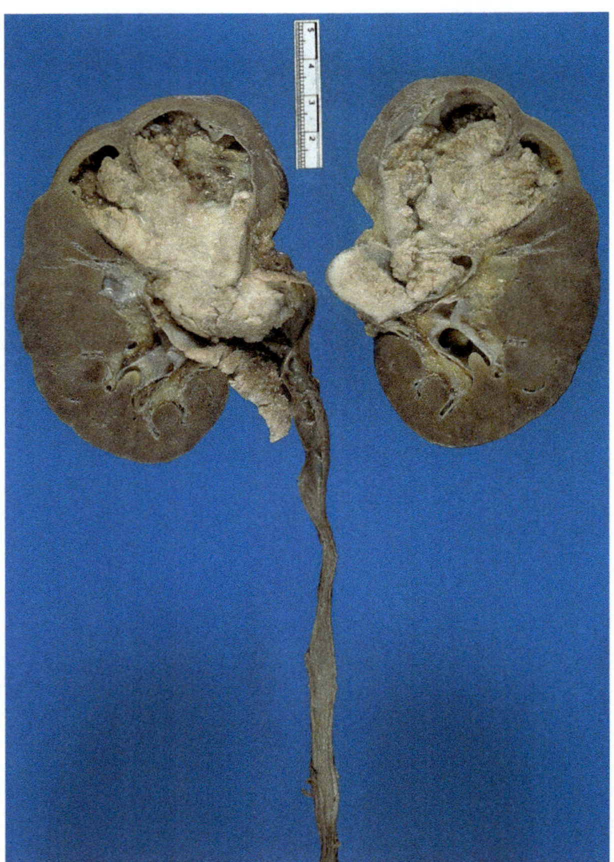

Answers to Case 2.17

1. Figure 2.17.1a is a retrograde pyelogram demonstrating a well-defined filling defect within the inferior aspect of the left renal pelvis. (Note that retrograde pyelogram images can be differentiated from IVU images as the kidneys and the renal parenchyma are not seen in an enhanced state in the former). Axial (Fig. 2.17.1b) and coronal (Fig. 2.17.1c) CT images demonstrate good contrast opacification of the renal collecting systems and confirm a mass-like filling defect within the left renal pelvis. There is no local infiltration.
2. The appearances are suspicious for transitional cell carcinoma, but the differential diagnosis for a filling defect within the collecting system includes a blood clot, radiolucent calculus, sloughed papilla, gas (from instrumentation or a gas forming organism) and pyeloureteritis cystica. The CT study shown has been performed in the excretory phase to optimally visualise the renal collecting system i.e. a CT urogram. Protocols vary between units, but the usual delay in scanning post-intravenous contrast is between 5 and 15 min. Longer imaging delays improve distension of the proximal urinary tract and may aid in visualisation of the lower segment of the ureter.
3. The diagnosis of upper tract TCC should be confirmed, either by urinary cytology or ideally by ureteroscopic biopsy, as this will better stage and grade the tumour. If this proves to be a localised tumour, with no contralateral upper tract tumour, then nephro-ureterectomy offers the best hope of cure. Endoscopic management may be used in selected patients with: smaller, low grade tumours; bilateral upper tract TCCs; a solitary kidney; chronic kidney disease.

   After a diagnosis of non-muscle invasive bladder cancer the incidence of upper tract TCC is 1.8%, the risk is 7.5% if the bladder tumour involves the trigone. The incidence of developing a bladder tumour after an upper tract TCC is 15–50% – these metachronous tumours occur most commonly within the first two years of diagnosis and are thought to be due either to tumour cell seeding or the pan-field effect.
4. The nephrectomy specimen demonstrates a papillary transitional cell carcinoma which is arising from and distending the renal pelvis and upper pole calyces and is associated with loss of renal parenchyma.

Further Reading

Babjuk M, Oosterlinck W, Sylvester R, Kaasinen E, Böhle A, Palou J, Rouprêt M. EAU guidelines on TaT1 (non-muscle invasive) bladder cancer. 2010.

Raman JD, Scherr DS. Management of patients with upper urinary tract transitional cell carcinoma. *Nat Clin Pract Urol.* 2007;4(8):432–443.

Vikram R, Sandler CM, Ng CS. Imaging and staging of transitional cell carcinoma: part 2, upper urinary tract. *AJR Am J Roentgenol.* 2009;192(6):1488–1493.

Case 2.18

This patient presented with a history of flank discomfort and weight loss.

1. Describe the findings on these CT images (Fig. 2.18.1a,b).
2. What is the diagnosis and what are the different patterns of renal involvement in this condition (an example is shown in Fig. 2.18.2a–c, from another patient)?
3. What is the likely prognosis?

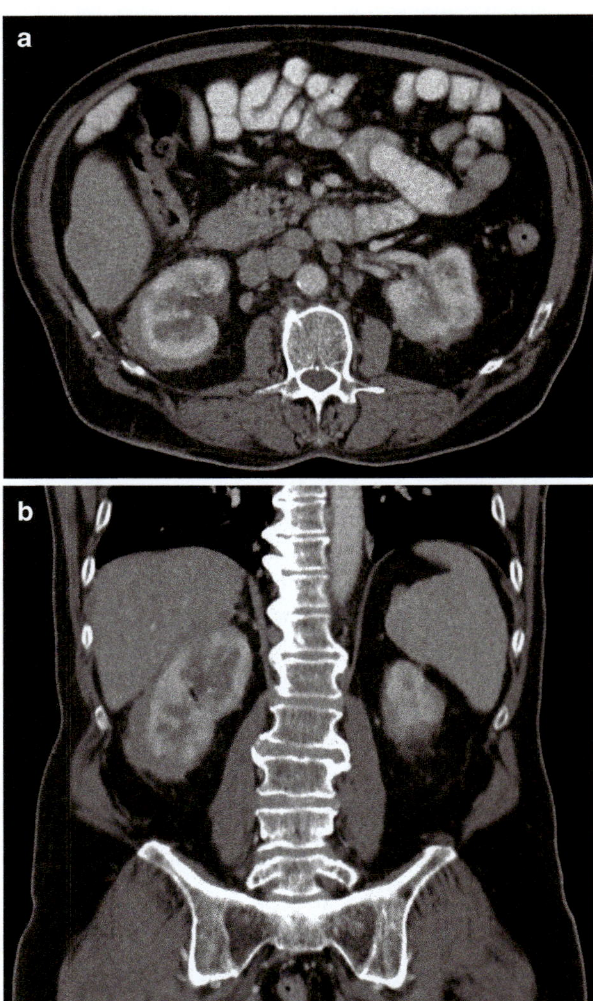

Fig. 2.18.1

Fig. 2.18.2

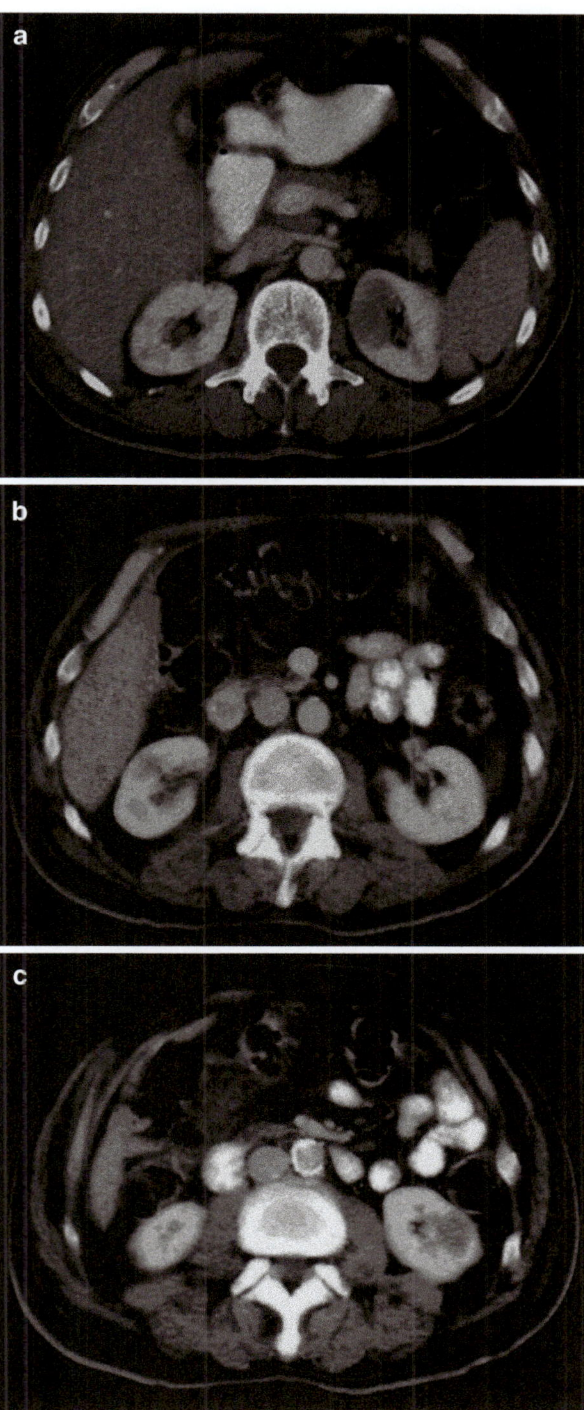

Answers to Case 2.18

1. Figure 2.18.1a,b are CT images showing poorly-enhancing soft tissue encasing both kidneys without parenchymal compression. There are no distinct renal masses seen, but the parenchymal enhancement pattern is irregular. Enlarged para-aortic lymph nodes are also seen.
2. These images demonstrate one of the described patterns of renal lymphoma, others relate to the different mechanisms of spread to the kidneys.
   - The most common CT manifestation (in 40–60%) is shown in Fig. 2.18.2a–c, with multiple bilateral ball-shaped renal masses which reflects haematogenous dissemination.
   - Solitary masses are less common (10–20%).
   - Contiguous invasion from retroperitoneal tissues (in 30%) is highly characteristic of renal lymphoma – typically a large, bulky retroperitoneal mass encases the renal vasculature and invades the renal hilum and parenchyma. Patients commonly present with hydronephrosis. This can be mimicked by retroperitoneal fibrosis.
   - Diffuse infiltrative disease (20%) is associated with lymphomatous proliferation within the interstitium of the kidney, which presents as global renal enlargement, with preservation of renal contour. This diagnosis is often subtle and may manifest as insidious loss of renal function.
   - Perirenal lymphoma as seen in Fig. 2.18.1a,b, in the absence of retroperitoneal nodes or parenchymal involvement is rare. This can present a diagnostic difficulty as rarely retroperitoneal fibrosis and extra-medullary haemopoiesis can present with similar CT findings.
3. The diagnosis is lymphoma with a poor prognosis as renal involvement usually indicates disseminated disease. Although only 3–8% of patients with lymphoma have CT evidence of renal involvement autopsy studies demonstrate infiltration in 34–68% of such patients. Primary renal lymphomas are rare and of these post transplant lymphoproliferative disorder is most frequently seen, thought to be the result of EBV infection during immunosuppressive therapy.

Further Reading

Urban BA, Fishman EK. Renal lymphoma: CT patterns with emphasis on helical CT. *Radiographics*. 2000;20(1):197–212.

Case 2.19

These are the images from three separate patients with the same condition. They all presented with microscopic haematuria.

1. Describe the findings on Fig. 2.19.1a,b.
2. Describe the finding on the Fig. 2.19.2a,b.
3. Describe the finding on Fig. 2.19.3.
4. Describe what you see in the close up of a renal papilla (Fig. 2.19.4). What is the diagnosis?

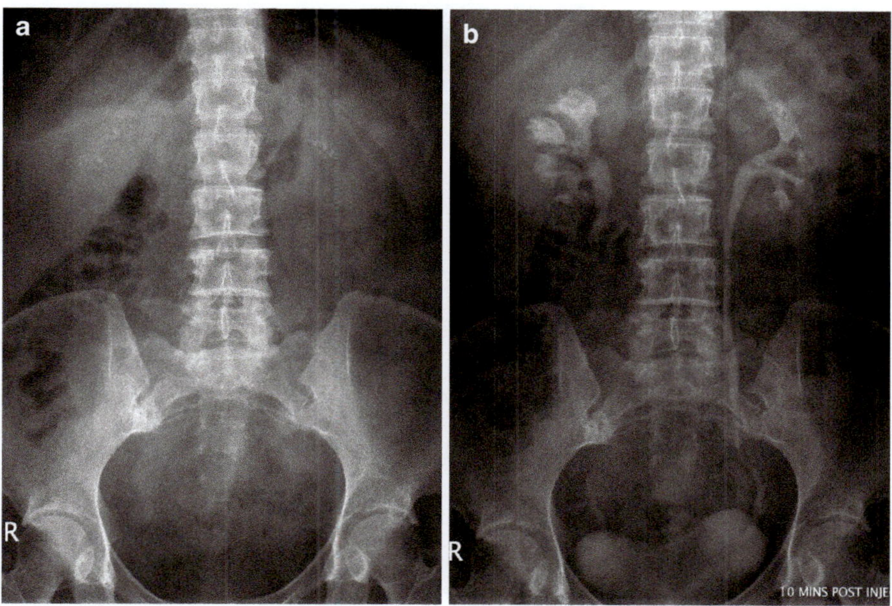

Fig. 2.19.1

Fig. 2.19.2

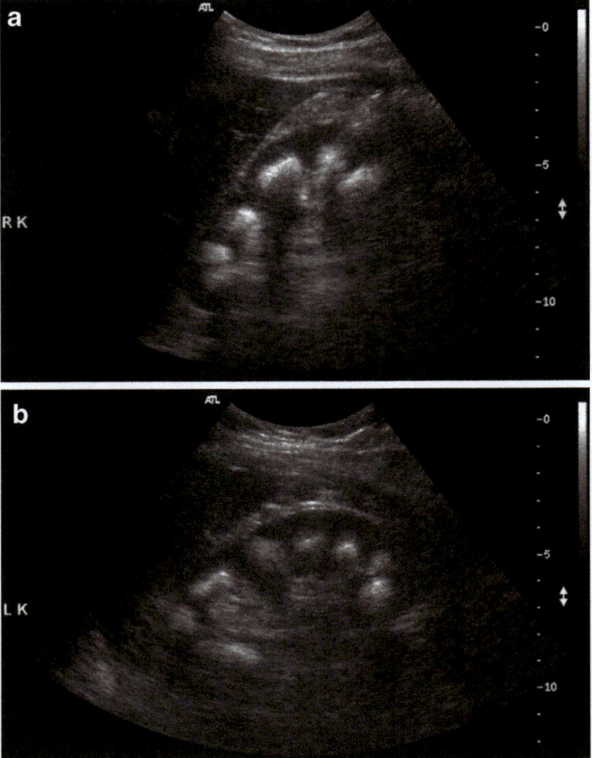

Fig. 2.19.3

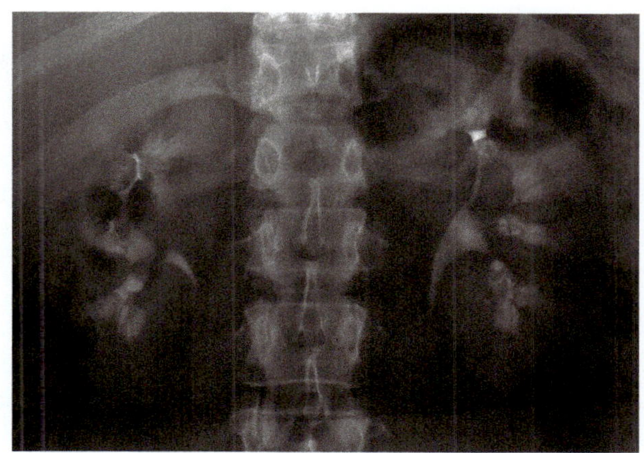

Fig. 2.19.4

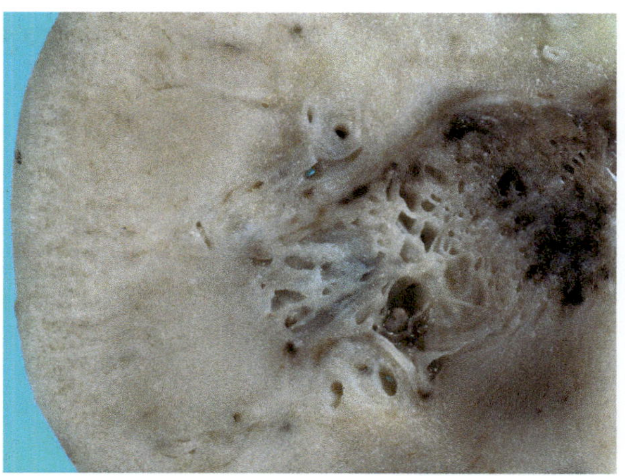

Answers to Case 2.19

1. Figure 2.19.1a is plain radiograph showing multiple clusters of calcification in both kidneys. The IVU post contrast film (Fig. 2.19.1b) demonstrates that although multiple calyceal calculi are possible, the calcification is relatively peripheral in location in the kidneys and likely to be parenchymal.
2. These ultrasound images (Fig. 2.19.2a,b) demonstrate symmetrical highly echogenic medullary pyramids, some seen to cast an acoustic shadow, and therefore represent multiple calcified renal pyramids. The reminder of the kidney is normal and there is no hydronephrosis. The appearances on this ultrasound image and the plain radiograph (Fig. 2.19.1) are the typical radiological appearances of nephrocalcinosis. More specifically it should be referred to as medullary nephrocalcinosis (to differentiate it from the much rarer pattern of cortical nephrocalcinosis). Nephrocalcinosis is a non-specific finding on plain radiography and the differential diagnosis includes hyperparathyroidism, renal tubular acidosis, medullary sponge kidney and, less commonly, primary hyperoxaluria and other causes for hypercalcaemia or hypercalciuria – milk-alkali syndrome, sarcoidosis, hypervitaminosis D.
3. The post-contrast film (Fig. 2.19.3) taken as part of an intravenous urogram series, demonstrates dense papillary blush with streaks of contrast material radiating from the medullary pyramids. The underlying calyces are broad and distorted.
4. The close up of the renal papilla (Fig. 2.19.4) shows ectasia and cyst-like cavities of the collecting ducts.

   The appearances of the radiological images (Fig. 2.19.3) and renal papilla are in keeping with medullary sponge kidney (MSK). MSK is usually bilateral, but may involve focal areas of a single kidney. MSK has been described as associated with many conditions, such as renal calculi, distal renal tubular acidosis, horseshoe kidney, renal artery stenosis, ureteric duplication, pyeloureteritis cystica, autosomal dominant polycystic kidney disease, Ehlers-Danlos syndrome and Beckwith-Wiedemann syndrome.

   IVU is currently the most accurate way of diagnosing MSK, though newer CT protocols show some promise. Early cases of MSK may not have any nephrocalcinosis, but the ectatic ducts will still be seen, as shown in Fig. 2.19.3.

Further Reading

Gambaro G, Feltrin GP, Lupo A, et al. Medullary sponge kidney (Lenarduzzi-Cacchi-Ricci disease): a Padua Medical School discovery in the 1930s. *Kidney Int.* 2006;69(4):663–670.

Gedroyc WM, Saxton HM. More medullary sponge variants. *Clin Radiol.* 1988;39(4):423–425.

Yendt ER. Medullary sponge kidney and nephrolithiasis. *N Engl J Med.* 1982;306(18):1106–1107.

Case 2.20

A 25-year-old male presents to the Emergency department with a 1 h history of left loin to groin pain. Microscopic haematuria is found on urine testing.

1. Describe the findings on the intravenous urogram.
2. Discuss the advantages and disadvantages of this investigation over alternative radiological modalities.
3. How would you manage and follow-up this patient?
4. Describe the macroscopic changes in the bisected nephrectomy specimen, what is the cause?

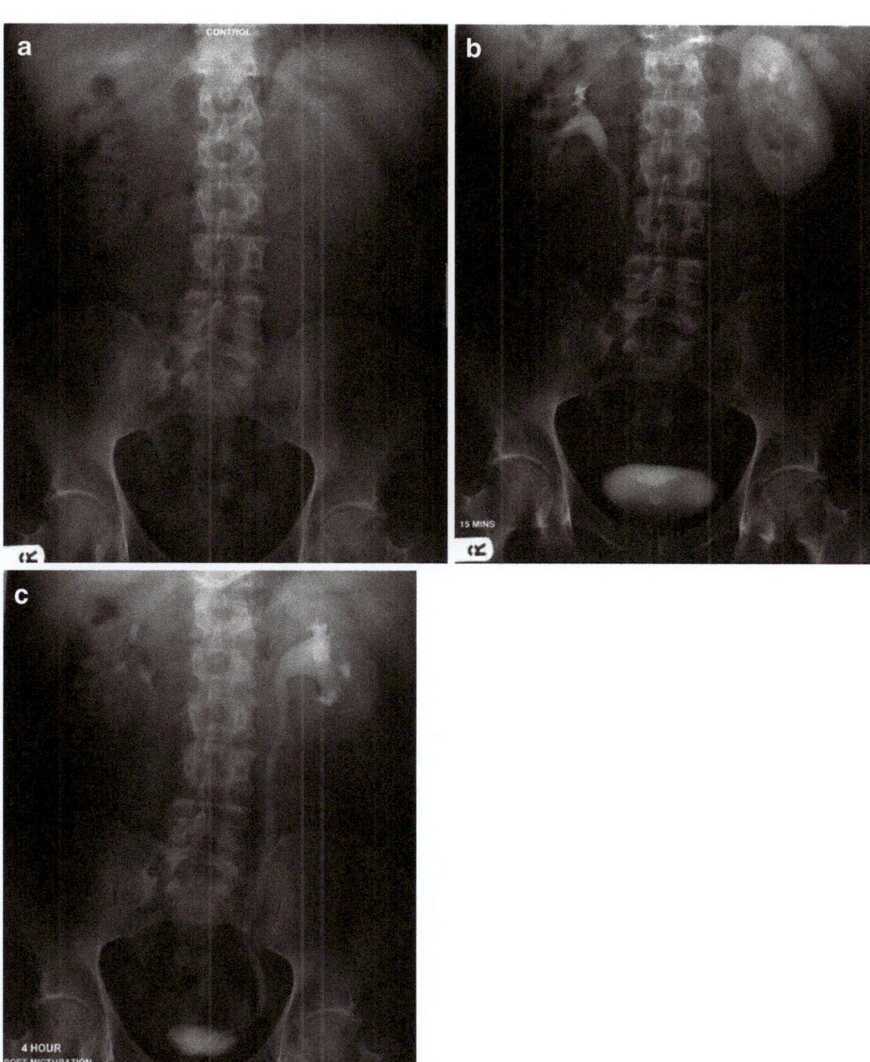

Fig. 2.20.1

Fig. 2.20.2

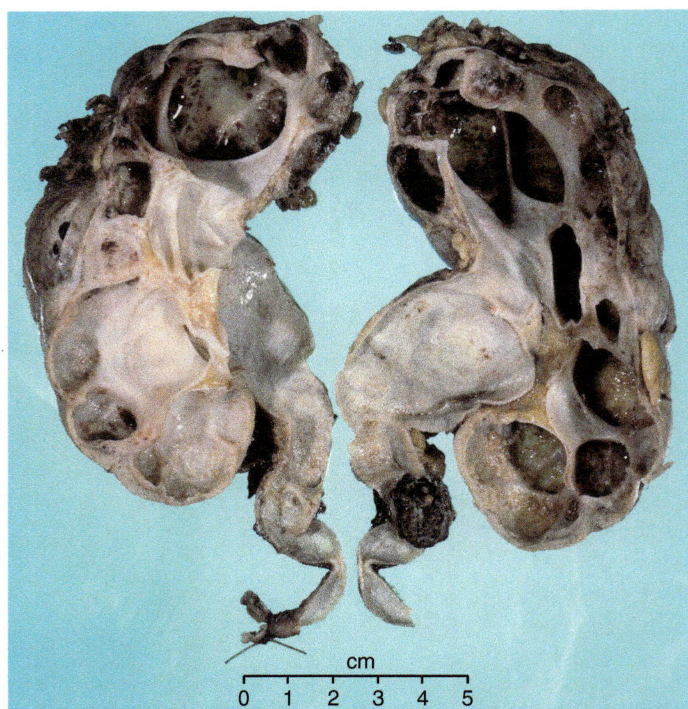

Answers to Case 2.20

1. Figure 2.20.1 is part of a limited IVU series, showing a control (a), 15-min (b) and 4-h postmicturition (c) film. On the control film, there is a small radio-opacity seen near the left VUJ, which is causing ureteric obstruction with a bright, delayed nephrogram on the 15-min film. By the 4-h film, the level of obstruction (i.e. the VUJ) has been demonstrated.
2. The advantages of the IVU for acute colic is that it is widely available at all hours and the images are easier to interpret as the collecting system anatomy is better demonstrated. Follow-up imaging, where a stone is visible, can be with a KUB radiograph. The modern alternative is a non contrast helical CT KUB. This has a superior accuracy, and iodinated contrast is not required. It is also very quick and radiolucent stones (e.g. uric acid stones) are also visualised. Furthermore, other intra-abdominal pathology may be diagnosed on CT. The radiation dose of an IVU is slightly lower than most CT KUBs. Neither is suitable as first line investigations for children or during pregnancy, for which an ultrasound and KUB are used, supplemented by MRU (magnetic resonance urogram) for the latter.
3. Immediate management is tailored according to clinical status. Pain control with a non-steroidal anti-inflammatory drug and hydration are paramount. Medical expulsive therapy with an alpha-blockers e.g. tamsulosin is recommended to expedite ureteric stone passage. Those with signs of infection may require renal de-obstruction (either a nephrostomy or stent placement). A patient with a single kidney, bilateral obstruction or poor renal function may also require de-obstruction. Later management is dependent on the size and site of the ureteric calculus, and also its likely composition. Large (>6–7 mm) ureteric calculi are unlikely to pass spontaneously and may require lithotripsy or ureteroscopic extraction. Follow-up of stone progress is generally best done with KUB (if the stone is opaque), unless it is located, as in this case, at the VUJ in which case bladder ultrasound may be more suitable.
4. Figure 2.20.2 demonstrates a bisected nephrectomy specimen in which function was poor. Chronic obstruction from an upper ureteric stone has caused hydroureter and hydronephrosis with extensive loss of renal parenchyma.

Further Reading

Smith RC, Verga M, McCarthy S, Rosenfield AT. Diagnosis of acute flank pain: value of unenhanced helical CT. *AJR Am J Roentgenol*. 1996;166(1):97–101.

Case 2.21

1. This KUB and CT scan is from a patient, taken on the same day, with a history of recurrent stones. Describe what is demonstrated.
2. Explain the discrepancy between the plain radiographic and CT findings.
3. Describe the clinical implication of this discrepancy.
4. Could drug therapy have a bearing on the discrepancy?

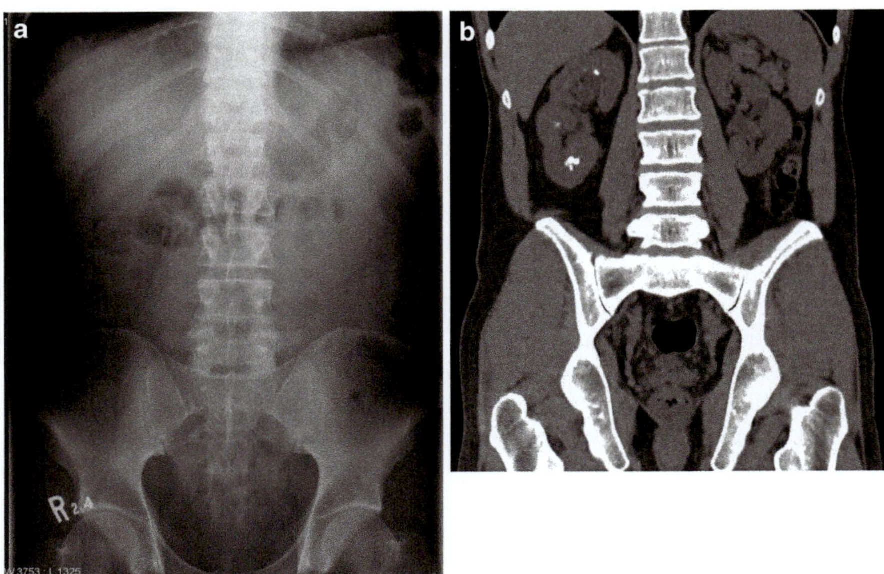

Fig. 2.21.1

Answers to Case 2.21

1. Right lower pole calculi are faintly visible on the KUB radiograph (Fig. 2.21.1a). On the CT however multiple right renal calculi are clearly visible (Fig. 2.21.1b).
2. Stones with a density <200 HU on CT are not visible on plain film. Calculi of >300 HU tend to be visible, although this is dependent on size. In this case the stones were cystine stones. Other calculi that may be radiolucent include uric acid stones, though these may become secondarily calcified and so visible, matrix and some magnesium ammonium phosphate (struvite) stones.
3. Cystine stones have a density of ~500 HU (cf. calcium phosphate stones = 850 HU), and smaller stones may not be visible on plain film. Radiological follow-up of stone patients with radiographically lucent or barely visible stones is problematic, as although renal stones will be visible on ultrasound, ureteric stones will not be.
4. Although many drugs have been said to cause urinary tract stones, in practice they are rare. Most contemporary cases are associated with anti-retroviral drugs (e.g. indinivir stones), the majority of which are lucent on all radiological modalities.

Further Reading

Ng CS, Streem SB. Medical and surgical therapy of the cystine stone patient. *Curr Opin Urol.* 2001;11(4):353–358.

Wu DS, Stoller ML. Indinavir urolithiasis. *Curr Opin Urol.* 2000;10(6):557–561.

Case 2.22

A 35-year-old lady presents with recurrent urinary tract infections.

1. Describe the US and CT findings.
2. What are the potential complications, as demonstrated in Fig. 2.22.2?
3. Describe the management of this condition.

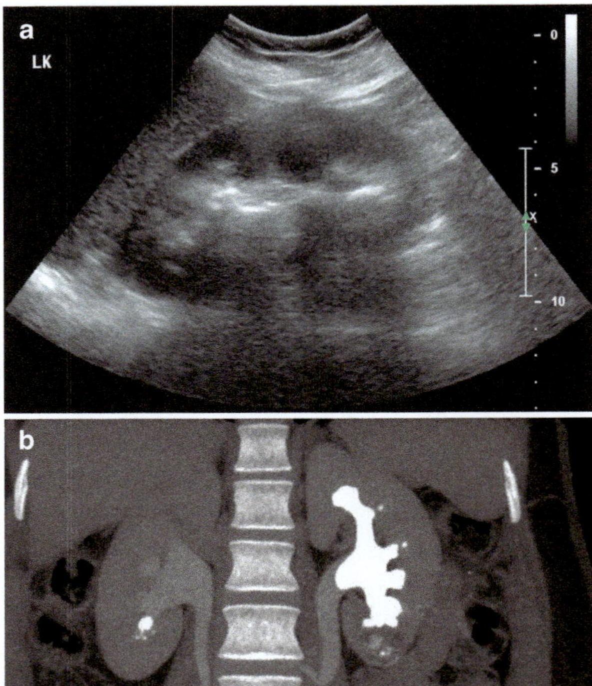

Fig. 2.22.1

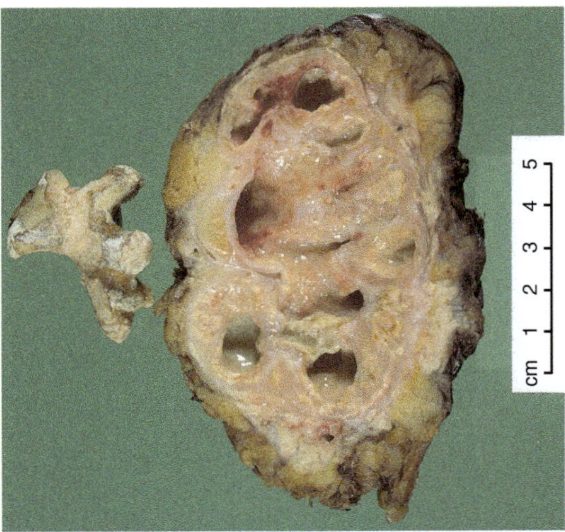

Fig. 2.22.2

Answers to Case 2.22

1. The ultrasound scan (Fig. 2.22.1a) demonstrates a large echogenic lesion occupying the central portion of the left kidney which casts an acoustic shadow. The coronal MIP* CT image (Fig. 2.22.1b) shows a large calcified stone which completely opacifies the left renal pelvicalyceal system. A small stone is also seen in the infundibulum to a lower pole calyx of the right kidney. The appearance on the left is of a staghorn calculus which is composed of calcium magnesium ammonium phosphate (struvite).
2. Complications of this are recurrent urinary tract infections which may lead to pyonephrosis or renal abscess formation. Renal obstruction and eventual renal loss may be seen. Patients may rarely progress to develop xanthogranulomatous pyelonephritis (XGP) as shown in Fig. 2.22.2, where the staghorn calculus has been removed from the surgical specimen in which the kidney had been extensively destroyed by a xanthogranulomatous inflammatory response.
3. Firstly the presence of infection should be excluded. If present it should be aggressively treated, the additional placement of a ureteric stent or nephrostomy to relieve any obstructive pyonephrosis may be required. The residual renal function should be measured (by a DMSA or MAG3 nuclear medicine test). Then depending on the patient's co-morbidities and the likelihood of recovery of renal function either percutaneous nephrolithotomy, open pyelolithotomy or nephrectomy are the main treatment options.

Further Reading

Preminger GM, Assimos DG, Lingeman JE, Nakada SY, Pearle MS, Wolf JS Jr. AUA nephrolithiasis guideline panel. Chapter 1: AUA guideline on management of staghorn calculi: diagnosis and treatment recommendations. *J Urol.* 2005;173(6): 1991–2000.

---

* MIP = Maximal intensity projection. This is a form of image post-processing, whereby the image settings are chosen to optimally visualise the maximal density in any given pixel, at the expense of all the lower densities. It is especially useful for highlighting structures/tissues etc. of intrinsically high density. In urology, it is useful for showing urinary tract stones or the collecting system on CT urographic studies.

Case 2.23

This woman presented with chronic pelvic and bilateral loin pain, which had cyclical variability. Microscopic haematuria was also noted.

1. Describe the findings on this image taken as part of an intravenous urogram.
2. Suggest a differential diagnosis and further investigations.

Fig. 2.23.1

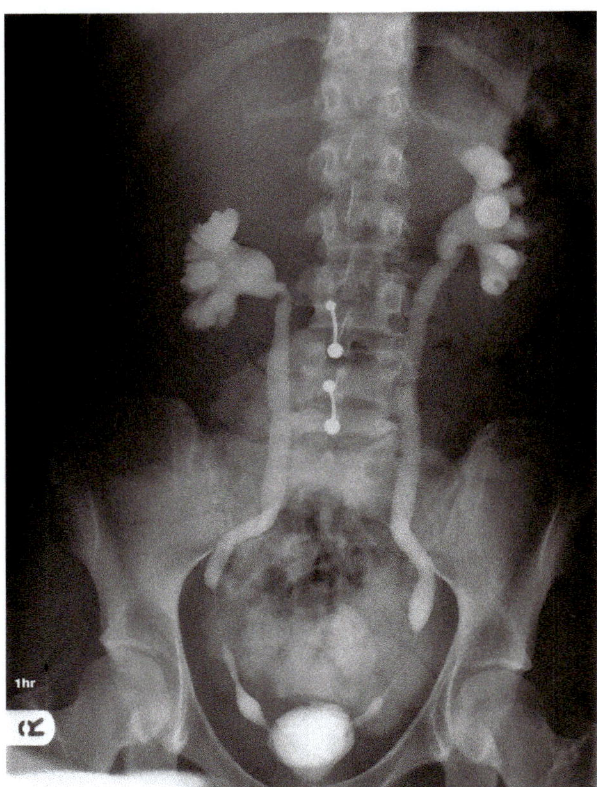

Answers to Case 2.23

1. Figure 2.23.1 is a postcontrast image from an IVU series showing smoothly narrowed distal ureters with dilatation of the more proximal ureters and pelvicalyceal systems. Contrast still passes into the bladder i.e. appearances are in keeping with partial obstruction. The upper tracts are dilated but otherwise normal. This patient proved to have bilateral endometriosis.
2. The smoothness of the mucosal outline of the strictures would suggest an extra luminal mass of benign aetiology. Possible causes are endometriosis, post radiation, retroperitoneal fibrosis, extra-luminal compression by pelvic masses (e.g. ovarian cysts) pelvic inflammatory disease, lymphadenopathy, collections or ischaemic strictures following pelvic surgery. Further investigations that may help are CT/MRI +/– biopsy. Ureteroscopy is unlikely to contribute other than to confirm the strictures, but occasionally the nodules of endometriosis may be seen in the wall. The diagnosis is often made at diagnostic laparoscopy.

Further Reading

Wong-You-Cheong JJ, Woodward PJ, Manning MA, Davis CJ. From the archives of the AFIP: Inflammatory and nonneoplastic bladder masses: radiologic-pathologic correlation. *Radiographics*. 2006;26(6):1847–1868.

Case 2.24

1. What is the likely diagnosis on this IVU series and MAG3 renogram?
2. What are the important causes of this condition?
3. Are any further investigation necessary or warranted?

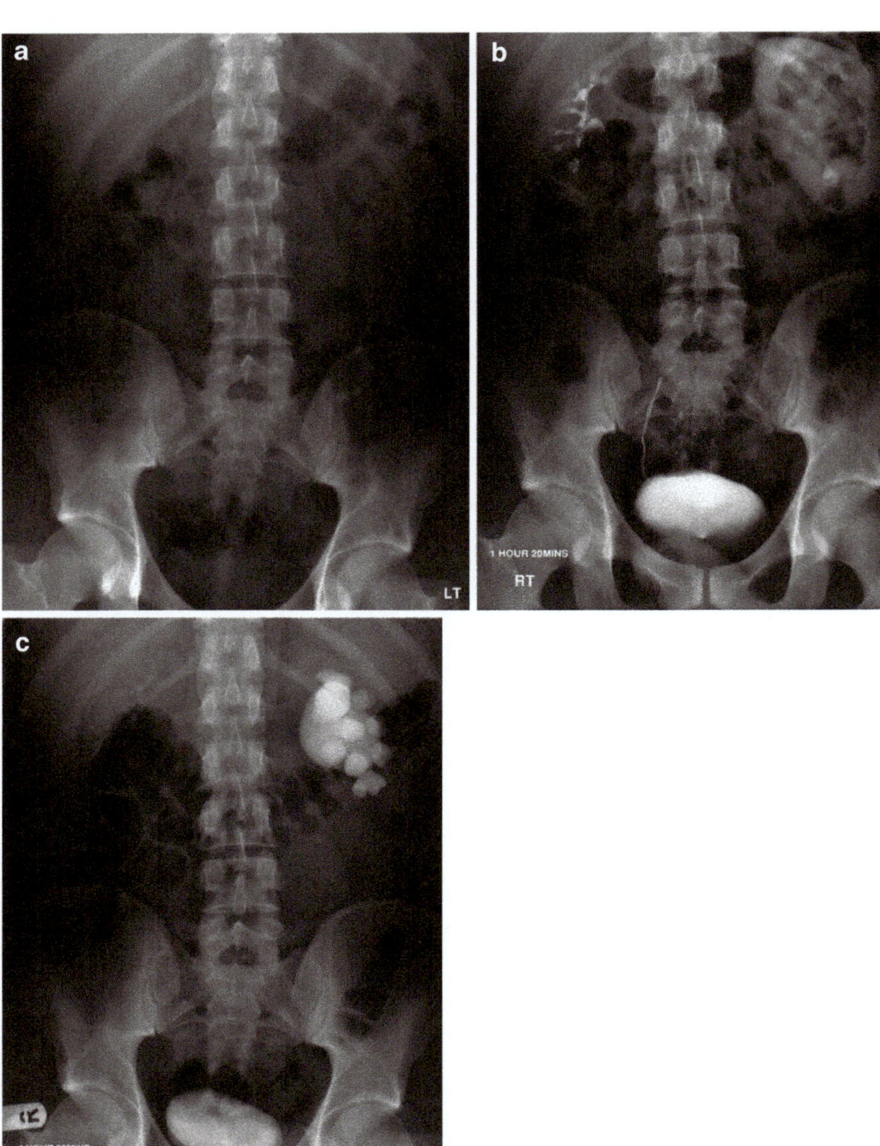

Fig. 2.24.1

DYNAMIC RENOGRAM [Composite] 08/03/2006
%
67
0
Left Kidney
Right Background
957K 128x128 Pix:4.8mm 99m Technetium
(B:0%,T:67%)
Table of Result Summary
Parameters Left Right Total
Split Function (%) 48.7 51.3
Kidney Counts (cpm) 25985 27354 53339
Time of Max (min) 9.169 2.335
Time of ½ Max (min) 9.146
Table of Patient Parameters
Parameters Values
Renal Protocol Generic(None)
Kidney Depth Method Standard
Patient Name BERRY, MARTIN
Patient ID J408630
Sex Male
Age 29
Reference BSA 1.73 m²
Split Uptake Interval (min) 2.0 - 3.0
Radiopharmaceutical 80.0 MBq 99m Technetium MAG3
Method Adult
Kidney
TMax-R
T½-R
40mg FRUSEMIDE AT F = 15
Counts/Second
Minutes
Flow
Counts/Second
Seconds

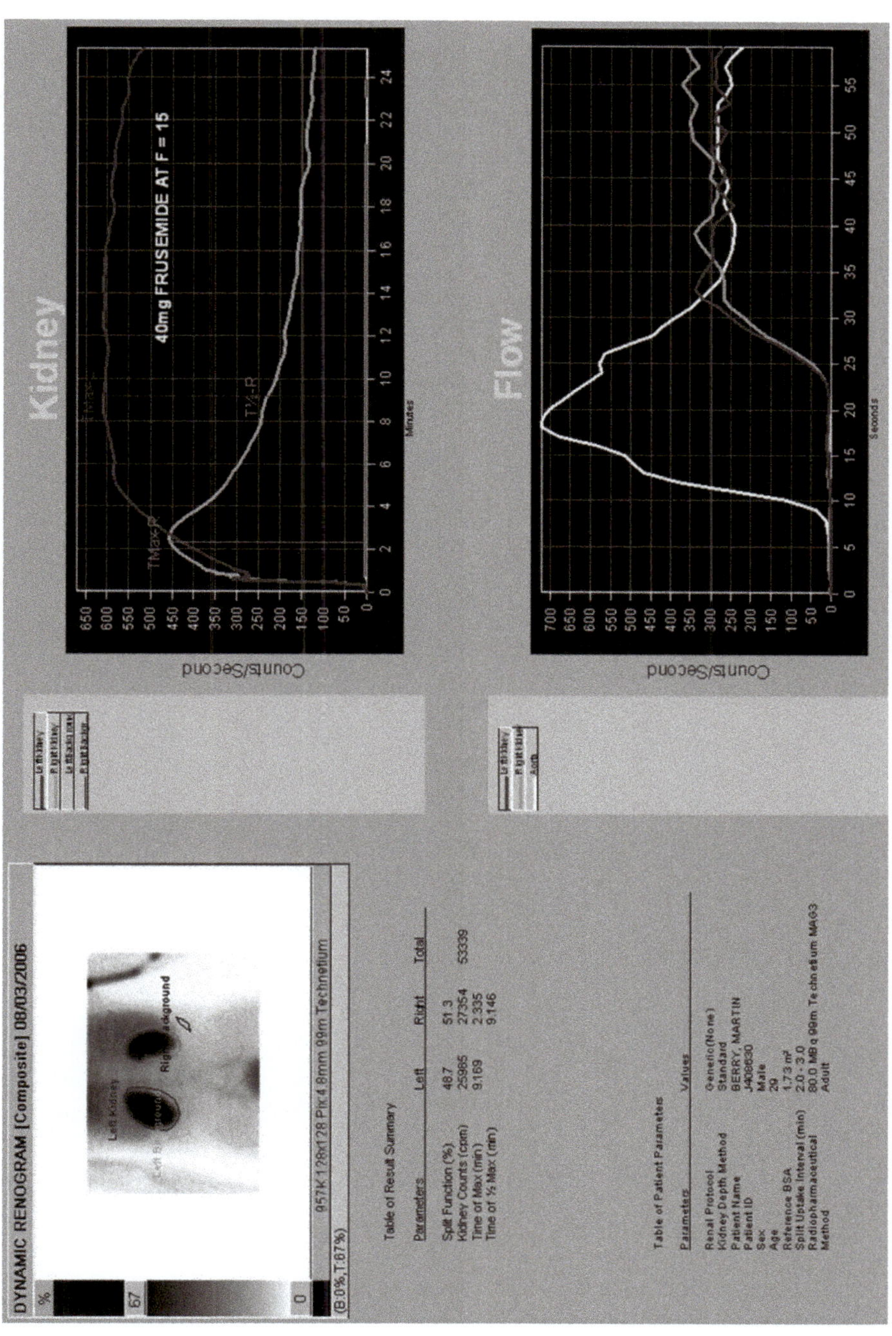

Fig. 2.24.2

Answers to Case 2.24

1. There are no calculi or any renal tract calcification on the control film (Fig. 2.24.1a). Post-contrast images show complete obstruction with a delayed nephrogram still evident at 80 min (Fig. 2.24.1b) and no drainage past the pelvi-ureteric junction at 260 min (Fig. 2.24.1c). Figure 2.24.2, the MAG-3 activity curve (graph marked 'KIDNEY') shows normal rapid uptake and exponential clearance in the right kidney. There is normal uptake in the left kidney, but the curve plateaus rather than decreasing despite administration of Frusemide at 15 min, in keeping with obstruction. Split function is still normal (LK=49%).
2. The causes are:
   - Idiopathic – more common in men and on the left (10% bilateral). Unknown aetiology, aberrant lower pole vessels are a frequent finding, other possible mechanisms include a persistent urothelial fold or obstruction secondary to discontinuity in the muscle which disrupts normal peristalsis.
   - Calculus – no calcification seen on the control film, but this could be a radiolucent calculus.
   - Tumour (e.g. TCC).
3. In patients with a typical clinical history and imaging findings, no further investigation is necessary. But in the elderly or those with haematuria, especially in smokers, ureteroscopy and/or CT may be necessary to exclude a ureteric tumour. Similarly if a stone is suspected then a CT KUB may be useful.

Case 2.25

A male neonate has a left sided abdominal mass.

1. What are the USS findings and the likely diagnosis?
2. What further imaging test could be performed to differentiate between this condition and alternative possibilities?
3. What are the clinical implications of this diagnosis?

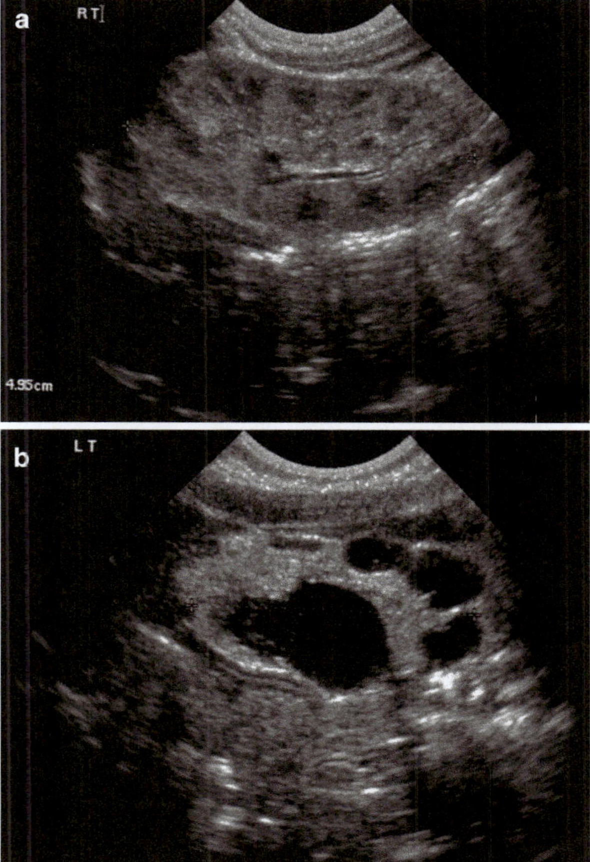

Fig. 2.25.1

Answers to Case 2.25

1. The ultrasound of the right kidney (Fig. 2.25.1b) shows normal corticomedullary differentiation and no hydronephrosis. The left kidney (Fig. 2.25.1b) demonstrates multiple hypoechoic cysts of variable shapes and size, with complete loss of corticomedullary differentiation. Other images from the USS confirmed that the cysts do not communicate. The appearances are suggestive of a multicystic dysplastic kidney.
2. Nuclear medicine studies (e.g. DMSA or MAG-3) are sensitive at detecting residual renal function in a hydronephrotic kidney in contrast to complete absence of function seen (MCDK).
3. Essentially the kidney is non-functional and by the time of adulthood the affected kidney may have undergone complete involution. Rare complications include hypertension, pain and suspicious enlargement after birth for which surgery is indicated. Malignant transformation is rare. The majority of complications relate to the contralateral kidney which has a relatively high risk of associated anomalies, most commonly PUJ obstruction, vesicoureteric reflux and ureteric anomalies. Bilateral MCDK is incompatible with life and affected individuals die in-utero or in the early post natal period.

Further Reading

Agrons GA, Wagner BJ, Davidson AJ, Suarez ES. Multilocular cystic renal tumor in children: radiologic-pathologic correlation. *Radiographics.* 1995;15(3): 653–669.

Hopkins JK, Giles HW Jr, Wyatt-Ashmead J, Bigler SA. Best cases from the AFIP: cystic nephroma. *Radiographics.* 2004;24(2):589–593.

Case 2.26

1. Describe the abnormalities in Figs. 2.26.1, 2.26.2, and 2.26.3 what are the diagnoses?
2. What are the associations and potential complications of these conditions?

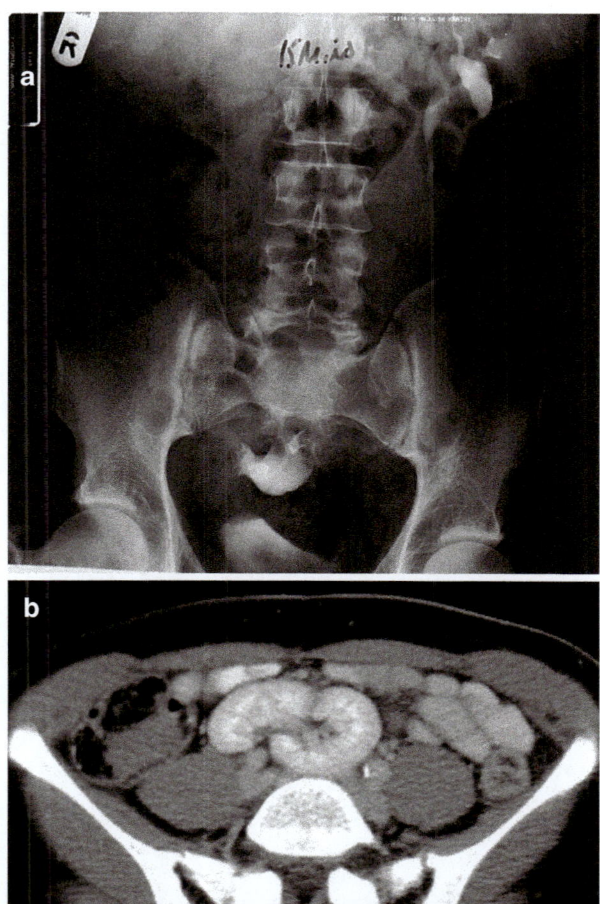

Fig. 2.26.1

Fig. 2.26.2

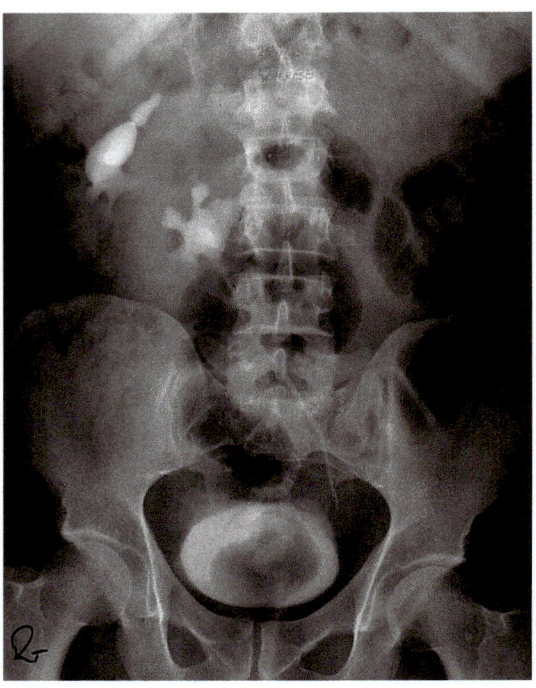

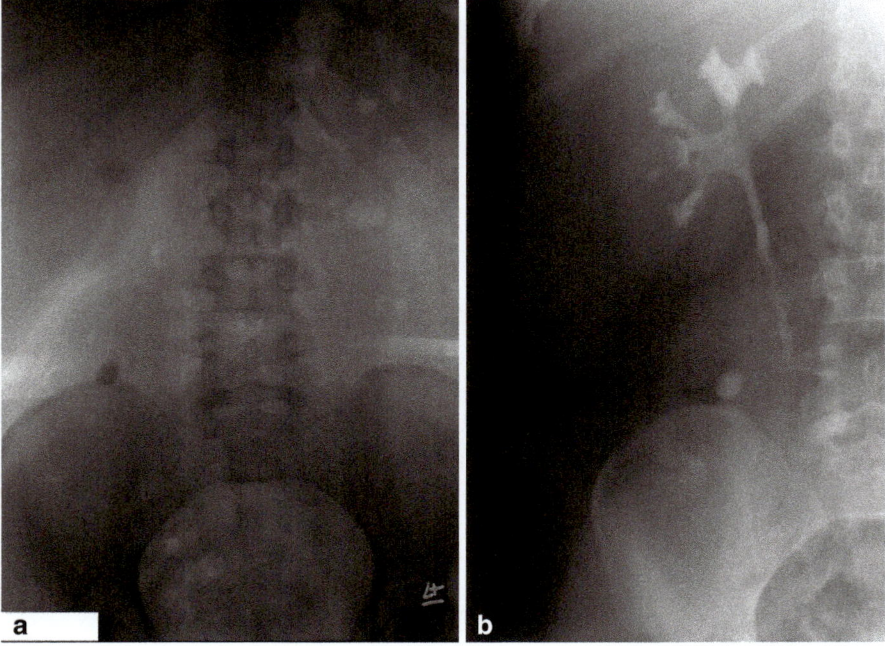

Fig. 2.26.3

Answers to Case 2.26

1. The first radiograph is a 15-min post contrast film from an IVU series (Fig. 2.26.1a) showing normal contrast opacification of the left renal collecting system, but no contrast opacification is seen at the expected location of the right kidney. However contrast opacifies a mal-ascended kidney in the pelvis. Figure 2.26.1b is a CT through the pelvis demonstrating a normal-sized right kidney lying centrally within the pelvis. Appearances are in keeping with a right pelvic kidney. Figure 2.26.2 is a single image from an IVU series showing opacification of two collecting systems on the right side of the abdomen. The ureter associated with the inferior 'crossed' kidney passes across the midline to insert into the trigone on the left side of the bladder. There is no left sided kidney. This is crossed fused ectopia and results from disordered renal ascent during embryogenesis, with subsequent partial fusion of the 'crossed' kidney to the inferior aspect of the normal kidney on this side. Renal arteries are usually anomalous, but as demonstrated in the above example the ureter inserts correctly into the trigone on the side of origin (i.e. the ureters are always heterotopic; distinguishing this condition from say an absent left kidney with a duplex right kidney and ureter). Figure 2.26.3a,b are a control film and 20 min post contrast film of a patient with crossed renal ectopia, the kidneys in this case have not fused. The control demonstrates two opacities in the right side of the abdomen. The 20 min film shows there to be stones in both collecting systems, and the lower kidney has poor function.
2. Both these conditions may be asymptomatic. Pelvic kidney may be associated with contralateral renal agenesis, nephrolithiasis, vesicoureteric reflux or PUJ obstruction. Crossed ectopia is associated with nephrolithiasis, recurrent infections, vesicoureteric reflux, hypospadias, urethral valves, cryptorchidism and multicystic dysplastic kidneys.

Further Reading

Patel TV, Singh AK. Crossed fused ectopia of the kidneys. *Kidney Int.* 2008;73(5):662.

Case 2.27

1. What is shown by the IVU and CT scans below?
2. In this condition, what is the additional diagnostic value of CT scanning?
3. What are the main clinical complications of this condition, one is shown in Fig. 2.27.2a,b?

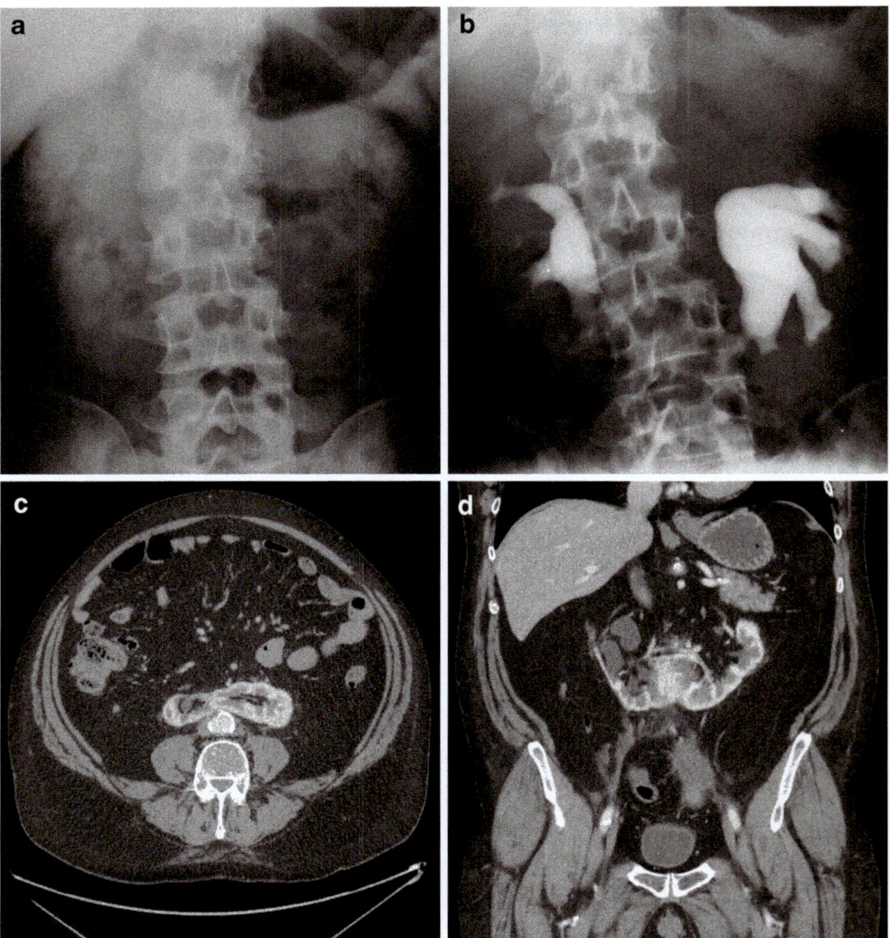

Fig. 2.27.1

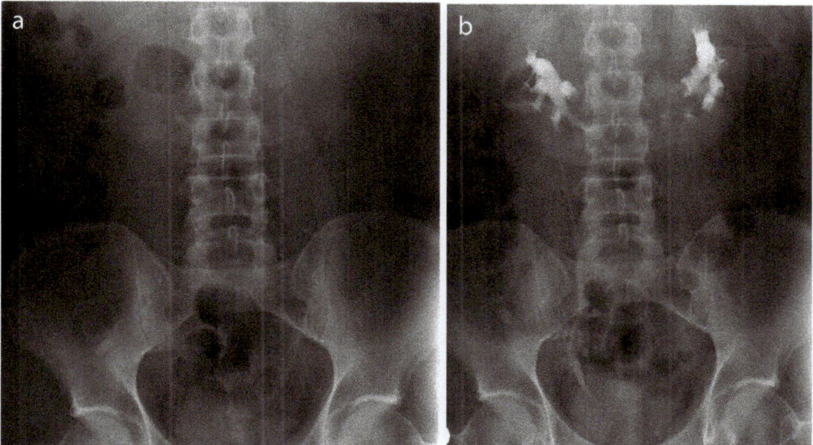

Fig. 2.27.2

Answers to Case 2.27

1. Figure 2.27.1a is the control film of an IVU, there is an abnormal central opacity in the abdomen. Following intravenous contrast (Fig. 2.27.1b), there is opacification of both renal collecting systems which appear medially positioned and malrotated. The IVU findings are highly suggestive of a horseshoe kidney but the isthmus is difficult to accurately characterise. This is where CT can be informative, as shown in Fig. 2.27.1c, d – CT confirms a functional parenchymal isthmus rather than a fibrous isthmus.
2. As well as better demonstrating the presence of a functional isthmus, CT will show the degree and site of fusion, the degree of malrotation, variant arterial anatomy particularly in the presurgical setting, renal calculi and associated renal parenchymal lesions such as scarring, cysts and tumours.
3. Figure 2.27.2a is a control film in a patient with a horseshoe kidney demonstrating an opacity adjacent to the third lumbar vertebra, the 20 min film (Fig. 2.27.2b) shows this to be a stone. As well as an increased risk of calculi there is increased risk of trauma due to the location of the isthmus anterior to the lumbar spine, PUJ obstruction and recurrent urinary tract infections. There is a reported increased relative risk of certain types of tumour including Wilm's tumour, transitional cell carcinoma and carcinoid tumour – however the risk is low.

Case 2.28

This abnormality was an incidental finding on ultrasound and further evaluated on CT.

1. Study the US and CT images and describe the findings.
2. What is the diagnosis? What are the diagnostic features?
3. What is its significance?

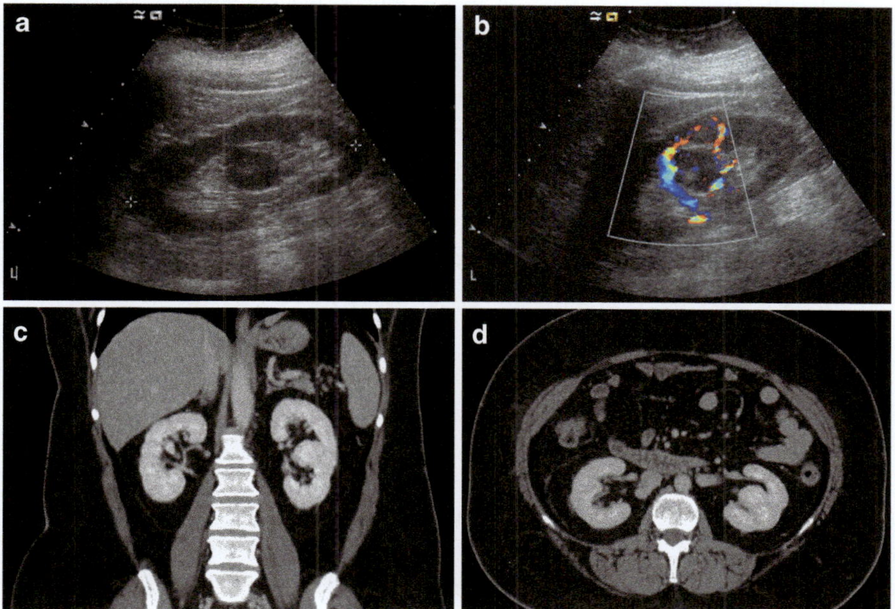

Fig. 2.28.1

Answers to Case 2.28

1. Greyscale (Fig. 2.28.1a) and colour Doppler (Fig. 2.28.1b) ultrasound images through the left kidney showing a hypoechoic region centrally within the interpolar region. This has a mass like appearance and on colour Doppler ultrasound, it has peripheral vascularity. There is no posterior acoustic enhancement in keeping with a solid composition. Coronal (Fig. 2.28.1c) and axial (Fig. 2.28.1d) postcontrast CT images through the upper abdomen which depict the region noted on ultrasound. Although it also has a mass like appearance, the renal outline is preserved although it does appear to bulge into the renal sinus fat. However, and critically, it demonstrates isodense enhancement when compared to the remainder of the renal parenchyma.
2. This is an example of junctional parenchyma, but more familiarly known as a hypertrophic column of Bertin. The diagnostic features include location between the overlapping portion of the upper and lower poles, and that it contains normal renal tissue that is continuous with the adjacent renal cortex. Being functionally normal, it shows normal echogenicity on US and normal enhancement and tracer uptake on CT/MRI and nuclear medicine, respectively.
3. This is due to unresorbed renal parenchyma where the embryological upper and lower pole moieties fuse. It is a normal variation and does not predispose to any complication. It's only clinical significance is that it closely mimics a centrally lying renal mass.

Further Reading

Lafortune M, Constantin A, Breton G, Vallee C. Sonography of the hypertrophied column of Bertin. *AJR Am J Roentgenol*. 1986;146(1):53–56.

Yeh HC, Halton KP, Shapiro RS, Rabinowitz JG, Mitty HA. Junctional parenchyma: revised definition of hypertrophic column of Bertin. *Radiology*. 1992;185(3): 725–732.

Case 2.29

1. Describe the congenital abnormalities on the left side of this patient.
2. There is a well-recognised general rule regarding the vesico-ureteric anatomy in this condition. What is the eponymous term for this rule and what does it state?
3. Describe the 'drooping lily' sign
4. Figure 2.29.2 relates to a 23-year-old patient who presented with several episodes of epididymo-orchitis. He was not sexually active. What is the likely cause shown on this MRI image?

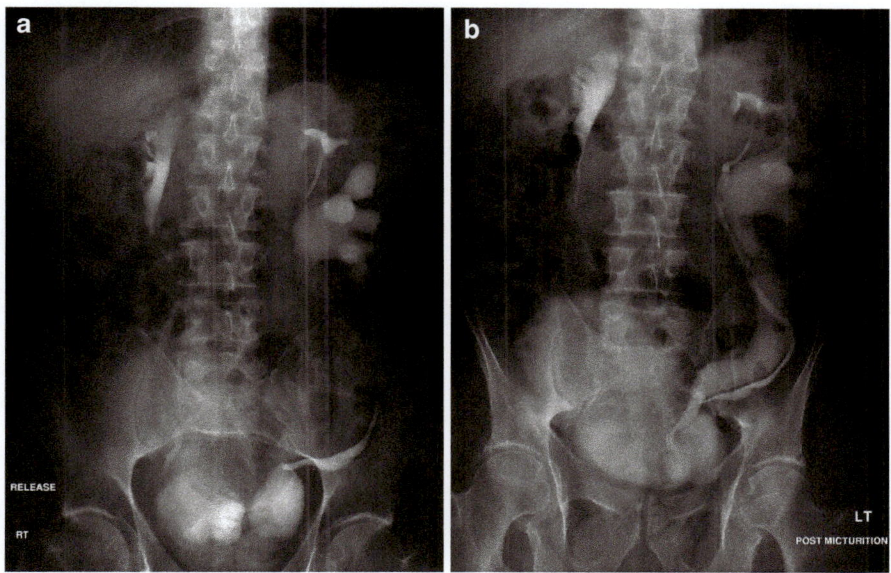

Fig. 2.29.1

Fig. 2.29.2

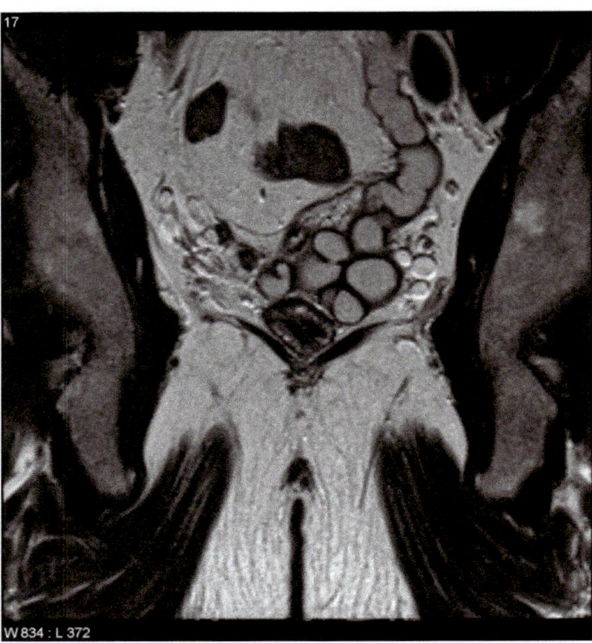

Answers to Case 2.29

1. Figure 2.29.1a,b are two postcontrast images from an IVU series. The left kidney is a complete duplex system, with completely separate ureteric insertions. There is also a Hutch diverticulum associated with the upper moiety ureter. The lower moiety pelvicalyceal system and ureter are distended.
2. The Weigert Meyer rule states that with a complete duplex system, the upper moiety ureter inserts more inferiorly and medially in the bladder than the lower moiety ureter. The lower moiety ureter is prone to reflux. In comparison, the upper moiety ureter is prone to obstruction at the vesicoureteric junction and may be associated with an ureterocoele.
3. This is a characteristic appearance on IVU. The upper moiety obstructs and therefore does not opacify, but it does increase in size thereby pushing the lower moiety downwards. Therefore only the 'drooping' lower moiety is seen on IVU.
4. Figure 2.29.2 is a coronal MRI showing the left ureter inserting into the left seminal vesicle. Ectopic ureters are usually associated with Duplex systems. They may be diagnosed prenatally due to hydronephrosis or dilation of an upper moiety and ureter. Ectopic ureters may arise in the bladder or in males in the seminal vesicles, ejaculatory ducts or vas, above the external sphincter, so continence is maintained. Epididymo-orchitis is a common presenting feature. An ectopic ureter in a female may insert into the urethra or vagina and cause continuous dribbling incontinence with normal voiding in between.

Further Reading

Dyer RB, Chen MY, Zagoria RJ. Classic signs in uroradiology. *Radiographics*. 2004 ;24 (Suppl 1):S247–S280.

Fernbach SK, Feinstein KA, Spencer K, Lindstrom CA. Ureteral duplication and its complications. *Radiographics*. 1997;17(1):109–127.

Horst M, Smith GH. Pelvi-ureteric junction obstruction in duplex kidneys. *BJU Int*. 2008;101(12):1580–1584. Epub 2008.

Case 2.30

1. Describe the images shown in this 23-year-old man with recurrent UTI and abdominal pains. What is the most likely diagnosis and what is the aetiology?
2. Figure 2.30.2 is the CT scan of a 16-year-old who presented with right loin pain and hamaturia, what is the diagnosis in this case and what operation was performed to rectify this congenital abnormality?

Fig. 2.30.1

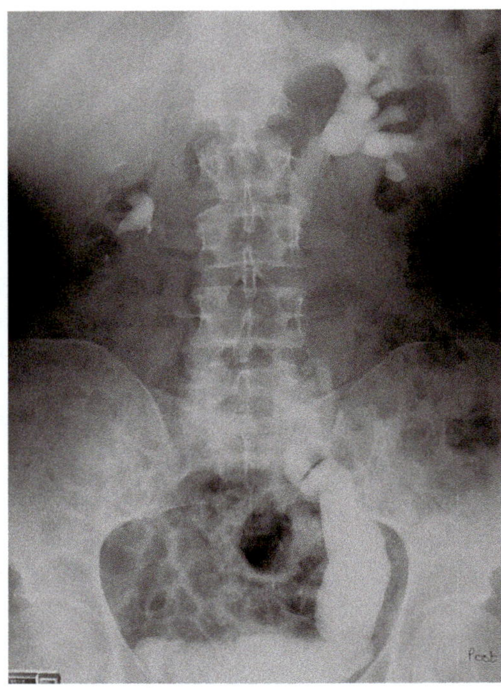

Fig. 2.30.2

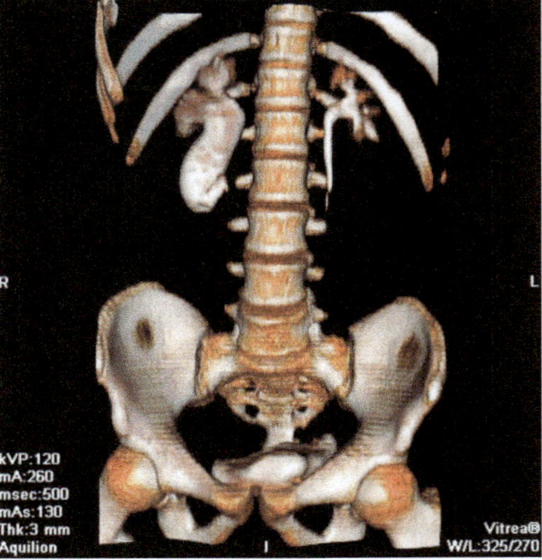

Answers to Case 2.30

1. Figure 2.30.1 shows marked localised dilatation of the lower third of the left ureter, with mild prominence of the collecting system proximally. The differential diagnosis includes chronic ureteric obstruction, vesicoureteric reflux, diabetes insipidus, psychogenic polydipsia or primary megaureter. This is primary megaureter, which is a congenital condition and is typically a unilateral process, occurring more frequently on the left and in males. The aetiology is abnormal muscle development within a segment of ureter near to the vesicoureteric junction. This leads to reduced peristalsis and subsequent dilatation of the distal ureter which tapers smoothly just proximal to the vesicoureteric junction. In rare cases the whole ureter and pelvicalyceal system may be dilated, i.e. megaureter with megacalycosis.
2. The CT reconstruction (Fig. 2.30.2) shows appearances in keeping with a retrocaval ureter. Retrocaval ureter is a rare congenital anomaly resulting from persistence of the posterior cardinal veins during embryologic development. It is more common in males and usually presents with loin pain, haematuria is often also present with or without proximal calculi. There is a classic S shaped bend in the upper ureter centred around the L3 vertebra. Cross sectional imaging is usually required to exclude other causes of medially placed ureters including retroperitoneal fibrosis and a retroperitoneal mass. In obstructed patients the Anderson Hynes pyeloplasty is performed, as originally described in 1949 for the retrocaval ureter, and now used more commonly for PUJ obstruction.

Further Reading

Avni FE, Hall M, Collier C, Schulman C. Anomalies of the renal pelvis and ureter. In: Baert AL, Sartor K eds. *Paediatric Uroradiology*. 1st ed. Berlin: Springer; 2002:61–90.

Dyer RB, Chen MY, Zagoria RJ. Classic signs in uroradiology. *Radiographics*. 2004 ;24 (Suppl 1):S247–S280.

Case 2.31

A 40-year-old female presented with 4 days pyrexia and right loin pain.

1. Describe the CT findings.
2. What is the differential diagnosis?
3. If there is uncertainty regarding the diagnosis, how would you investigate this further with imaging?
4. Is repeat imaging necessary and why?

Fig. 2.31.1

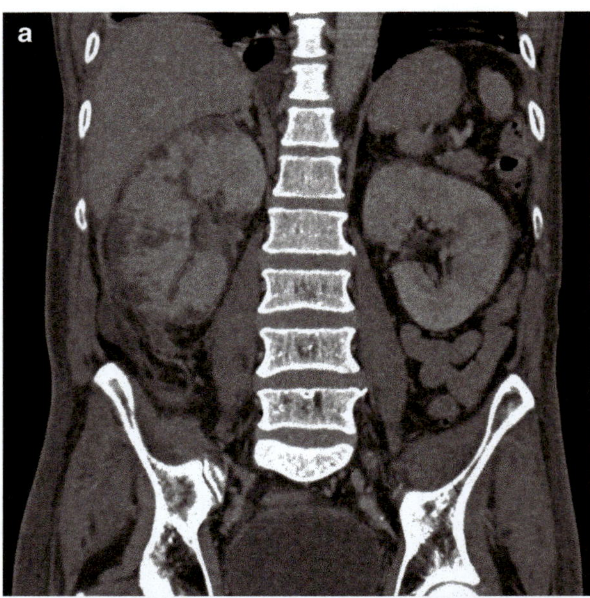

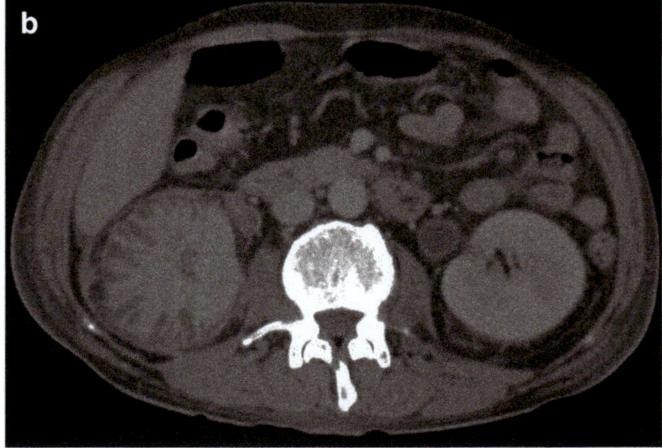

Answers to Case 2.31

1. Postcontrast coronal (Fig. 2.31.1a) and axial (Fig. 2.31.1b) CT images through the upper abdomen. Multiple wedge-shaped peripheral low attenuation lesions are seen throughout the right kidney. The right kidney is larger than the left and there is marked perinephric fat stranding. The urothelium of the upper right ureter also enhances and is thickened (Fig. 2.31.1b).
2. The main differential diagnosis is between infection and infarction, as the appearances can be very similar. The presence of the perinephric changes and the global changes favour acute pyelonephritis. In comparison, solitary or few focal, wedge shaped defects with a normal perinephric space would implicate infarction. Either can be bilateral. Infiltrative disease such as diffuse malignancy or lymphoma is unlikely because of the peripheral preponderance of the changes.
3. Further imaging at this time is unlikely to be of help. For example, DMSA/MAG3 will show defects in all these conditions, and MRI appearances will be similar. Clinical correlation is often the most helpful.
4. Routine repeat imaging is not necessary, but if there is poor clinical response to antibiotics, then early repeat imaging is necessary to exclude abscess formation. This can take the form of US, CT or MRI, but the latter two would be more accurate.

Further Reading

Craig WD, Wagner BJ, Travis MD. Pyelonephritis: radiologic-pathologic review. *Radiographics*. 2008; 28(1):255–277; quiz 327–328.

Case 2.32

This was an incidental finding on a CT scan. The patient is asymptomatic with normal urinalysis.

1. Describe the findings in Fig. 2.32.1a–c.
2. What are the predisposing factors for this condition?
3. What procedure has been performed in image Fig. 2.32.1d?

Fig. 2.32.1

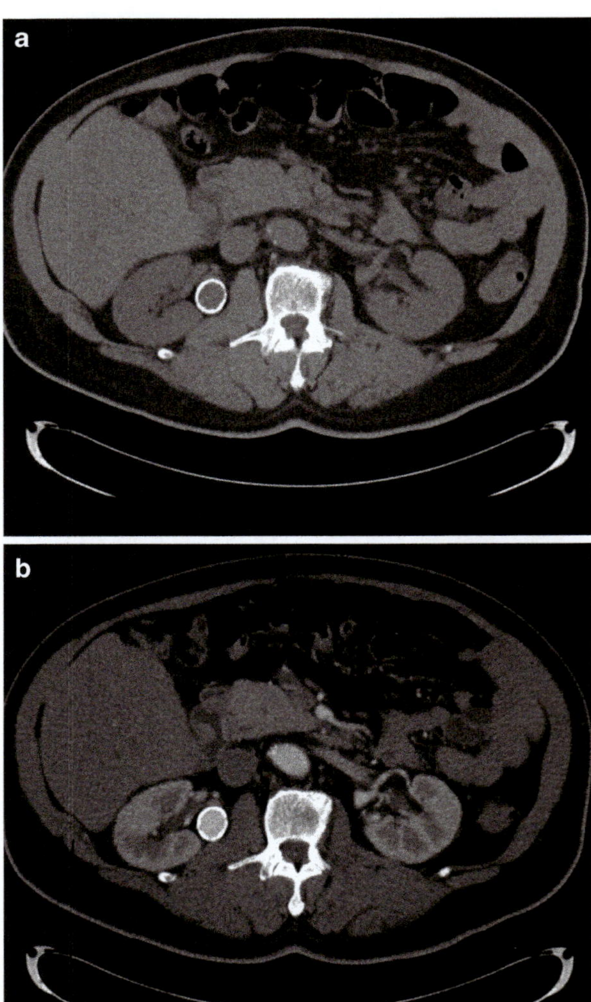

Fig. 2.32.1 (continued)

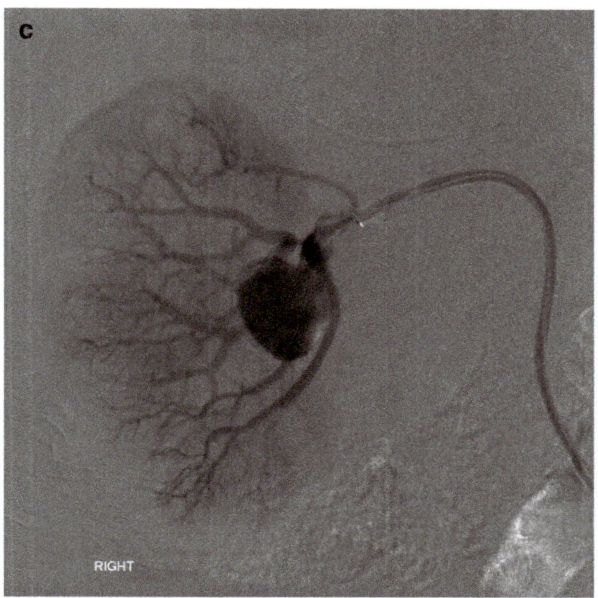

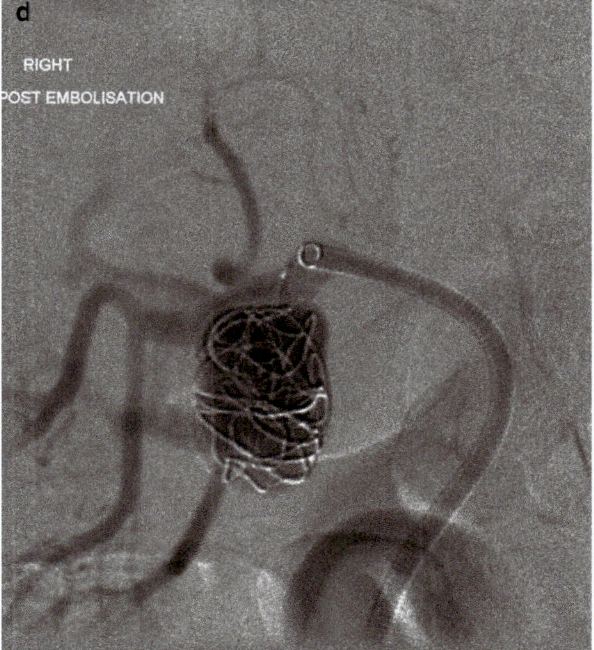

Answers to Case 2.32

1. The CT (Fig. 2.32.1a,b) shows a ring-calcified enhancing lesion lying just medial to the right renal hilum. The mass is located outside the kidney, and it enhances synchronously with the aorta (Fig. 2.32.1b). Thus it is either a vascular mass or a well vascularised extra-renal tumour. Some tumours can be richly enhancing, but they would be more heterogeneous in enhancement and the renal angiogram (Fig. 2.32.1c) confirms that this is a saccular renal artery aneurysm.
2. Some predisposing factors or associations are:
   - Fibromuscular dysplasia
   - Ehlers-Danlos syndrome
   - Mycotic (i.e. infection)
   - Kawasaki's disease
   - Polyarteritis nodosa
   - TB
   - Trauma/dissection/iatrogenic
3. In Figure 2.32.1d percutaneous renal artery aneurysm embolisation is being undertaken. Coils or thrombogenic material is introduced into the saccular aneurysm, with care taken not to thrombose the main renal artery or infarct non-target renal parenchyma.

Further Reading

Eskandari MK, Resnick SA. Aneurysms of the renal artery. *Semin Vasc Surg*. 2005; 18(4):202–208.

Case 2.33

These three patients underwent renal transplantation. Patient 1 made an uneventful postoperative recovery (Fig. 2.33.1a,b). Patient 2 was anuric immediately after the operation (Fig. 2.33.2a,b). Patient 3 became oliguric 48 h after surgery and was tender over the graft site (Fig. 2.33.3a,b).

1. What is the diagnosis in all three patients?
2. What is the aetiology of these complications, how do they present and what are the likely sequelae?

Fig. 2.33.1

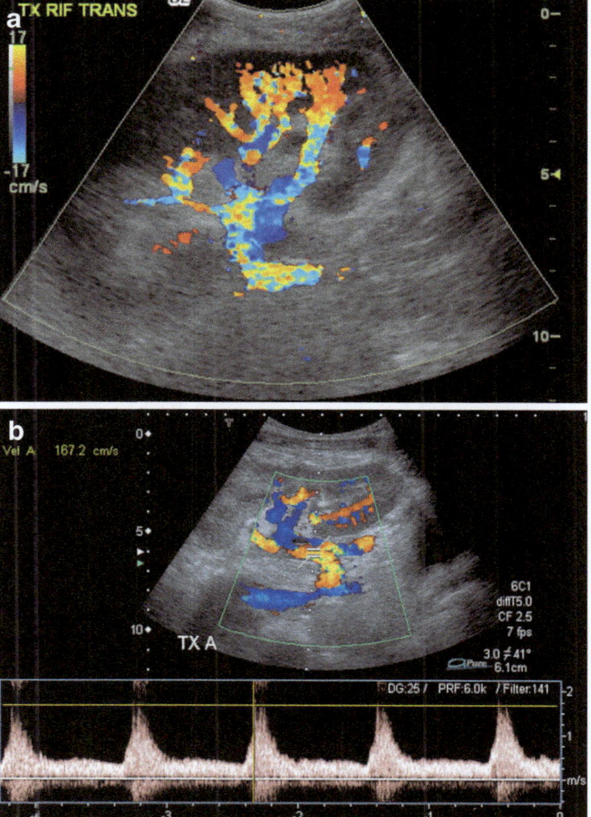

a
RIF TX
b
ANTERIOR
RT
Ph:2 Fr:13-42 Duration: 300sec 99m Technetium
ANTERIOR
Ph:2 Fr:43-72 Duration: 300sec 99m Technetium
ANTERIOR
Ph:2 Fr:73-102 Duration: 300sec 99m Technetium
ANTERIOR
Ph:2 Fr:103-132 Duration: 300sec 99m Technetium
ANTERIOR
Ph:2 Fr:133-162 Duration: 300sec 99m Technetium
ANTERIOR
Ph:2 Fr:163-192 Duration: 300sec 99m Technetium
ANTERIOR
Ph:2 Fr:193-222 Duration: 300sec 99m Technetium

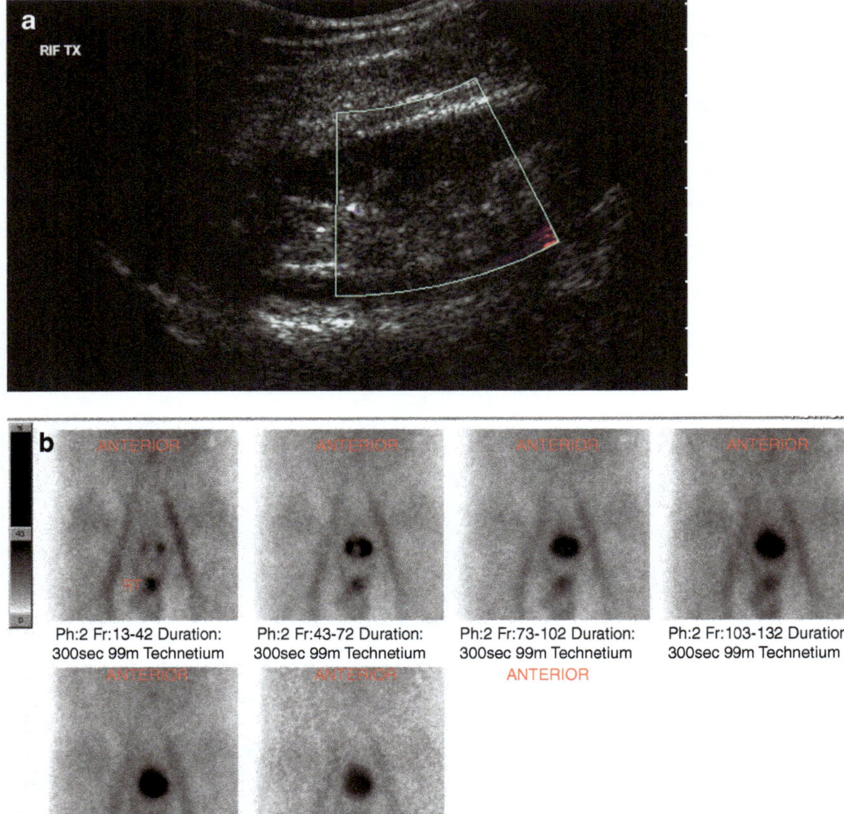

Fig. 2.33.2

Fig. 2.33.3

a
LIF TX
b
1 Vs 27.91 cm/s
Vd 3.38 cm/s
RI 1.12
-20
cm/s
LIF TX
AC 44
80
60
40
20
[cm/s]
-20
0
5
10
-4
-3
-2
-1
0

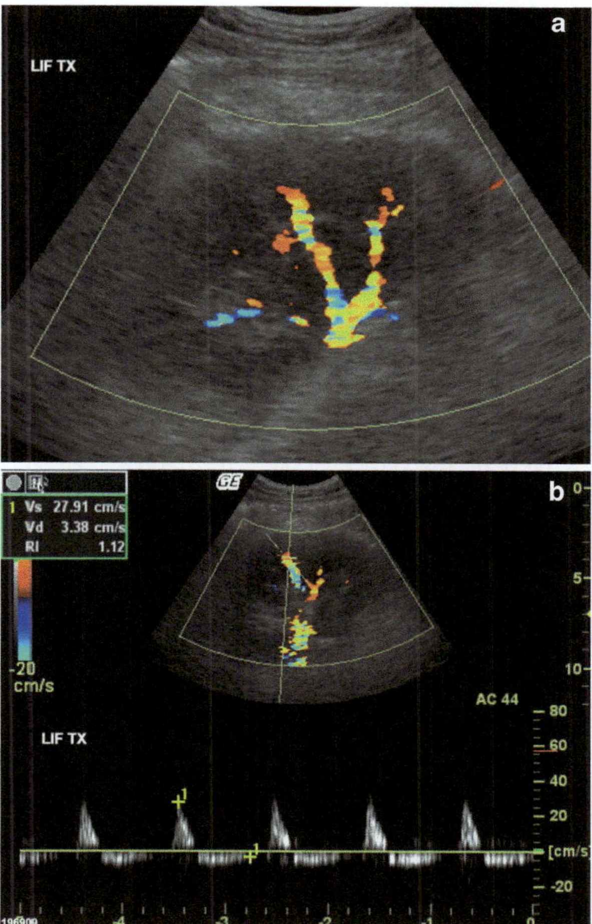

Answers to Case 2.33

1. Patient 1 has a normal post transplant US (Fig. 2.33.1a,b), and the entire organ is well vascularised with normal ostium. In comparison, in patient 2 the colour Doppler ultrasound (Fig. 2.33.2a) shows no parenchymal flow within the transplanted kidney. MAG-3 nuclear medicine scan (Fig. 2.33.2b) shows flow within the iliac arteries, but not the transplant artery – there is no renal uptake. Appearances are consistent with renal artery thrombosis. In patient 3, the colour Doppler ultrasound scan (Fig. 2.33.3a) shows reduced vascularity in the transplant kidney due to absence of venous flow back towards the renal hilum. Spectral Doppler examination of the segmental artery shows a raised resistive index of 1.12 (i.e. over 0.70) with diastolic flow reversal on the trace. The latter finding is highly suggestive of renal vein thrombosis.
2. Renal artery thrombosis is a rare complication (<1%) due to the creation of an intimal flap during donor nephrectomy or perfusion. Other causes include vessel size discrepancy/misalignment/torsion/kinking, atherosclerosis, hyperacute rejection or prothrombogenic conditions. Presentation is in the intraoperative or early postoperative period, it is usually painless and there is a sudden cessation of urine output. Arterial thrombosis usually results in transplant loss (unless it is discovered prior to skin closure), due to prolonged warm ischaemia. Some groups have tried anticoagulation and thrombolysis, but the risk of haemorrhage is high. Renal vein thrombosis is an infrequent complication (1–5%) and is due to: kinking either as a result of an excessively long renal vein or a mobile graft, extrinsic compression of the renal vein or iliac vein, poor surgical technique, hypovolaemia and prothrombogenic conditions. Patients usually present in the first postoperative week with oliguria, haematuria, graft tenderness and swelling. Late thrombosis is rare and usually associated with thrombophilic states. Early detection and treatment is critical to prevent venous infarction and rupture, urgent surgical exploration is the treatment of choice though thrombolysis may be attempted, particularly when the diagnosis is delayed.

Further Reading

Irshad A, Ackerman SJ, Campbell AS, Anis M. An overview of renal transplantation: current practice and use of ultrasound. *Semin Ultrasound CT MR.* 2009;30(4):298–314.

Sandhu C, Patel U. Renal transplantation dysfunction: the role of interventional radiology. *Clin Radiol.* 2002;57(9):772–783.

Case 2.34

A routine post transplant USS was performed on this patient 2 weeks following his surgery. The transplant is functioning normally, and the patient is well.

1. Describe the findings.
2. What is the differential diagnosis?
3. How should this be managed?

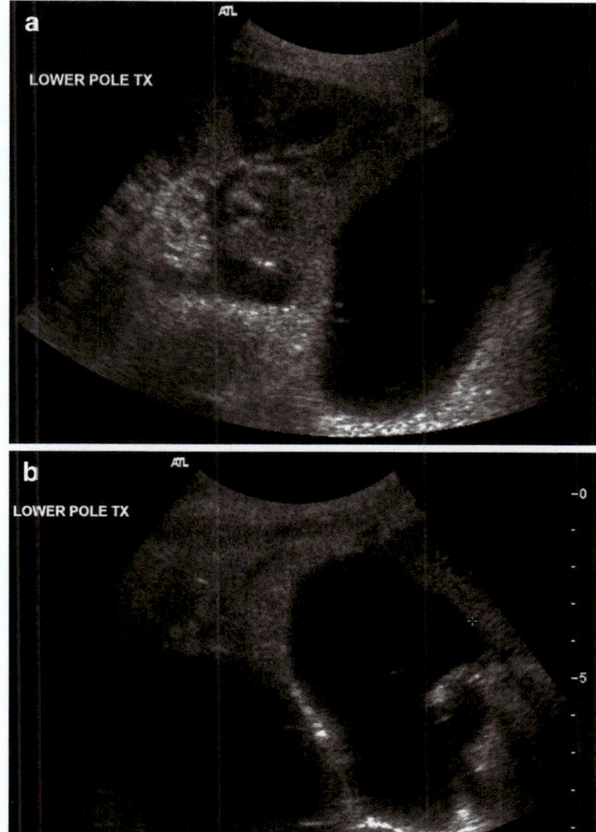

Fig. 2.34.1

Answers to Case 2.34

1. These ultrasound images (Fig. 2.34.1a,b) through the lower pole of the renal transplant show a fluid collection below the renal hilum.
2. This may represent:
   - Urinary bladder (may lie adjacent to a transplant kidney)
   - Urinoma
   - Lymphocoele (5–15% of patients)
   - Abscess
   - Haematoma (tends to be more echogenic)
3. The need for intervention (radiological or surgical) is dependent on the clinical status. In this case the collection should be followed on ultrasound as most post transplant collections resolve naturally. A few may compress or obstruct the ureter, become infected, rarely compress the kidney itself ('Page' kidney) or even more rarely compress the iliac veins. Drainage can usually be performed percutaneously under ultrasound guidance, but simple drainage is not always curative and surgical exclusion may be required. Regarding surgery, if this proves to be a lymphocoele then surgical marsupialisation is required.

Case 2.35

These are ultrasound images from a patient with deteriorating renal function 12 days post renal transplant.

1. Describe the findings.
2. What is the differential diagnosis?
3. What are the indications for treatment and what are the treatment options?

Fig. 2.35.1

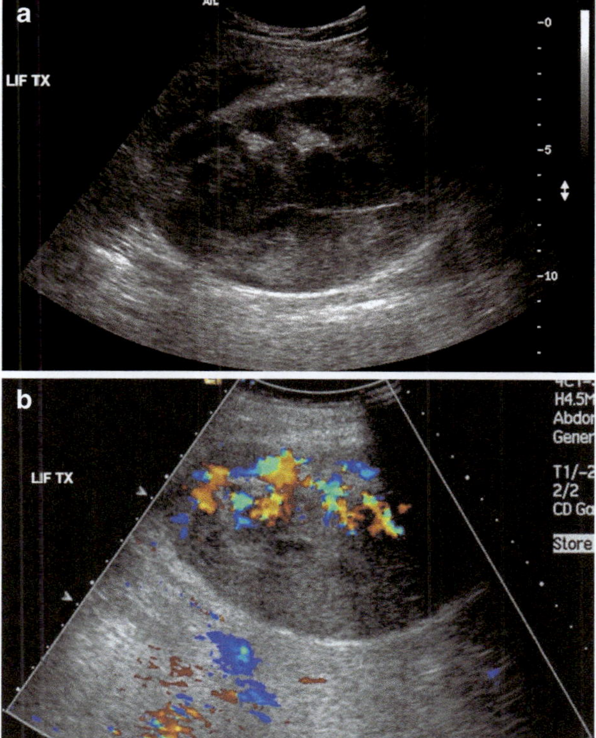

Answers to Case 2.35

1. The greyscale (Fig. 2.35.1a) and colour Doppler images (Fig. 2.35.1b) show a mildly hyperechoic lesion lying adjacent and deep to the transplant kidney. This lesion broadly follows the outline of the kidney but there is no vascularity demonstrated in this region. In comparison, normal vascularity is seen within the kidney.
2. This is most likely to represent subcapsular haematoma. This is usually secondary to renal biopsy or local trauma. Lymphocoele or urinoma is usually anechoic but both of these will be external to the kidney, not subcapsular.
3. Indications for treatment include:
   - Mass effect causing compression of the renal parenchyma leading to hypertension due to a 'Page' kidney (this was the case here).
   - Less commonly urinary obstruction.
   - Rarely infection of the haematoma.

   The haematoma may be too thick to completely drain percutaneously, but sufficient evacuation may occur such that the compression is relieved and the haematoma allowed to resolve naturally. Otherwise surgical drainage is necessary.

Further Reading

Page IH, McCubbin JW. Renal vascular and systemic arterial pressure responses to nervous and chemical stimulation of the kidney. *Am J Physiol.* 1953;173(3): 411–419.

Case 2.36

These are the 2-week and 1 year follow-up post-renal transplant US scans. The nephrostogram was undertaken after a therapeutic intervention.

1. Describe the findings.
2. What is the significance of these appearances?
3. How is it treated?

Fig. 2.36.1

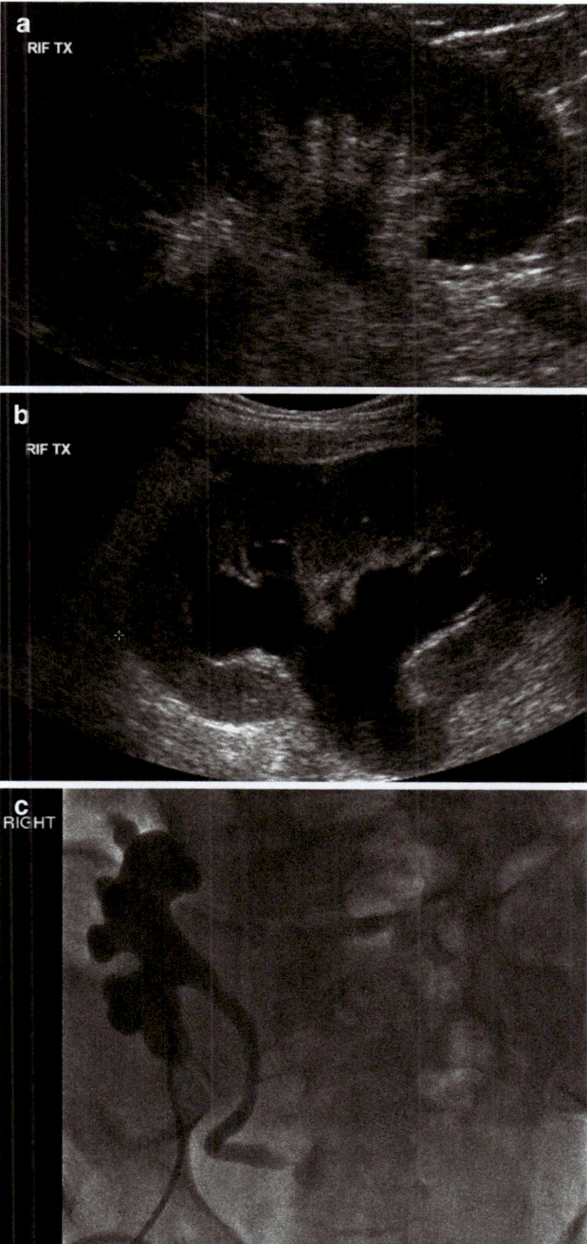

Answers to Case 2.36

1. The 2-week postoperative USS (Fig. 2.36.1a) shows essentially normal appearances of the right iliac fossa and transplant kidney. The USS undertaken 1 year later demonstrates pelvicalyceal dilatation (Fig. 2.36.1b). A nephrostomy tube was inserted and the nephrostogram shows obstruction at the ureteric anastomosis, just above the vesicoureteric junction (Fig. 2.36.1c).
2. Post-transplant pelvicalyceal dilatation is not always significant. The ureteric anastomosis is prone to reflux and may cause pelvicalyceal prominence. This prominence tends to decrease post-micturition. Serial scanning maybe useful, and worsening pelvicalyceal dilatation, together with deteriorating renal function can be an indicator of obstruction, which occurs in 5% of renal transplants. Most causes of obstruction are due to anastomotic stenosis (80%) though high bladder pressure or urinary retention can also lead to increasing upper tract dilatation and decompensation.
3. Nephrostomy may be needed in an emergency to protect renal function. Long-term, the stricture will require correction. Balloon dilatation, either antegrade or retrograde, is curative in about half the cases, the rest require either long term stenting (which may be with a long term metal stent) or anastomotic revision. If the dilatation is due to bladder outflow obstruction, it will require surgical relief.

Further Reading

Kobayashi K, Censullo ML, Rossman LL, Kyriakides PN, Kahan BD, Cohen AM. Interventional radiologic management of renal transplant dysfunction: indications, limitations, and technical considerations. *Radiographics*. 2007;27(4): 1109–1130.

Case 2.37

1. The USS is a routine follow-up scan of a transplanted kidney. Describe the findings. What is the diagnosis?
2. How do transplant recipients develop tumours and what are the more common sites?

Fig. 2.37.1

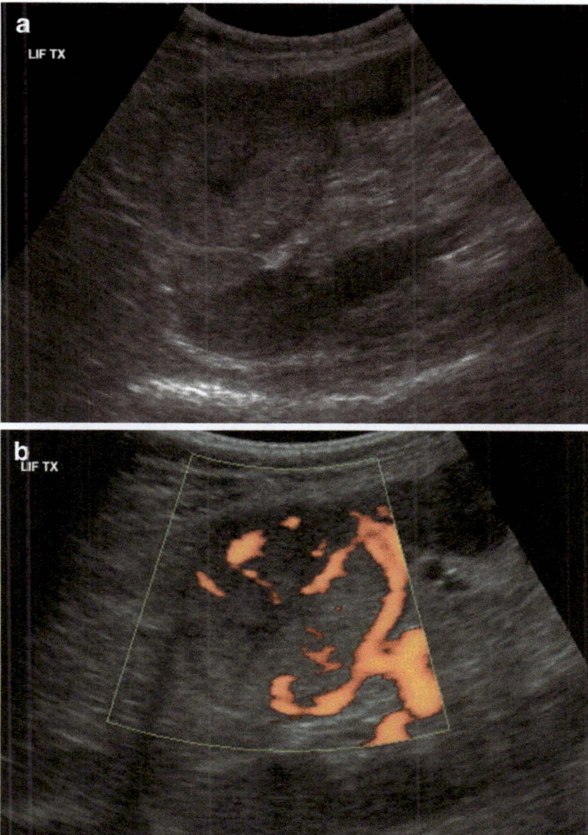

Answers to Case 2.37

1. Greyscale (Fig. 2.37.1a) US image of the left iliac fossa transplant kidney shows a solid mass in the upper pole which demonstrates some vascularity on colour Doppler imaging (Fig. 2.37.1b). Appearances are suggestive of a tumour in the transplant kidney.
2. Transplant recipients are at higher risk of all tumours. Tumours may arise de novo, or be transmitted in the transplant. Tumours transmitted from the donor are rare, and are thought to occur in 0.2% of renal transplants. Some tumours are not a contraindication to kidney donation. Skin basal cell carcinoma, low grade brain tumours and CIS in the cervix or larynx do not exclude kidney donation, some even propose organ donation from donors with small renal carcinomas following excision of the lesion and informed consent.

   The presence of active malignancy in the recipient is an absolute contraindication to kidney transplant. In patients with a previous history of malignancy a balance must be weighed between the risk of tumour recurrence (site, grade, stage, duration recurrence free) and the age and quality of life of the potential recipient without a transplant. Patients with a prior history of malignancy need closer follow-up and the immunotherapy may be tailored accordingly.

   The risk of de novo tumours after transplant is several times higher than the general population and malignancy is one of the commonest causes of death after transplantation. The commonest tumours are skin cancers (50%) – by 20 years post transplant 50% of patients will have developed a skin cancer and 50% of these are squamous cell carcinomas. Annual dermatological checks and the use of total UV sunblock are recommended.

   Post transplant lymphoproliferative disease (PTLD) is increasing with current immunosuppressive agents and is potentially life threatening. PTLD usually presents within the first year post transplant and is characterised by non-Hodgkin's lymphomas and EBV-infected B-lymphocytes. Treatment involves reduction or even cessation of immunosuppressive therapy, the remission rate is 50–68%.

   Other sites in which malignancy occurs in transplant individuals more than in the general population include the cervix, due to reactivation of the HPV virus, the urothelium and the native and transplanted kidney. The evidence for increased malignancy in other common sites including the bowel, lung and prostate remains controversial and surveillance of these sites is less well defined.

Further Reading

Kälble T, Alcaraz A, Budde K, Humke U, Karam G, Lucan M, Nicita G, Süsal C. EAU guidelines: renal transplantation. 2009.

The Adrenal

3

Anwen Newland, Dan Berney, and Andrea G. Rockall

Case 3.1

These are images of normal adrenal glands.

1. What is the size of the normal adrenal gland?
2. What is the arterial supply and venous drainage of the right and left adrenal gland?
3. Name the different layers of the adrenal gland shown in Fig. 3.1.3, their embryonic derivation and the main hormones produced within each.

S. Bott et al. (eds.), *Images in Urology*,
DOI 10.1007/978-0-85729-769-3_3,

Fig. 3.1.1

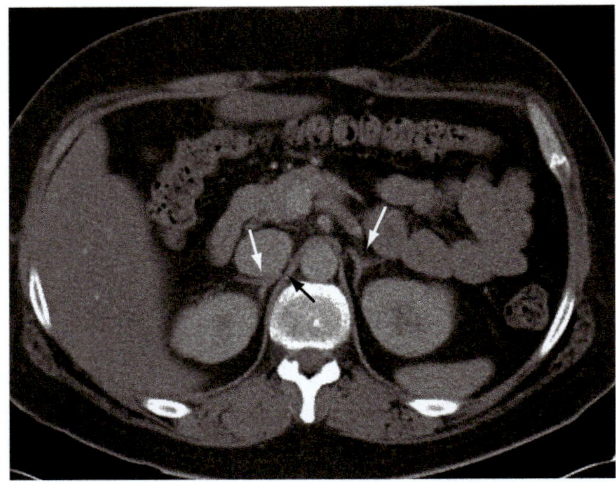

Fig. 3.1.2

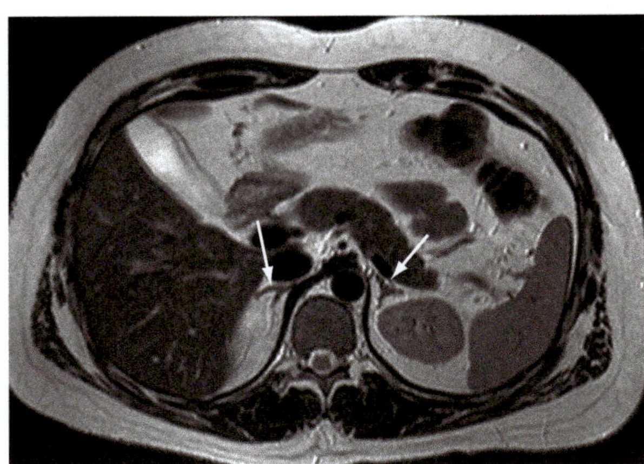

Fig. 3.1.3

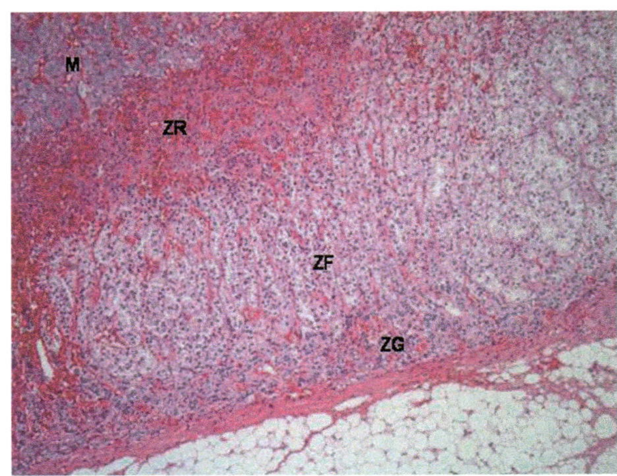

Answers to Case 3.1

1. Figure 3.1.1 is an axial contrast-enhanced CT, and Fig. 3.1.2 is a T2-weighted MR image of the upper abdomen. Both demonstrate normal adrenal glands (white arrows). The maximum width of the right adrenal gland is 0.6 cm (SD ± 0.2) and of the left is 0.8 cm (SD ± 0.2). The maximum width of each limb of the gland is approximately 0.3 cm (SD ± 0.1). As a rough guide, the limbs of the adrenal gland are of similar width to the crus of the diaphragm (black arrow).
2. Each adrenal gland is supplied via the superior adrenal artery (from the inferior phrenic artery), middle adrenal artery (from the aorta) and inferior adrenal artery (from the renal artery). The right adrenal vein drains into the IVC and the left adrenal vein into the left renal vein.
3. Figure 3.1.3 is an H&E stain of the normal adrenal gland. The adrenal cortex is derived from the mesoderm and is composed of the outer zona glomerulosa (ZG – producing mostly aldosterone), the zona fasiculata (ZF – producing mostly cortisol) and the inner zona reticularis (ZR – producing some androgens). The adrenal medulla (M) is derived from the neural crest and produces epinephrine and norepinephrine.

Further Reading

Mayo-Smith WW, Boland GW, Noto RB, Lee MJ. State-of-the-art adrenal imaging. *Radiographics*. 2001;21:995–1012.

Vincent JM, Morrison ID, Armstrong P, Reznek RH. The size of normal adrenal glands on computed tomography. *Clin Radiol*. 1994;49:453–455.

Case 3.2

Study these four images of an adrenal lesion

1. What is the difference between the cellular distribution of fat within a lipid-rich adenoma and a myelolipoma (Figs. 3.2.1 and 3.4.1)?
2. What is the appearance of a lipid rich adenoma on the CT in Fig. 3.2.2?
3. What is the MRI sequence shown in Fig. 3.2.3a,b, and what does the lesion demonstrate?

Fig. 3.2.1

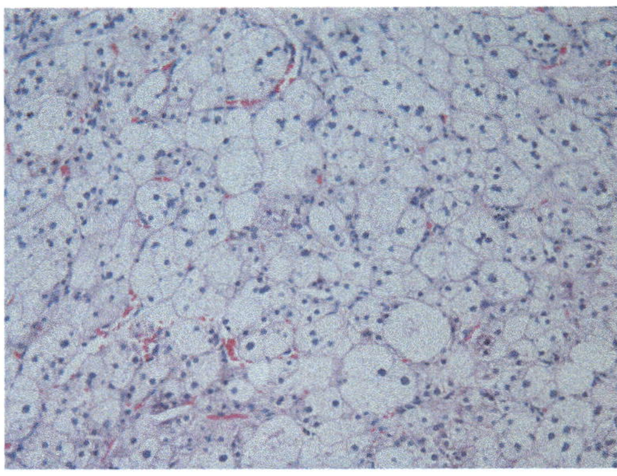

Fig. 3.2.2

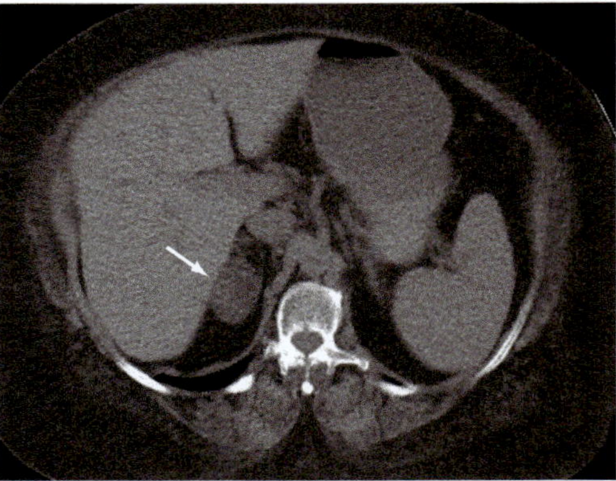

Fig. 3.2.3

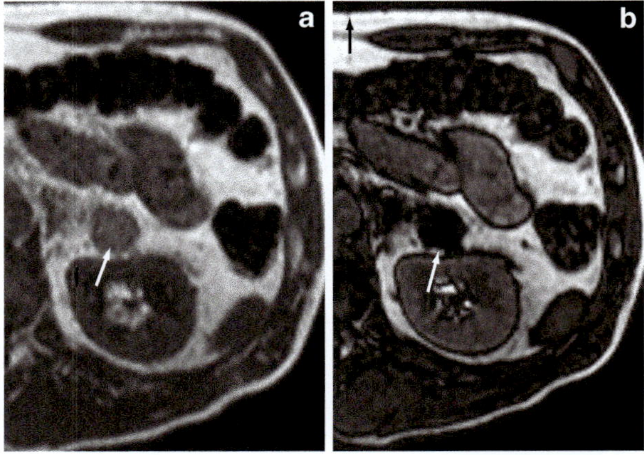

Answers to Case 3.2

1. Figure 3.2.1 is an H&E stain of a lipid-rich adrenal adenoma, demonstrating abundant intracytoplasmic lipid droplets within the adrenocortical cells and resembling zona fasciculata. This differs from a myelolipoma, where the fat lies within adipose tissue cells (adipocytes). Adrenal adenomas are very common lesions at autopsy and as incidental findings on cross-sectional abdominal imaging.
2. Figure 3.2.2 is an axial non-contrast CT image demonstrating a low-attenuation (−12HU) right adrenal lesion. An attenuation value of <10HU indicates the presence of intracellular lipid within the lesion and confirms the diagnosis of a benign cortical adenoma. The lesion is also less than 3 cm in size, consistent with a benign lesion. Therefore no further imaging is required, though is sometimes undertaken (see below). Functional and endocrinological assessment can also be helpful. A lesion greater than 5 cm is unlikely to be benign and carcinoma should be suspected.
3. Figure 3.2.3a and b are in- and out-of-phase MRI images respectively. The left adrenal lesion loses signal on the out-of-phase images (white arrow), confirming the presence of intracellular lipid. In this sequence loss of signal intensity only occurs when soft tissue and lipid occur within the same voxel. Note that subcutaneous fat does not lose signal intensity (black arrow). A fat-saturated sequence will not result in signal drop-out in the case of a lipid-rich adenoma, whereas a fat-saturation sequence will result in signal loss where there are adipocytes and radiologically visible fat, as seen in a myelolipoma.

Further Reading

Boland GW, Lee MJ, Gazelle GS, et al. Characterization of adrenal masses using unenhanced CT: an analysis of the CT literature. *AJR Am J Roentgenol.* 1998;171:201–204.

Lack EE. *Tumours of the Adrenal Glands and Extraadrenal Paraganglia 2007.* Washington: ARP Press; 2007: chap 3, pp 57–97.

Lee MJ, Hahn PF, Papanicolaou N, Egglin TK, et al. Benign and malignant adrenal masses: CT distinction with attenuation coefficients, size and observer analysis. *Radiology.* 1991;179:415–418.

Mayo-Smith WW, Boland GW, Noto RB, Lee MJ. State-of-the-art adrenal imaging. *Radiographics.* 2001;21:995–1012.

Case 3.3

Study the images and answer the questions below:

1. What percentage of adrenal cortical adenomas are lipid-poor?
2. How do they differ from lipid-rich adenomas on imaging?
3. How can lipid-poor cortical adenomas be characterised?

Fig. 3.3.1

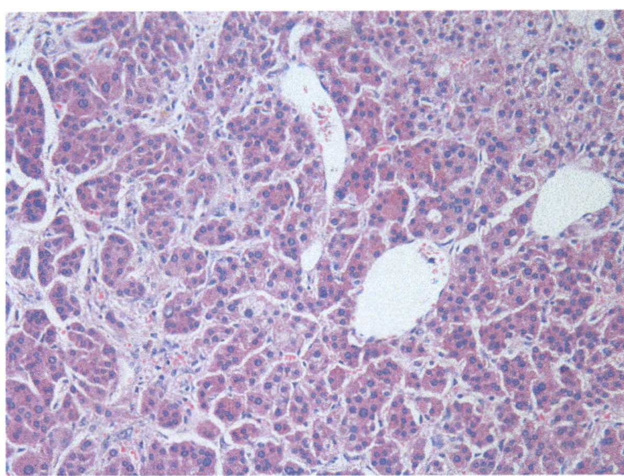

Fig. 3.3.2

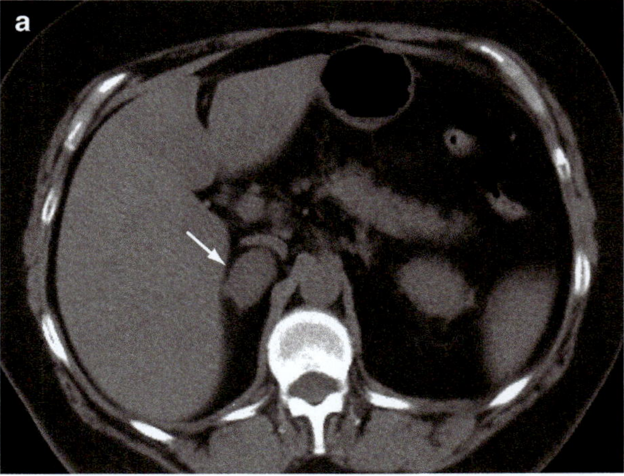

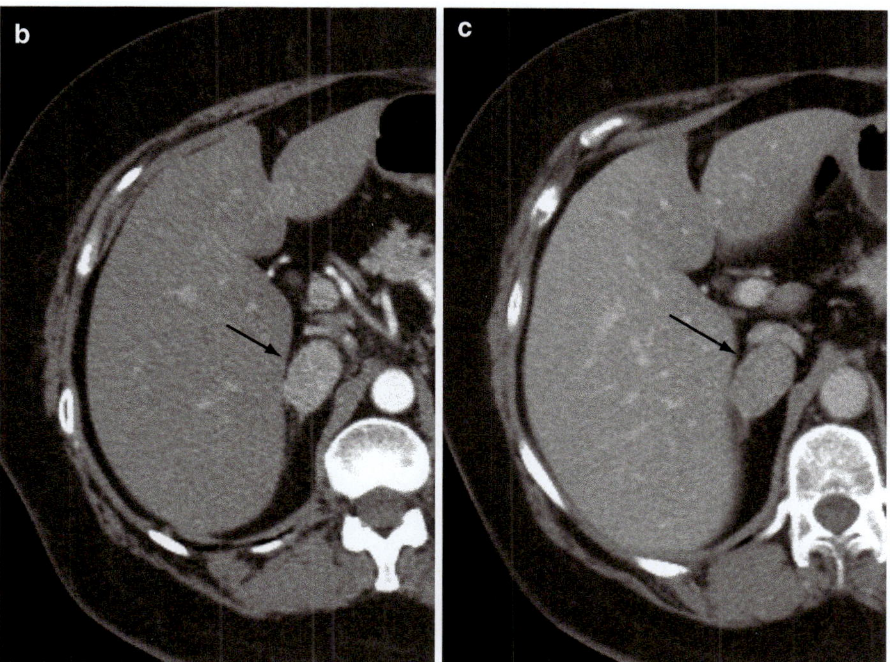

Fig. 3.3.2 (continued)

Answers to Case 3.3

1. Lipid-poor adenomas account for up to 30% of adrenal adenomas. Figure 3.3.1 is an H&E stain of a lipid-poor adenoma; it is composed of eosinophilic (oncocytic) cytoplasm and resembling zona reticularis with no intracellular lipid.
2. Figure 3.3.2a is an axial non-contrast CT image demonstrating a right adrenal mass with an attenuation value of >34HU. A lesion with an attenuation value of >10HU is not a lipid-rich adenoma and requires further characterisation, to exclude a metastatic deposit in the adrenal gland or a primary adrenal malignancy. If the lesion is between 10 and 30HU, in- and out-of-phase MRI may be helpful. If the attenuation is >30HU, there will be no signal drop out on MRI and a CT contrast 'wash-out' study is indicated. Adenomas show more rapid washout of contrast than adrenal metastases.
3. Figure 3.3.2b and c are late arterial-phase and delayed (15 min post-contrast injection) CT images, respectively, demonstrating the contrast enhancement and washout of the adrenal lesion. Absolute washout (AWO) of >60% confirms the diagnosis of an adenoma (calculation of absolute washout requires a pre-contrast CT). Relative washout can be assessed without a pre-contrast scan; washout of >40% is needed to confirm the lesion is an adenoma.

Further Reading

Dunnick NR, Korobkin M. Imaging of adrenal incidentalomas: current status. *AJR Am J Roentgenol.* 2002;179:559–568.

Case 3.4

Examine the images below and then answer these questions:

1. What is the composition of a myelolipoma?
2. How can the presence of fat be confirmed on CT?
3. What are these MRI sequences and what do they demonstrate?
4. What are the complications of a myelolipoma?

Fig. 3.4.1

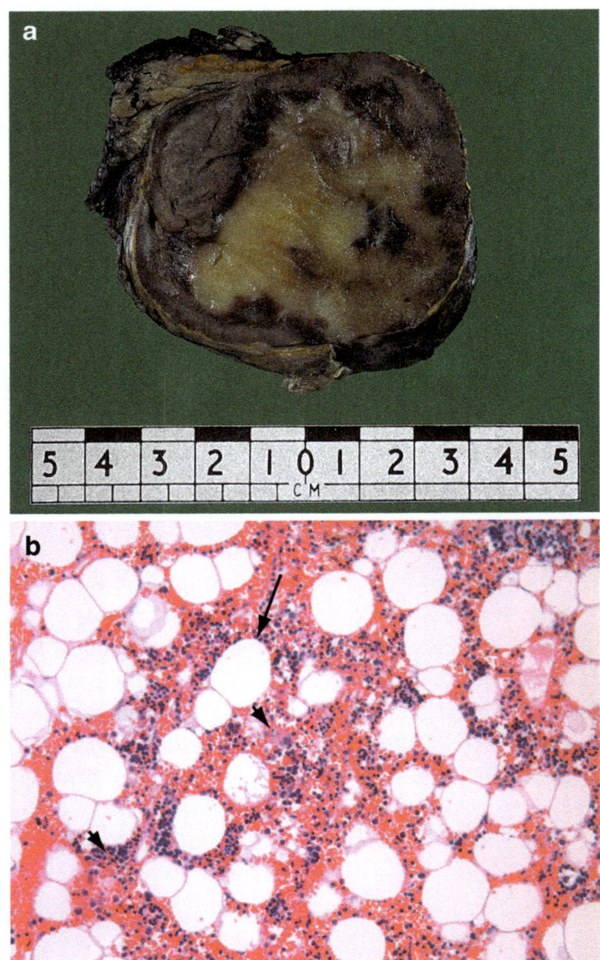

Fig. 3.4.2

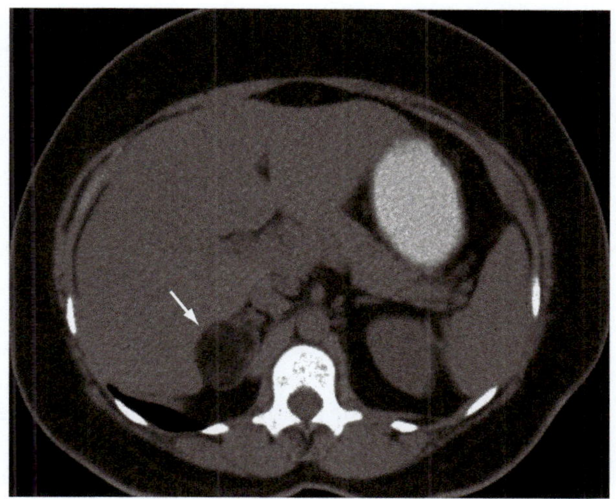

Fig. 3.4.3

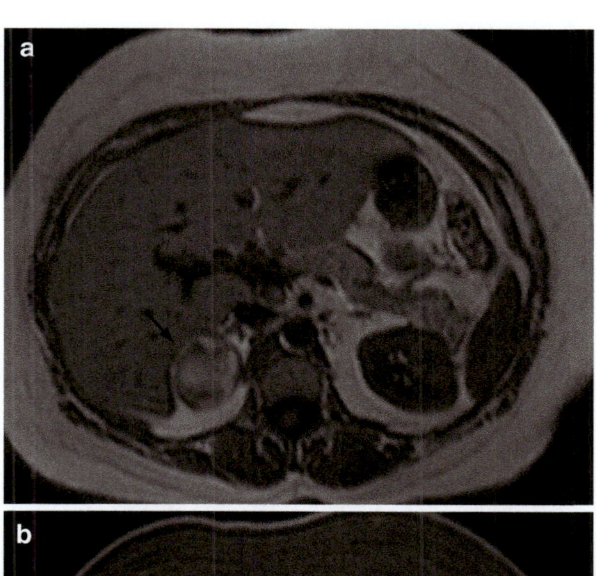

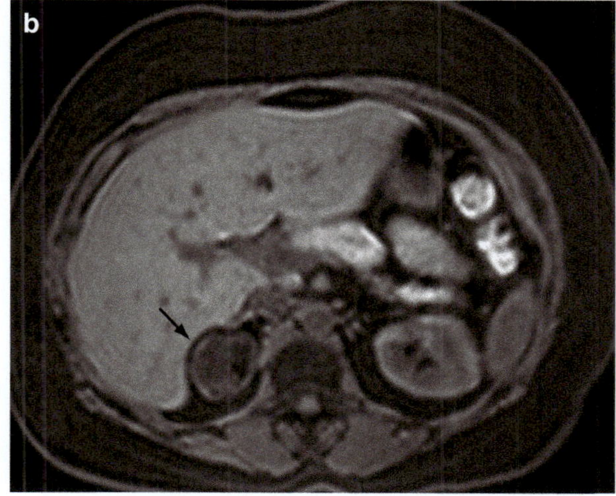

Answers to Case 3.4

1. Figure 3.4.1a shows the macroscopic appearance of an adrenalectomy containing a fatty and vascular mass, typical of myelolipoma. The normal adrenal tissue is compressed, best seen on the left of the specimen. Myelolipomas are seen in 0.2–0.4% of the population. Figure 3.4.1b shows the microscopic features in which adipocytes (long arrow), erythroid and myeloid components (arrowheads) are all present.
2. Figure 3.4.2 is an axial non-contrast CT demonstrating a well-defined low attenuation lesion in the right adrenal gland with an attenuation value of less than –50HU, consistent with fat. Twenty percent of lesions may also demonstrate calcification on CT.

   If the lesion is entirely fatty on imaging, the diagnosis is myelolipoma and no further investigation is needed. If there is a focal soft tissue component, the possibility of a 'collision' tumour should be considered, where two separate tumours abut one another. The soft tissue component may be adenomatous, but if this is large, malignancy cannot be excluded. Rarely, no macroscopic fat is demonstrated within a myelolipoma on imaging, precluding a preoperative diagnosis, as differentiation from a sarcoma or carcinoma cannot be made.
3. Figure 3.4.3a is a T1-weighted MRI sequence demonstrating high-signal intensity within the lesion. Fat also appears as high-signal intensity on T2-weighted sequences. Figure 3.4.3b is a T1 fat-saturated MR image which demonstrates signal drop-out within the lesion, confirming the presence of macroscopic fat. (Note that the subcutaneous and intra-abdominal fat has also lost signal.)
4. Large lesions may rarely undergo spontaneous haemorrhage and may require prophylactic resection.

Further Reading

Dunnick NR, Korobkin M. Imaging of adrenal incidentalomas: current status. *AJR Am J Roentgenol.* 2002;179:559–568.

Elsayes KM, Mukundan G, Narra VR et al. Adrenal masses: MR imaging features with pathological correlation. *Radiographics.* 2004;24:S73–S86.

Mayo-Smith WW, Boland GW, Noto RB, Lee MJ. State-of-the-art adrenal imaging. *Radiographics.* 2001;21:995–1012.

Case 3.5

The following five images are from different patients. Study these and then attempt the questions.

1. How does primary hyperaldosteronism present and what are the two most common causes?
2. Why is it important to differentiate between the two causes?
3. What procedure can be performed to confirm the diagnosis in equivocal cases?
4. What specific histological feature of Conn's adenoma can occasionally be identified?

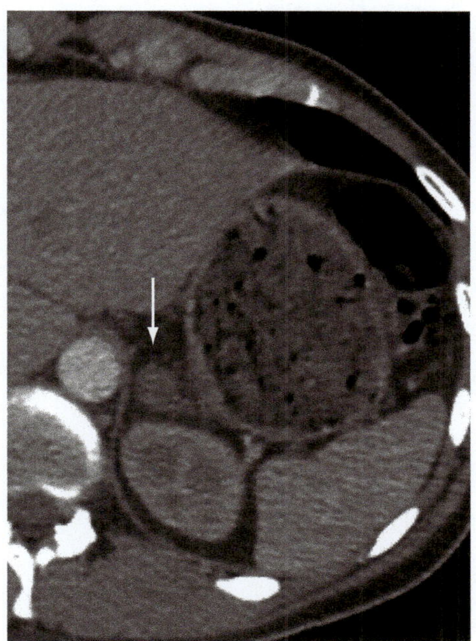

Fig. 3.5.1

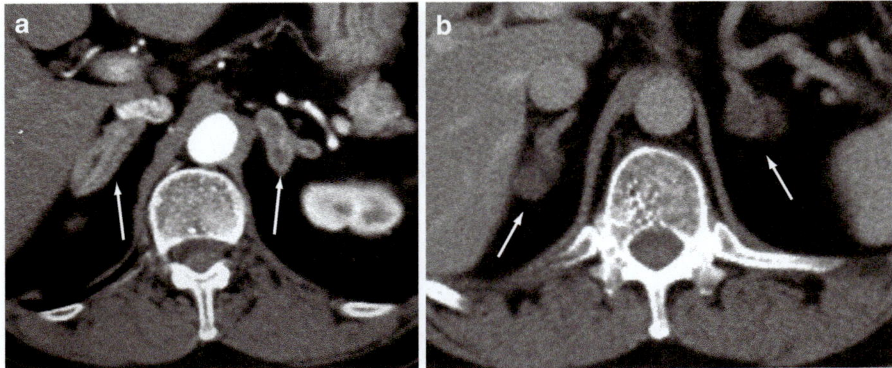

Fig. 3.5.2

Fig. 3.5.3

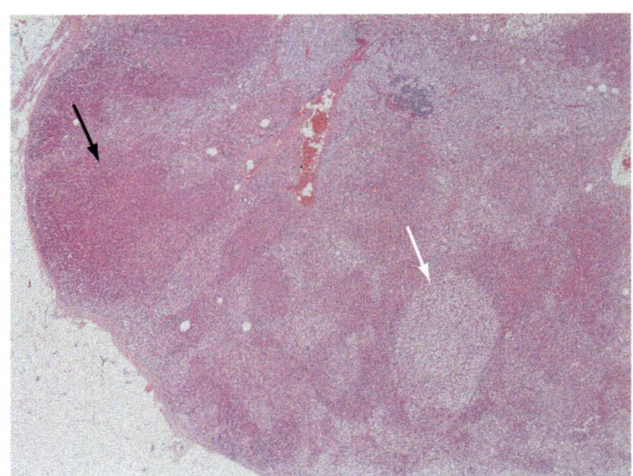

Fig. 3.5.4

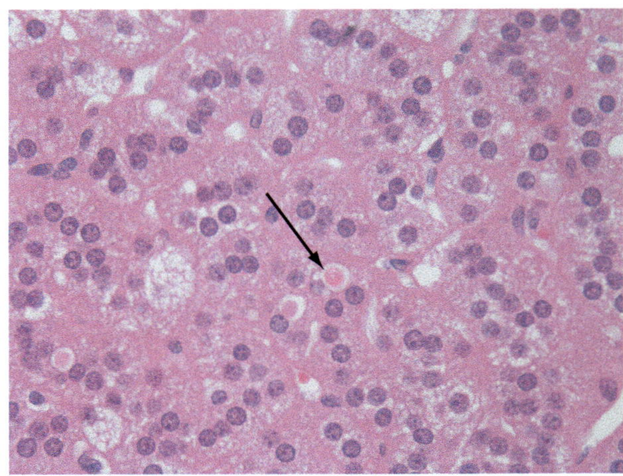

Answers to Case 3.5

1. Hyperaldosteronism most commonly presents with hypertension. The two common causes are a unilateral aldosterone-producing adenoma (Conn's adenoma) (Fig. 3.5.1) and bilateral adrenal hyperplasia, each accounting for 33% and 66% of cases, respectively. Bilateral hyperplasia may be smooth and micronodular (Fig. 3.5.2a) or macronodular (Fig. 3.5.2b) in appearance. Other rare causes include unilateral adrenal hyperplasia, adrenal carcinoma and familial hyperaldosteronism. Aldosterone-producing adenomas tend to be found in younger patients (<40 years) and bilateral hyperplasia in older patients (>40 years).
2. Adrenal adenomas are managed surgically, with 30–60% of patients becoming normotensive after surgery. Bilateral hyperplasia is managed with medical therapy. A mean adrenal limb thickness of 5 mm or greater has been shown to be highly specific for bilateral adrenal hyperplasia. Figure 3.5.3 demonstrates a case of adrenocortical hyperplasia with both lipid-rich (white arrow) and lipid-poor nodules (black arrow). A small Conn's adenoma may not be visualised on cross-sectional imaging.
3. The gold-standard for establishing a cause for hyperaldosteronism is adrenal vein sampling performed under radiological guidance.
4. Figure 3.5.4 demonstrates an H&E stain of a Conn's adenoma with a classic lamellated spironolactone body (arrow). These are only seen in patients pre-treated with spironolactone.

Further Reading

Lingam RK, Sohaib SA, Vlahos I, et al. CT of primary hyperaldosteronism (Conn's syndrome): the value of measuring the adrenal gland. *AJR Am J Roentgenol.* 2003;181:843–849.

Patel SM, Lingam RK, Beaconsfield TI, et al. The role of radiology in the management of primary aldosteronism. *Radiographics.* 2007;27:1145–1157.

Case 3.6

1. Where do ganglioneuromas occur?
2. What are their appearances on imaging?
3. Are they associated with any other tumour types?

Fig. 3.6.1

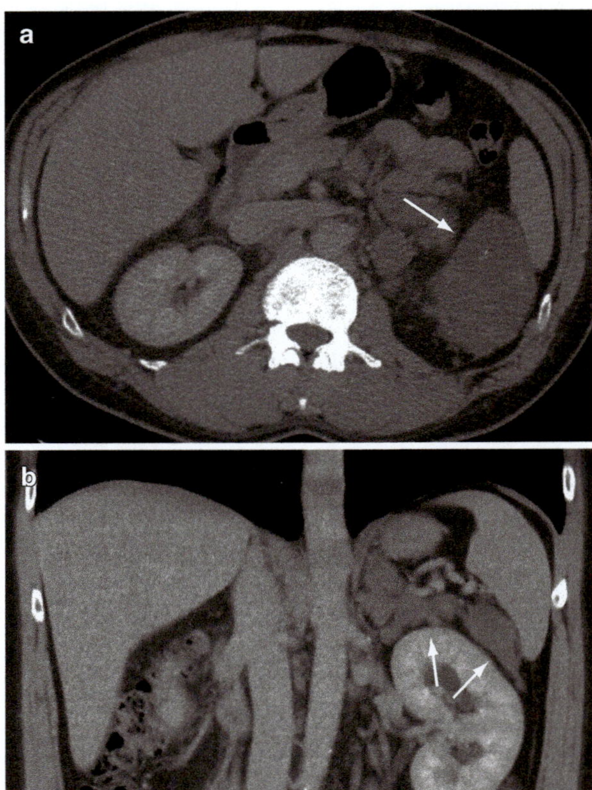

Fig. 3.6.2

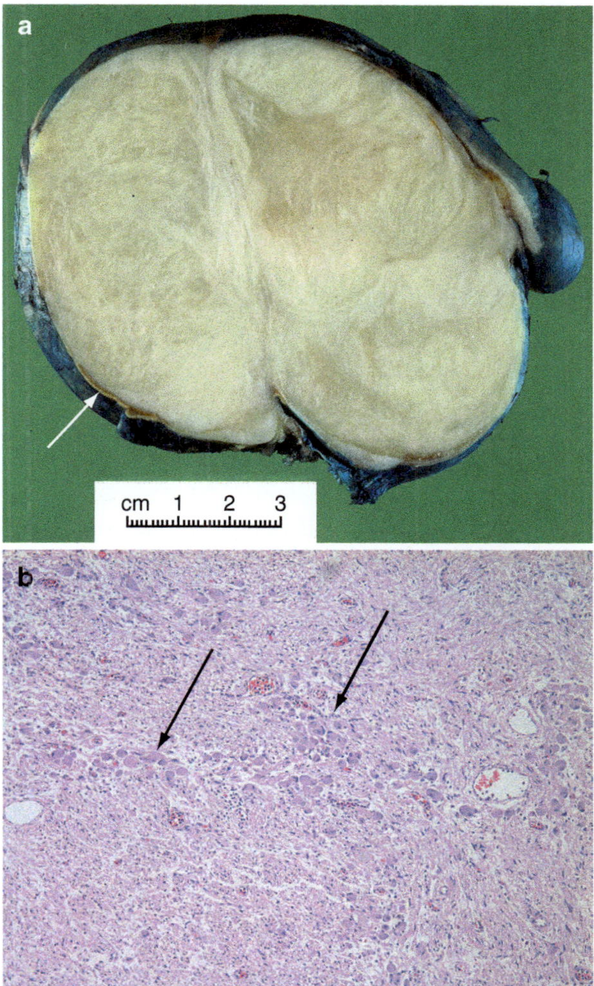

Answers to Case 3.6

1. Ganglioneuromas are benign tumours of the sympathetic nervous system and can occur anywhere along the paravertebral sympathetic plexus. Common sites include the adrenal gland (20–30%), retroperitoneum, posterior mediastinum, head and neck. Adrenal ganglioneuromas are usually non-secretory.
2. Figures 3.6.1a and b are axial and coronal post-contrast CT images of a left ganglioneuroma. This lobulated lesion demonstrates some of the specific features which suggest the diagnosis, namely the presence of calcification and absence of vascular invasion. Ganglioneuromas also demonstrate a low non-enhanced attenuation value of <40HU. On MRI they demonstrate low T1- and slightly high and heterogeneous T2-weighted signal intensity. They show late and gradual dynamic enhancement on MRI, occasionally with a whorled pattern. Ganglioneuromas may be difficult to differentiate from adrenal carcinoma on imaging. Catecholamine levels should always be checked prior to biopsy or surgical excision.
3. Thorough pathological assessment is required to exclude the possibility of a composite tumour which would include associated phaeochromocytoma or primitive neuroblastic elements that confer a worse prognosis. Figure 3.6.2a is the cut surface of an adrenal ganglioneuroma (the external surface painted with blue dye). The compressed adrenal cortex is seen intermittently at the circumferential limits, especially on the lower left of the specimen (arrowed). Figure 3.6.2b is a micrograph of a ganglioneuroma with bland neuronal tissue and clusters of ganglia (arrows).

Further Reading

Dunnick NR, Korobkin M. Imaging of adrenal incidentalomas: current status. *AJR Am J Roentgenol.* 2002;179:559–568.

Longergan JG, Schwab CM, Suarez ES, Carlson CL. Neuroblastoma, ganglioneuroblastoma and ganglioneuroma: radiologic-pathologic correlation. *Radiographics.* 2002;22:911–934.

Maweja S, Materne R, Detrembleur N, et al. Adrenal ganglioneuroma. *Am J Surg.* 2007;194:683–684.

Case 3.7

These four images are from different patients.

1. What are the different appearances of a phaeochromocytoma on CT and T2-weighted MRI?
2. What other imaging study, shown in Fig. 3.7.3, may be helpful in their assessment?
3. What histological features suggest malignancy in a phaeochromocytoma?

Fig. 3.7.1

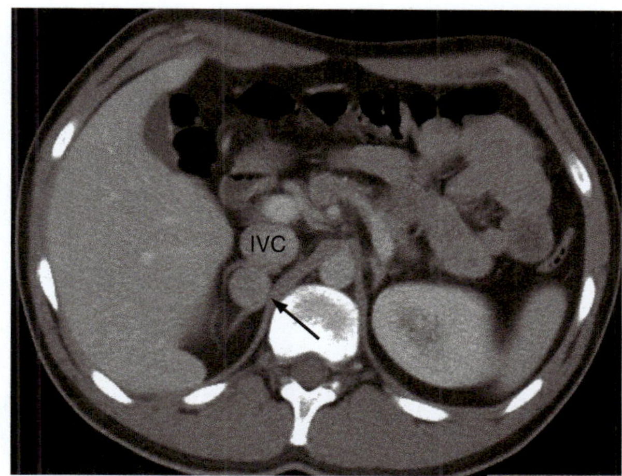

Fig. 3.7.2

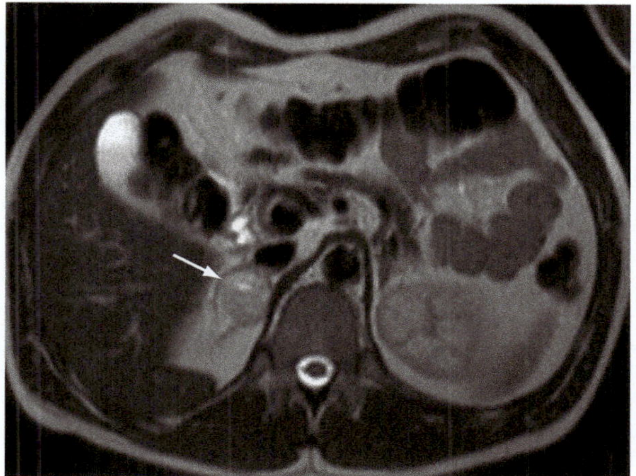

Fig. 3.7.3

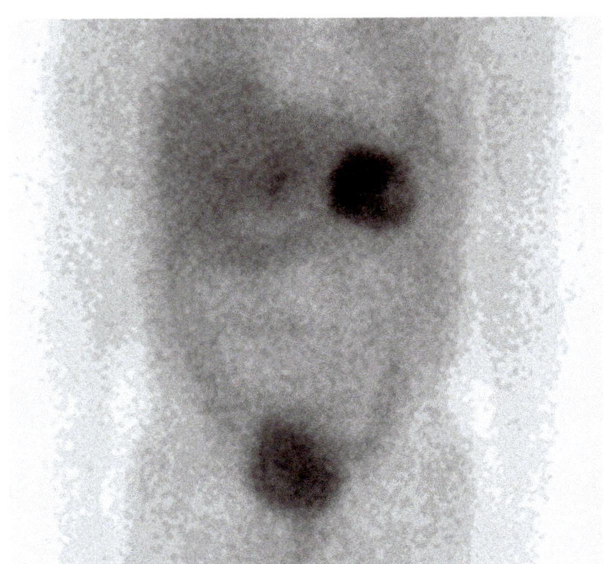

Fig. 3.7.4

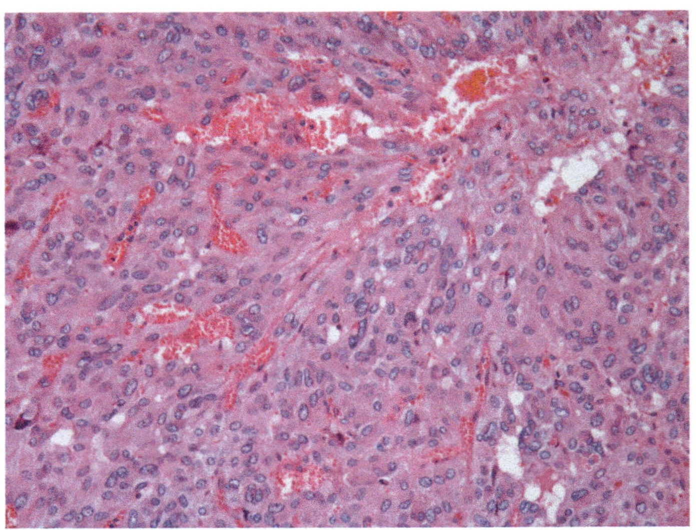

Answers to Case 3.7

1. Figure 3.7.1 is a contrast-enhanced CT of a right-sided phaeochromocytoma (IVC = inferior vena cava). Phaechromocytomas do not contain lipid and enhance avidly after contrast on CT. Figure 3.7.2 is a T2-weighted MR image demonstrating the most common appearance, with multiple 'pockets' of high T2 signal in a right-sided phaeochromocytoma. They may also appear 'classical' (the same signal as CSF), 'intermediate' (signal intensity between that of spleen and CSF) or 'marbled' (swirled areas of mixed intensity).
2. Figure 3.7.3 is a radionucleotide-labelled metaiodobenzylguanidine (MIBG) study showing uptake in a large left adrenal mass. This study is sensitive and highly specific for detecting phaeochromocytomas as MIBG is taken up by their catecholamine storage granules. Phaeochromocytomas may be malignant or bilateral in 10%.
3. Figure 3.7.4 shows a phaeochromocytoma with dense amphophillic (stains acid and base dyes to give a red/blue colour) cytoplasm. There are no reliable histological features to distinguish benign from malignant lesions.

Further Reading

Dunnick NR, Korobkin M. Imaging of adrenal incidentalomas: current status. *AJR Am J Roentgenol.* 2002;179:559–568.

Jacques AE, Sahdev A, Sandrasagara S, et al. Adrenal phaeochromocytoma: correlation of MRI appearances with histology and function. *Eur Radiol.* 2008;18:2885–2892.

Mukherjee JJ, Peppercorn PD, Reznek RH, et al. Pheochromocytoma: effect of nonionic contrast medium in CT on circulating catecholamine levels. *Radiology.* 1997;202:227–231.

Case 3.8

1. Study Fig. 3.8.1a. What features of this right adrenal mass on CT are suggestive of a malignant lesion?
2. What MRI sequence (Fig. 3.8.1b) is this and what imaging features are demonstrated?
3. In a separate patient what additional feature does Figure 3.8.2a demonstrate?
4. What is the imaging technique used in Fig. 3.8.2b and what does it show?
5. What histological features suggest malignancy in Fig. 3.8.3?

Fig. 3.8.1

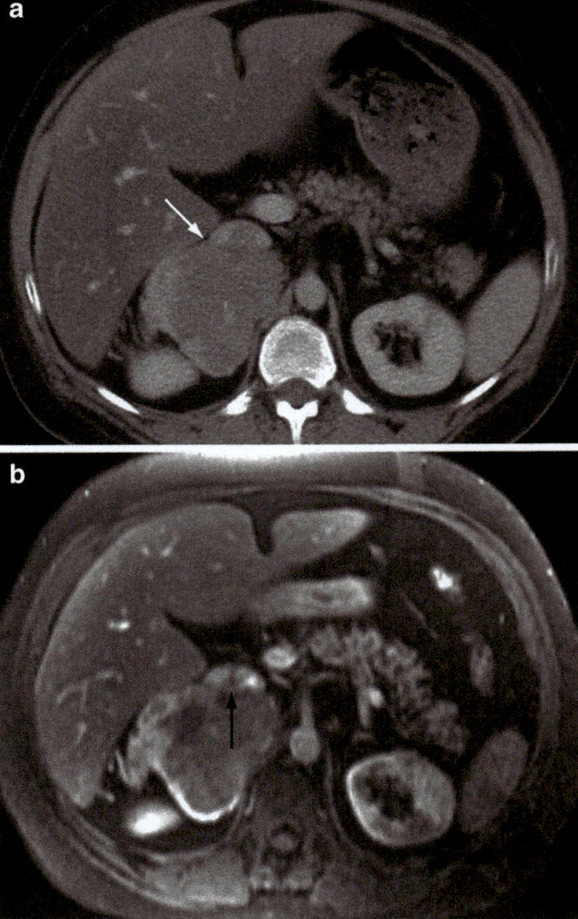

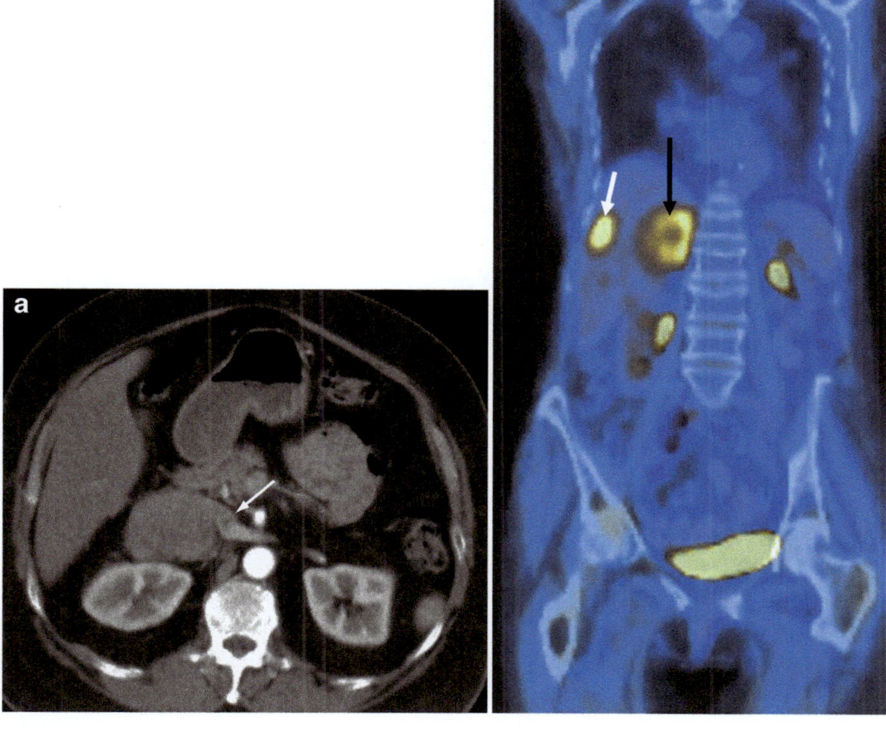

Fig. 3.8.2

Fig. 3.8.3

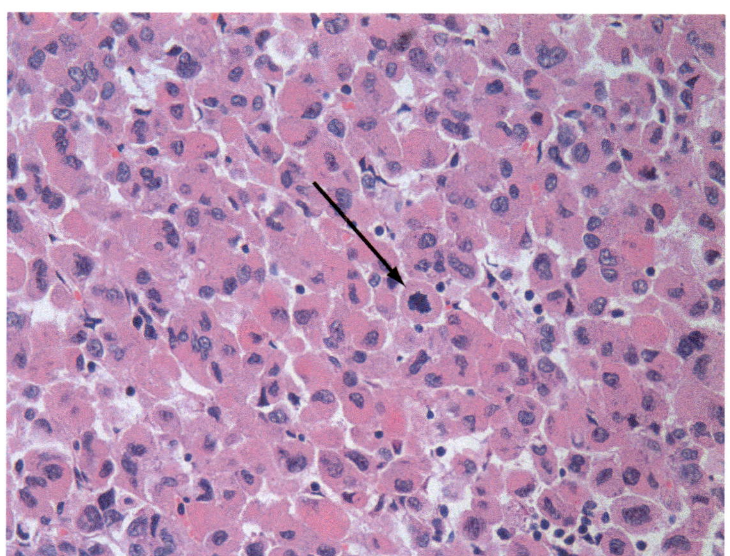

Answers to Case 3.8

1. Figure 3.8.1a is a portal venous phase contrast-enhanced CT image showing a right adrenal carcinoma. It is large (70% are >6 cm), has an irregular margin, shows small areas of calcification (seen in 30%) and is mildly heterogeneous (they commonly contain areas of necrosis and haemorrhage). This image demonstrates diffuse low attenuation of the liver indicating fatty infiltration, suggesting the patient may be Cushingoid. Adrenal carcinomas are bilateral in 10%, and as they are highly malignant, metastases are commonly seen. Half are functioning, most commonly producing cortisol.
2. Figure 3.8.1b is a post-contrast, fat-saturated T1-weighted MR image. There is heterogeneous enhancement of the mass. Heterogeneity and high T1- and T2-weighted signal intensity are often seen in cases of adrenal carcinoma. There is also invasion of the posterior wall of the IVC (arrow). Vascular invasion is another recognised feature of carcinoma.
3. Figure 3.8.2a is a post-contrast CT image of a different patient demonstrating tumour extension from the right adrenal gland into the IVC and extending into the left renal vein, also a common feature.
4. Figure 3.8.2b is a fused FDG-PET/CT image from the same patient as Fig. 3.8.2a, some time later, demonstrating the FDG-avid primary lesion (black arrow) and multiple liver metastases (white arrow).
5. Figure 3.8.3 demonstrates the increased mitotic activity (arrow) seen in an adrenal carcinoma. Other pathological features suggestive of malignancy include size of mass, invasiveness, vascular or capsular invasion, necrosis, pleomorphism and clear cell change. Scoring systems such as the Weiss criteria are used to assess these.

Further Reading

Babar S, Reznek RH. In: Husband JE, Reznek RH, eds. *Imaging in Oncology*, 2nd ed. London: Taylor and Francis; 2004.

Dunnick NR, Korobkin M. Imaging of adrenal incidentalomas: current status. *AJR Am J Roentgenol*. 2002;179:559–568.

Rockall AG, Babar SA, Sohaib SA, et al. CT and MR imaging of the adrenal glands in ACTH-independent cushing syndrome. *Radiographics*. 2004;24:435–452.

Weiss LM. *Adrenal Corticocarcinoma in Pathology and Genetics of Tumours of Endocrine Organs*. Lyon, France: IARC Press; 2004.

Case 3.9

Study the images below and answer the following questions

1. What features on CT are suggestive of an adrenal metastasis rather than a benign lesion?
2. What are the diagnostic features on MRI?
3. What other imaging techniques can be used to characterise metastases?

Fig. 3.9.1

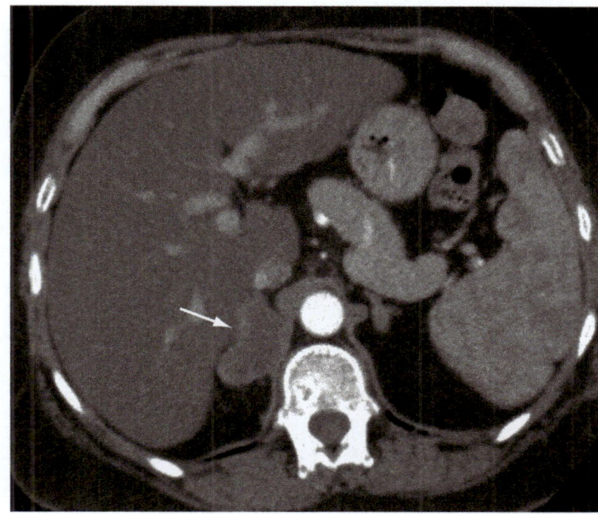

Fig. 3.9.2

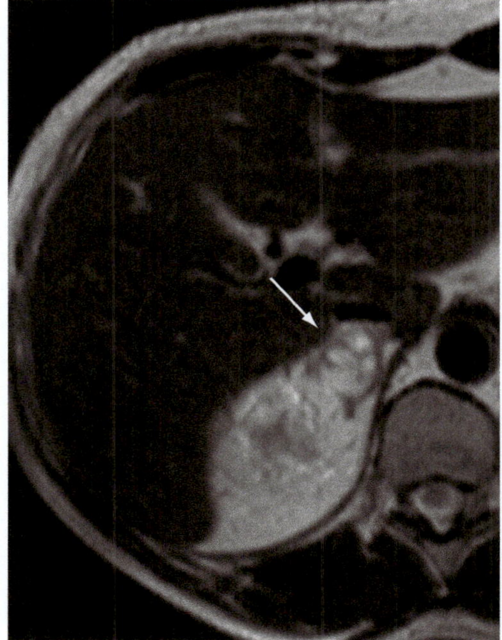

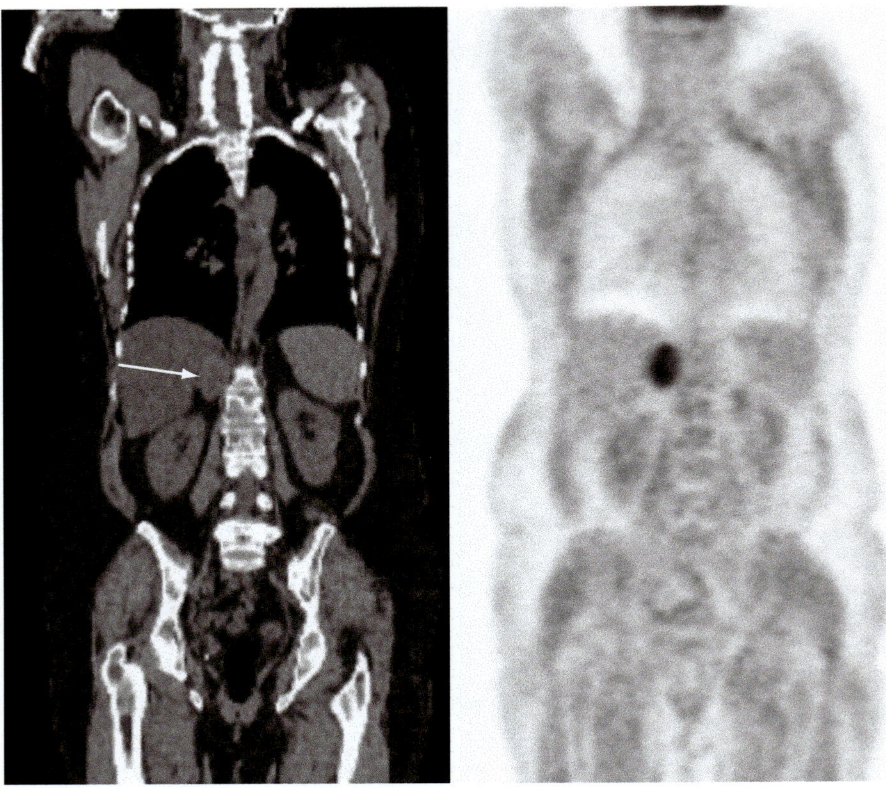

Fig. 3.9.3

Answers to Case 3.9

1. Figure 3.9.1a is a contrast-enhanced axial CT demonstrating a metastasis from ovarian cancer to the right adrenal gland. It has an attenuation value >10 HU, is greater than 5 cm in size and does not show rapid washout of contrast on delayed imaging. All these features indicate adrenal metastasis.
2. Figure 3.9.2 is a T2-weighted MR image. A right adrenal metastasis demonstrates high T2 signal intensity. Metastases do not demonstrate signal drop-out on in- and out-of-phase sequences.
3. Figure 3.9.3 is an FDG-PET/CT image demonstrating a large right adrenal mass which is strongly FDG avid on the PET image, indicating a malignant lesion. Adrenal metastases may be unilateral or bilateral. Haemorrhage and central necrosis may occur, but calcification is a rare finding. The adrenal gland is the fourth most common site of metastases, after the lung, liver and bone. The most common primary sites that metastasise to the adrenal glands are the lung, breast, skin melanoma, kidney thyroid and colon. No imaging technique can reliably differentiate a metastasis from a primary adrenal carcinoma. Clinical findings and the identification of a primary lesion on imaging assist in the diagnosis.

Further Reading

Boland GW, Hahn PF, Pena C, Mueller PR. Adrenal masses: characterization with delayed contrast-enhanced CT. *Radiology*. 1997;202:693–696.

Katz RL, Shirkhoda A. Diagnostic approach to incidental adrenal nodules in the cancer patient. Results of a clinical, radiologic and fine-needle aspiration study. *Cancer*. 1985;55:1995–2000.

The Retroperitoneum

4

Axel Martin and S. Aslam Sohaib

Case 4.1

These CT images (Fig. 4.1.1a,b) are from two separate patients

1. What is the tumour shown in each case?
2. Which descriptive term has been given to the radiological appearance in Fig. 4.1.1a?
3. What is the risk of de-differentiation of this tumour?
4. What is the main treatment modality?

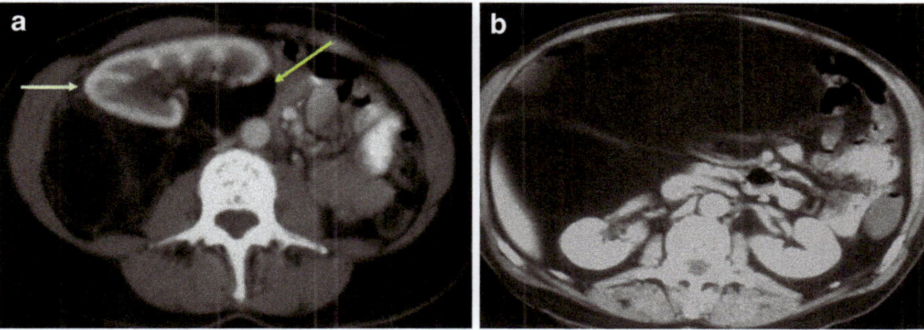

Fig. 4.1.1

S. Bott et al. (eds.), *Images in Urology*,
DOI 10.1007/978-0-85729-769-3_4,

Answers to Case 4.1

1. Figure 4.1.1a and b both show a well-differentiated liposarcoma. Sarcomas are rare tumours accounting for <1% of all malignancies. Liposarcoma was first described by Virchow in the 1860s and represents the most common soft tissue sarcoma. They usually arise *de novo* from deep seated stromal tissue in the retroperitoneum, limbs and rarely the spermatic cord, rather than from malignant transformation of a pre-existing lipoma. Five subtypes are described: well-differentiated, de-differentiated, myxoid, round cell and pleomorphic. The well- and de-differentiated subtypes are the subtype usually found in the retroperitoneum. These tumours characteristically contain fat density tissue on CT. Although the distinction between well-differentiated liposarcoma and an atypical lipoma is not always possible, de-differentiated tumours contain a soft tissue component and myxoid liposarcoma have a typical 'hazy' component on CT.
2. Figure 4.1.1a shows the 'floating kidney sign' and signifies that the tumour does indeed arise from the retroperitoneum. Note that the right kidney is displaced rather than invaded. However, the envelopment of renal hilar structures (arrows) suggests that a nephrectomy will be required for a complete resection of the tumour.
3. The risk of de-differentiation has been estimated at 15% in retroperitoneal liposarcomas. De-differentiation will, on average, occur after 7–8 years.
4. Surgery is the mainstay of treatment with no proven role for other treatment modalities.

Further Reading

Dei Tos AP, Pedentour F. Atypical lipomatous tumour/well differentiaed liposarcoma. Pathology and Genetics tumours of soft tissue and bone. IARC 2002

Weiss SW, Goldblum JR. Liposarcoma. *Enzinger and Weiss Soft Tissue Tumors*. 5th ed. St Louis: Mosby Elsevier Eds 2008:chap 16, pp.477–516.

Weiss SW, Rao VK. Well-differentiated liposarcoma (atypical lipoma) of deep soft tissue of the extremities, retroperitoneum, and miscellaneous sites. A follow-up study of 92 cases with analysis of the incidence of "dedifferentiation". *Am J Surg Pathol*. 1992;16(11):1051–1058.

Case 4.2

1. What is this lesion shown in the CT scan and resected specimen from a different patient and what is the most common presenting symptom?
2. Which anatomical structure is indicated by the arrow?
3. What is the local recurrence rate following resection?

Fig. 4.2.1

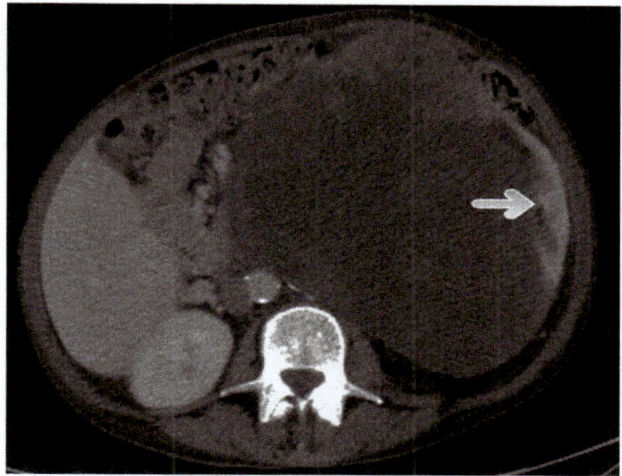

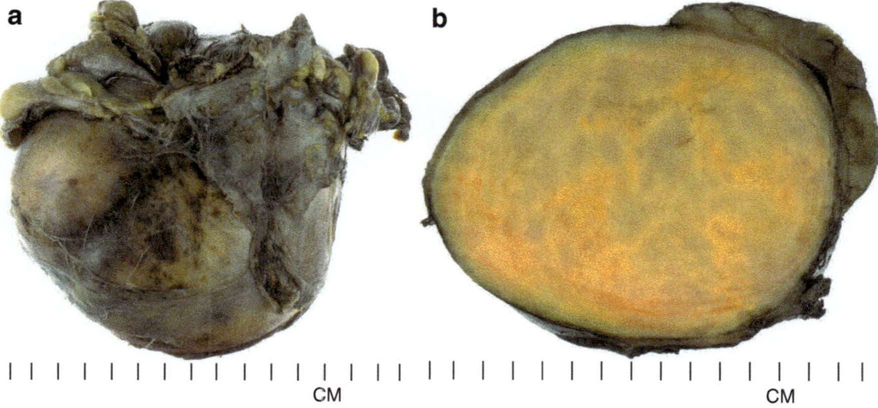

Fig. 4.2.2

Answers to Case 4.2

1. Figure 4.2.1 is an axial CT scan through the abdomen showing a de-differentiated liposarcoma. Figure 4.2.2a is the outer surface of a liposarcoma with normal retroperitoneal adipose tissue attached to the upper border. Figure 4.2.2b is the cut surface showing a heterogeneous yellow and white tissue mass with attached adipose tissue (upper right). Microscopy showed areas of de-differentiation in a liposarcoma.

   The most common presenting symptom is as a painless mass and this explains why the mean size at presentation is 20 cm. Most occur in late adult life.
2. The left kidney (arrow) is invaded, rather then displaced, attesting to the more aggressive nature of this tumour (*cf.* well-differentiated liposarcoma).
3. Surgical resection is the mainstay of treatment, though due to their size it can be difficult to achieve clear surgical resection margins. Local recurrence rates are reported as of 41–52%, distant metastases in 15% and there is a 30% disease-related mortality rate. The timing of recurrence is a predictor of disease-specific survival: patients in whom the tumour recurs after more than 13 months following resection have a better prognosis. Overall survival in patients with incomplete resection margins is less than 50% at 5 years.

Further Reading

Nascimento AG. Dedifferentiated liposarcoma. *Semin Diagn Pathol.* 2001;18(4):263–266.

Tateishi U, Hasegawa T, Beppu Y, Satake M, Moriyama N. Primary dedifferentiated liposarcoma of the retroperitoneum. Prognostic significance of computed tomography and magnetic resonance imaging features. *J Comput Assist Tomogr.* 2003;27(5):799–804.

Case 4.3

1. What is the lesion shown in Figs. 4.3.1a, b and 4.3.2 and what is the differential diagnosis of this lesion?
2. What is the significance of the central low attenuation area?
3. What is the frequency of metastases, and the most common sites affected?

Fig. 4.3.1

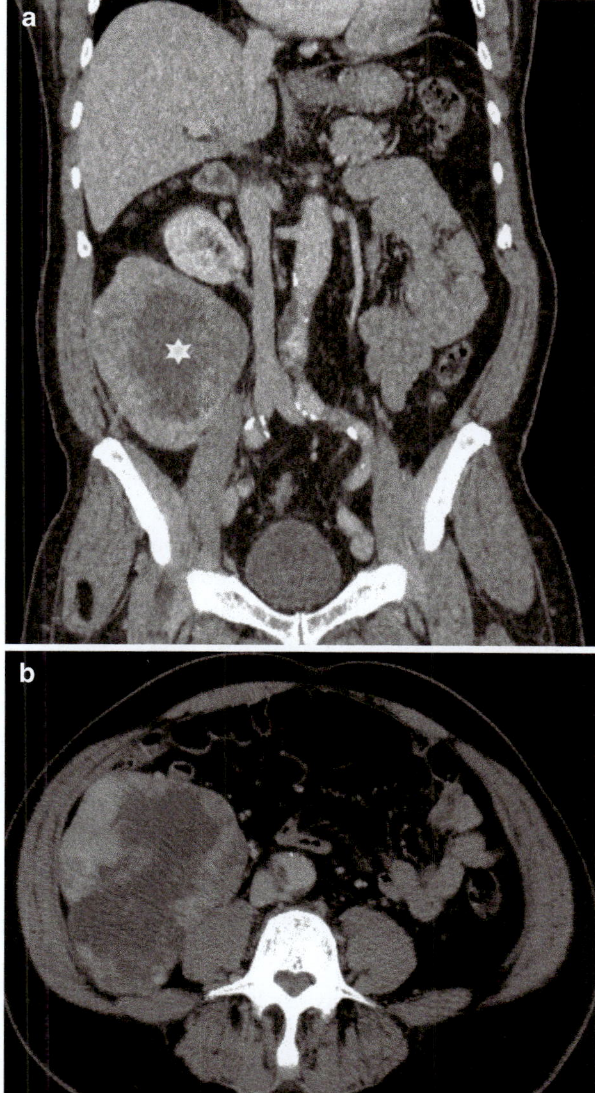

Fig. 4.3.2

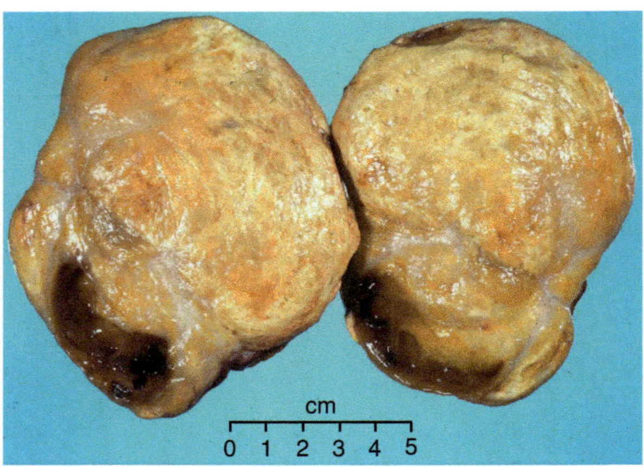

Answers to Case 4.3

1. These CT images (Fig. 4.3.1a,b) and macro histopathology image (Fig. 4.3.2) from a different patient with the same condition are of a leiomyosarcoma. The outer aspect of the resected specimen appears smooth, the cut surface is whorled and shows an area of cystic degeneration at the lower edge, rather than in the more typical central location. The differential diagnosis on CT includes paraganglioma, gastro-intestinal stromal tumours (GIST) and large non-Hodgkin's lymphoma masses (most commonly diffuse large B-cell lymphoma) which may all give a similar appearance. Retroperitoneal leiomyosarcomas have a non-specific presentation of weight loss, a mass or backache. They occur more commonly in females (2F:1M), and although the median age at presentation is in the sixth decade they may be found in the paediatric population up to the ninth decade of life. Surgical resection of the primary tumour improves long-term prognosis, if surgical clearance is not possible the prognosis is poor.
2. Central degeneration and necrosis (star) are commonly seen in large non-lipomatous primary tumours of the retroperitoneum. It is not indicative of malignancy.
3. Retroperitoneal leiomyosarcomas metastasise in 40–50%, most commonly to liver and lung.

Further Reading

O'Sullivan PJ, Harris AC, Munk PL. Radiological imaging features of non-uterine leiomyosarcoma. *Br J Radiol.* 2008;81(961):73–81.

Case 4.4

1. What is the tumour shown in these three images and from which great vessel does it arise?
2. Describe the radiological features seen on the enhanced axial CT image (Fig. 4.4.1a). What is indicated by the arrows? What feature of this tumour seen on the CT image will make it more difficult to obtain clear margins?
3. Does this tumour have a gender predilection?
4. Where in the body does this type of tumour preferentially occur?

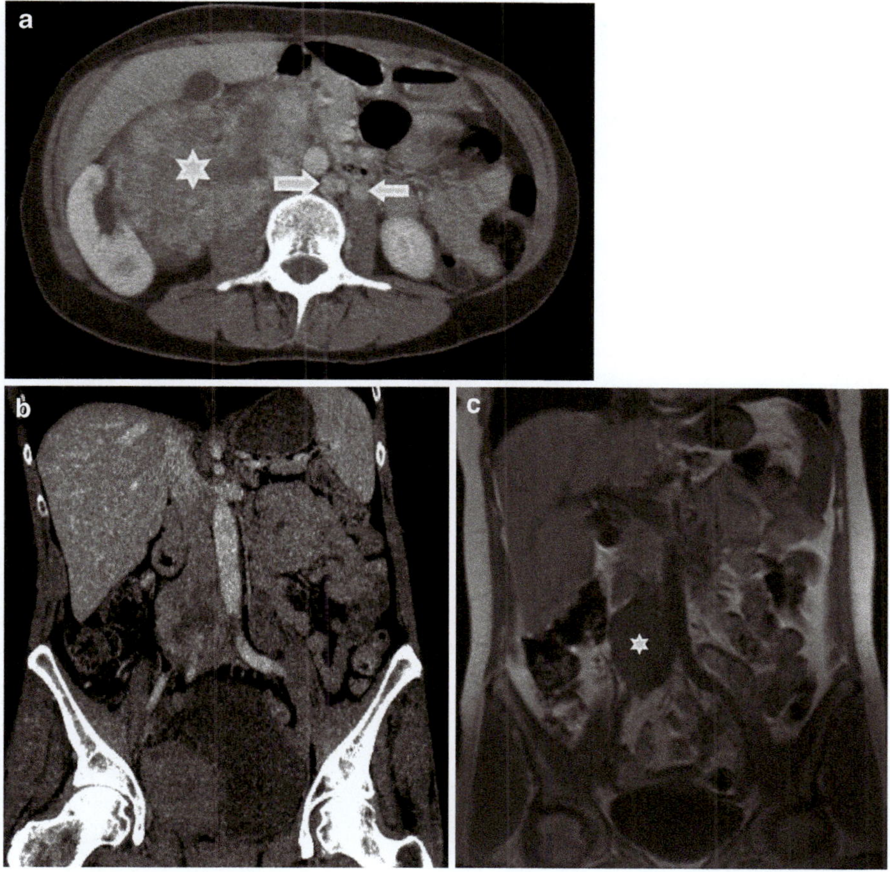

Fig. 4.4.1

Answers to Case 4.4

1. Figures 4.4.1a–c show a leiomyosarcoma of the inferior vena cava.
2. There is a large, heterogeneously enhancing tumour arising from the inferior vena cava (star). Mild right hydronephrosis is present. There is extensive left-sided venous collateralisation through the gonadal and hemi-azgos veins (arrows). Invasion of the right psoas muscle (Fig. 4.4.1a) makes resection surgically challenging.
3. IVC leiomyosarcoma is the only blood-vessel-associated leiomyosarcoma to have a pronounced gender preference, occurring almost exclusively in females.
4. Venous leiomyosarcomata almost always affect the IVC or lower extremity vessels, they are extremely rare in the upper limbs.

Further Reading

Dzsinich C, et al. Primary venous leiomyosarcoma: a rare but lethal disease. *J Vasc Surg*. 1992;15(4):595–603.

Case 4.5

1. Figure 4.5.1a–c show a paraganglioma. At which extra-adrenal sites may this tumour also be found?
2. Which radiological finding is considered to be a sign of malignancy? Which radiological features would indicate a benign pathology?
3. What proportion of retroperitoneal paragangliomas are functioning and therefore take up which radionuclide tracer (Fig. 4.5.1c)?

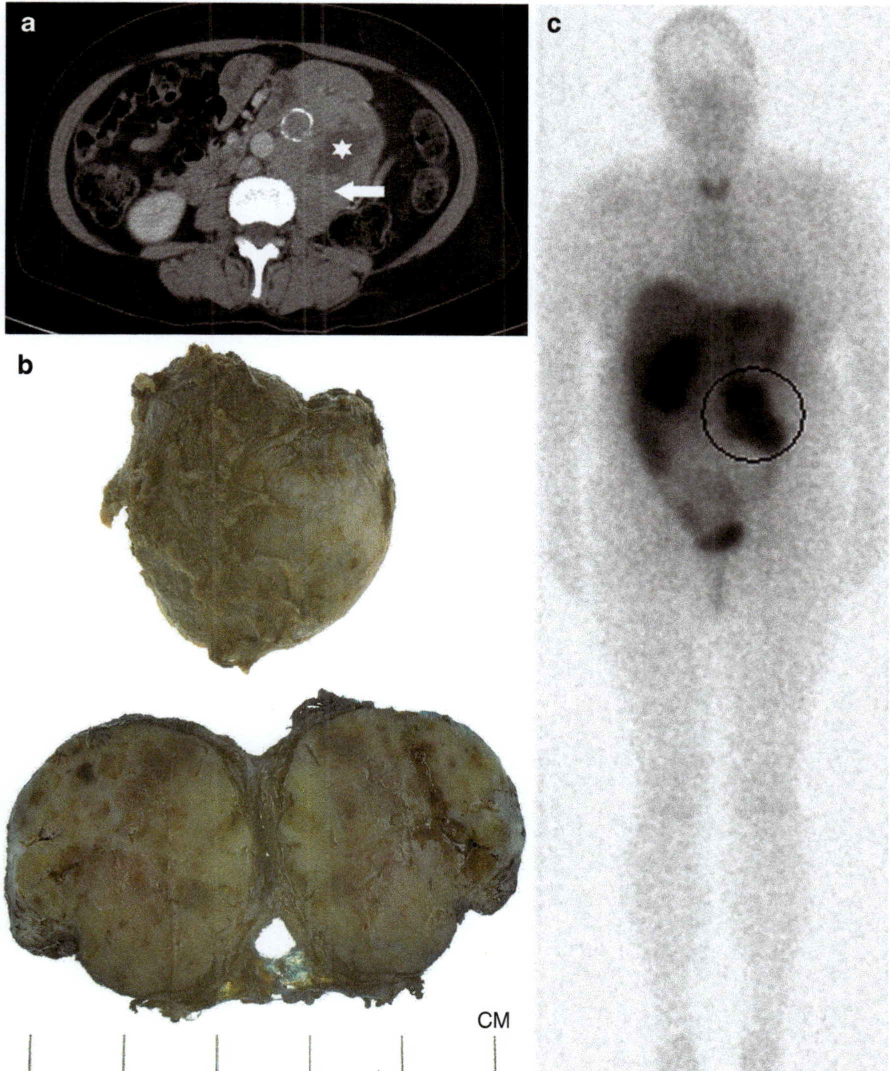

Fig. 4.5.1

Answers to Case 4.5

1. Extra adrenal paragangliomata are most frequently found in the abdomen (85%), most commonly arising from the organs of Zuckerkandl (as in this case – starred in Fig. 4.5.1a; the arrow points to the psoas muscle). Approximately 50% of these are malignant. Other extra adrenal sites include intrathoracic (12%) and cervical (3%) regions. Figure 4.5.1b shows the outer surface and the cut surface of a circumscribed, bisected mass composed of nodular grey tissue with areas of haemorrhage and cystic change. Microscopy showed a typical paraganglioma.
2. The only generally accepted radiological sign of malignancy is the presence of metastatic disease – most commonly to liver and lung. The presence of multiple paragangliomata (in 7–10% of patients) should not be confused with metastatic adenopathy which is very uncommon in this tumour. Benign paragangliomas are typically well-defined, enhance avidly and commonly contain a cystic component.
3. The reported incidence of symptoms from catecholamine production varies widely from 20 to 65%. Functioning tumours take up I-131 Metaiodobenzylguanidine (MIBG) and In-111 Octreotide (indicated in Fig. 4.5.1c).

Further Reading

Sahdev A, Sohaib A, Monson JP, Grossman AB, Chew SL, Reznek RH. CT and MR imaging of unusual locations of extra-adrenal paragangliomas (pheochromocytomas). *Eur Radiol.* 2005;15(1):85–92.

Sharon Weiss, John R. *Goldblum. Enziger's and Weiss' Soft-Tissue Tumours.* 4th ed. St Louis: Mosby; 2001.

van Gils AP, Falke TH, van Erkel AR, Arndt JW, Sandler MP, van der Mey AG, Hoogma RP.MR imaging and MIBG scintigraphy of pheochromocytomas and extraadrenal functioning paragangliomas. *Radiographics.* 1991;11(1):37–57.

Case 4.6

1. What are the findings on this patient's coronal (Fig. 4.6.1a) and axial CT (Fig. 4.6.1b)?
2. This tumour is grouped together with two eponymous tumours, name them and their common genetic characteristics.
3. What predicts survival in these patients?

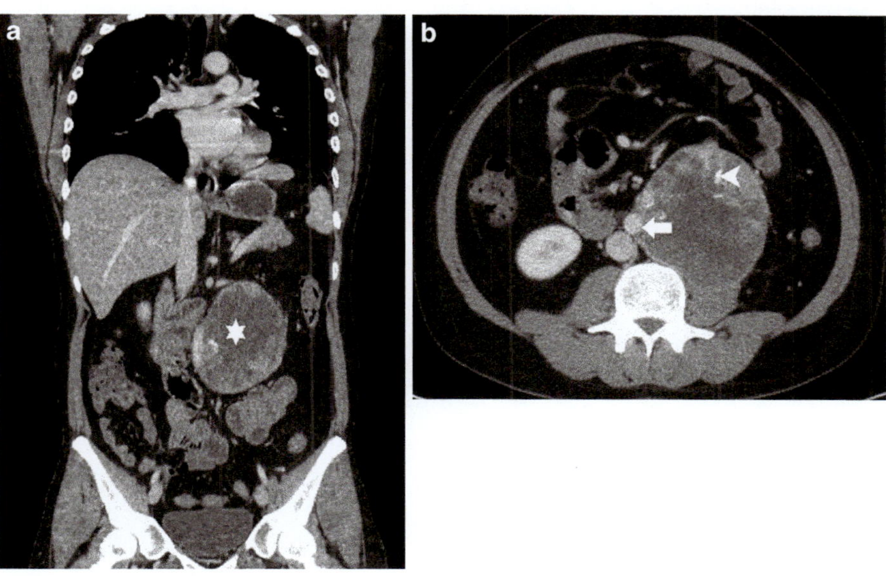

Fig. 4.6.1

Answers to Case 4.6

1. This patient's CT images (Fig. 4.6.1a,b) show a large heterogeneous left retroperitoneal mass which contains flecks of calcification (arrowhead) and displacement and partial encasement of the abdominal aorta (arrow). Surgico-pathological finding showed this was a primitive neuroectodermal tumour (PNET). Coarse calcification is mainly described in PNET tumours, though they may be found in other retroperitoneal tumours including liposarcomata.
2. The two eponymous tumours are extra-skeletal Ewing's sarcoma and Askin sarcoma, and both also have a reciprocal translocation of the long arms of chromosomes 11 and 22.
3. The size of the tumour, evidence of necrosis and the presence of metastatic disease are the main adverse prognostic factors.

Further Reading

Scurr M, Judson I. How to treat the Ewing's family of sarcomas in adult patients. *Oncologist*. 2006;11(1):65–72.

Case 4.7

1. Which stigmata of neurofibromatosis Type 1 (NF-1) are evident from this CT coronal reformat (Fig. 4.7.1)? What is the significance of the retro-peritoneal lesion? What is indicated by the curved arrow?
2. What is the risk of malignant transformation? Name the malignant entity?
3. What other tumours are associated with NF-1?

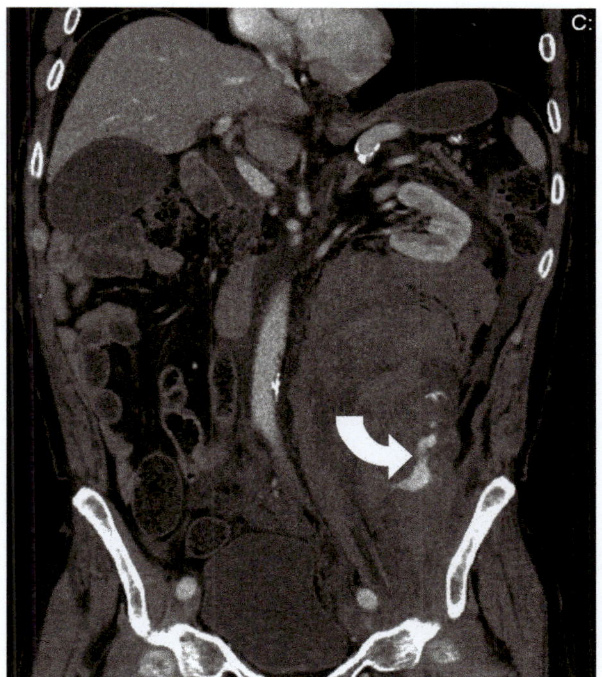

Fig. 4.7.1

Answers to Case 4.7

1. Figure 4.7.1 shows multiple skin-tags representing cutaneous neurofibromata (best seen as areas of subtle cutaneous and subcutaneous thickening along the extreme edge of the right lateral abdominal wall). The retroperitoneal tumour is a plexiform neurofibroma. This is considered pathognomic for NF-1. Haemorrhage into a plexiform NF (curved arrow) is a rare but potentially life-threatening event, because surgical options are limited.
2. The risk of malignant transformation is less than 10%. The resultant cancer is called Malignant Peripheral Nerve Sheath Tumour (MPNST).
3. Other tumours associated with NF-1 are:
   - Neurogenic (e.g., neurofibroma, ganglioneuroma);
   - Neuroendocrine (e.g., carcinoid, phaeochromocytoma);
   - Non-neurogenic GI mesenchymal neoplasms (e.g., GI stromal tumour [GIST]);
   - Embryonal tumour (e.g., Wilm's tumour, neuroblastoma)

Further Reading

Arun D, Gutmann DH. Recent advances in neurofibromatosis type 1. *Curr Opin Neurol*. 2004;17(2):101–105.

Case 4.8

1. Describe the four significant findings on these two coronal CT reformatted images of this 62-year-old lady, who was referred with a provisional diagnosis of retroperitoneal sarcoma (Fig. 4.8.1b is the more posterior located image of the same series).
2. What would be the most useful next investigation?
3. What is the likely diagnosis which would explain all these features?

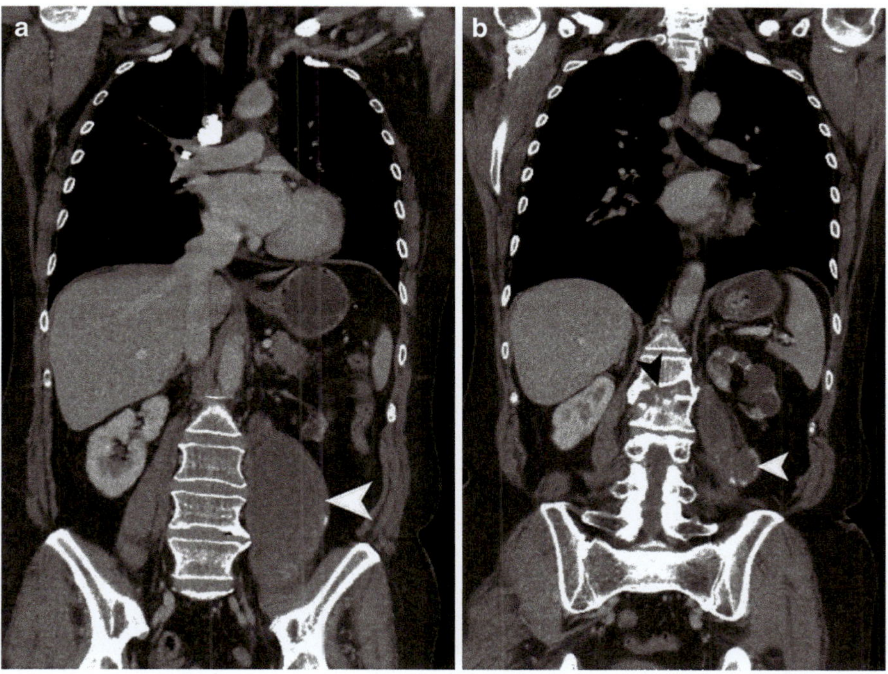

Fig. 4.8.1

Answers to Case 4.8

1. Figure 4.8.1a demonstrates a large low-density mass arising from the left psoas muscle (white arrowhead). There is a focus of wall calcification. Also note the presence of right hilar and paratracheal lymph node calcification. Figure 4.8.1b shows the sequelae of infective discitis at the L1/2 level (black arrowhead) and replacement of the left renal cortex by low-density cystic lesions associated with calcification, suggesting previous renal involvement.
2. CT-guided aspiration/biopsy of the psoas mass.
3. Post-primary extra-pulmonary tuberculosis is the unifying diagnosis. Aspiration of fluid from the psoas abscess demonstrated the presence of acid-fast bacilli.

Case 4.9

1. This patient was diagnosed with a non-seminomatous germ cell tumour (NSGCT) stage 1 and treated with radical orchidectomy. Pre-surgical CT was unremarkable. The CT image (Fig. 4.9.1) below is from a surveillance scan obtained 3 months later. Tumour markers (αFP and β-HCG) were within normal limits. What is the starred abnormality?
2. What is the relapse rate of patients with stage 1 NSGCT treated by orchidectomy alone?
3. What are the findings at retroperitoneal lymph node dissection in patients with metastatic NSGCT with residual masses following chemotherapy, as indicated in Fig. 4.9.2a, b)?

Fig. 4.9.1

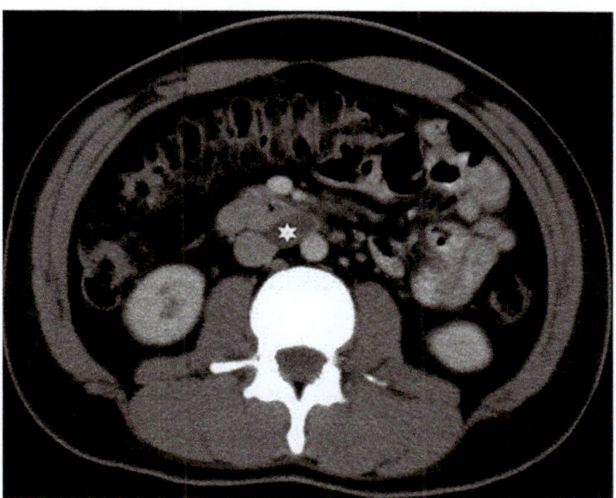

Fig. 4.9.2

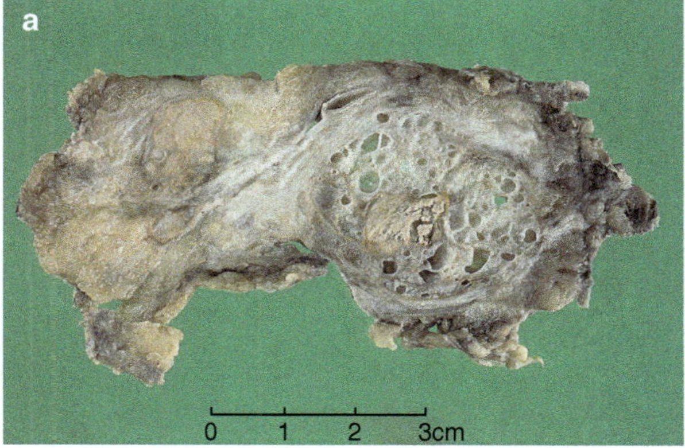

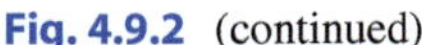

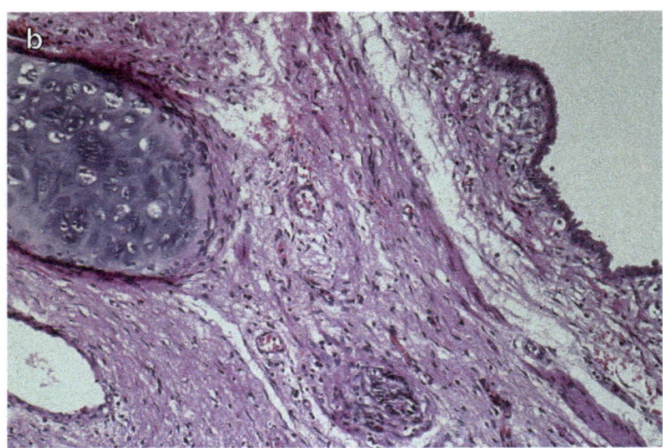

Fig. 4.9.2 (continued)

Answers to Case 4.9

1. In the axial CT, Fig. 4.9.1, there is low-density adenopathy in the aortocaval groove (star) measuring in excess of 2 cm but less than 5 cm. A retroperitoneal lymph node dissection revealed this lesion to be a teratoma differentiated (TD).
2. At diagnosis 55% of patients with NSGCT are stage 1 (compared with 75–80% of men with seminoma). The overall relapse rate after orchidectomy alone in stage 1 NSGCT is approximately 30%: 80% relapse in the first, 12% the second and 6% the third year. In patients with clinical stage 1 NSGCT the relapse rate increases to 50% if lymphovascular invasion is present in the primary tumour versus 15–20% in the absence of lymphovascular invasion. Other less significant predictors of relapse include proliferation rate and percentage of embryonal carcinoma.
3. In patients with residual retroperitoneal masses post-chemotherapy only 10% have viable tumour, 50% contain mature teratoma (Fig. 4.9.2a, b) and 40% necrotic tissue only. Imaging investigations including PET are unable to distinguish between these three pathological outcomes so RPLND is recommended in all cases.

Further Reading

Albers P, Albrecht W, Algaba F, Bokemeyer C, Cohn-Cedermark G, Fizazi K, Horwich A, Laguna MP. EAU Guidelines on testicular cancer 2010. Available at: http://www.uroweb.org/gls/pdf/Testicular%20Cancer%202010.pdf. Accessed October 21, 2010.

Sohaib SA, Koh DM, Husband JE. The role of imaging in the diagnosis, staging, and management of testicular cancer. *AJR Am J Roentgenol*. 2008;191(2):387–395.

Case 4.10

1. This 25-year-old man presented with a lump in his testis. Describe the findings on these three CT images.
2. How many men with germ cell tumours have elevated tumour markers at presentation?
3. This patient had a serum α-FP of 2172 ng/ml and a β-HCG of 786 IU/l. What is this patient's prognosis according to the International Germ Cell Tumor Consensus Conference Classification in the absence of any other metastatic disease?

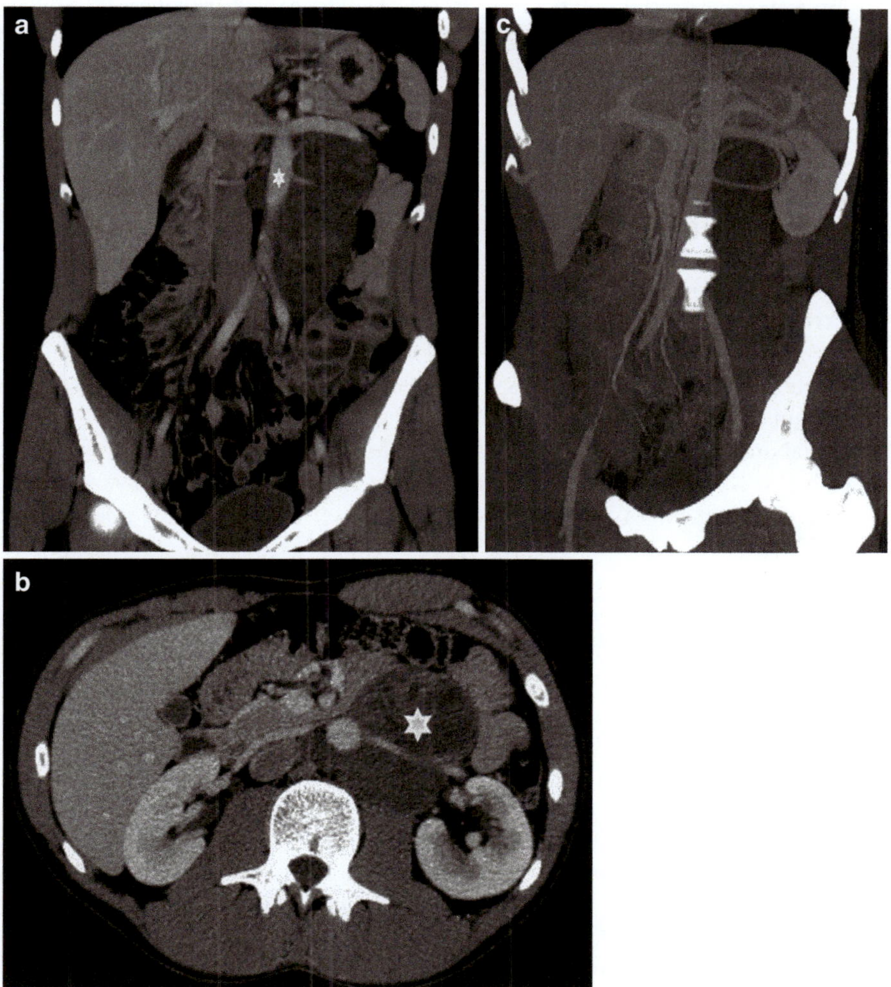

Fig. 4.10.1

Answers to Case 4.10

1. Figure 4.10.1a is a coronal CT reformatted image demonstrating a heterogeneous, mainly low-density lymph node mass extending behind the abdominal aorta, nodal stage N3. Figure 4.10.1b shows the mass (starred) encasing a vessel originating from the infrarenal aorta and Fig. 4.10.1c is a coronal oblique thick-slice reconstruction showing this vessel to be an accessory renal artery. This information assists in surgical planning.
2. Alpha-fetoprotein (α-FP) increases in 50–70% of patients with non-seminomatous germ cell tumour (NSGCT), and a rise in β-human chorionic gonadotropin (β-HCG) is seen in 40–60% of patients with NSGCT. In total 90% of NSGCT are associated with raised α-FP or β-HCG. (Up to 30% of patients with seminomas can present or develop an elevated β-HCG level during the course of their disease.) Lactate dehydrogenase (LDH) is a less specific marker, and its concentration is proportional to tumour volume. LDH levels are raised in 80% of men with advanced testis cancer.
3. The significantly raised α-FP means this patient has an intermediate prognosis according to the International Germ Cell Tumor Consensus Conference Classification (75% progression free and 80% overall 5-year survival).

Further Reading

International Germ Cell Consensus Classification: a prognostic factor-based staging system for metastatic germ cell cancers. International Germ Cell Cancer Collaborative Group. *J Clin Oncol.* 1997;15:594–603.

Sohaib SA, Koh DM, Husband JE. The role of imaging in the diagnosis, staging, and management of testicular cancer. *AJR Am J Roentgenol.* 2008;191(2): 387–395.

Case 4.11

1. What is the main difference in the CT appearances (Figs. 4.11.1 and 4.11.2) of the retroperitoneal adenopathy in these two patients with lymphoma? What is illustrated in Fig. 4.11.3?
2. From this can you draw any conclusions about the histology and biological behaviour?
3. Which of the two would be considered potentially curable?

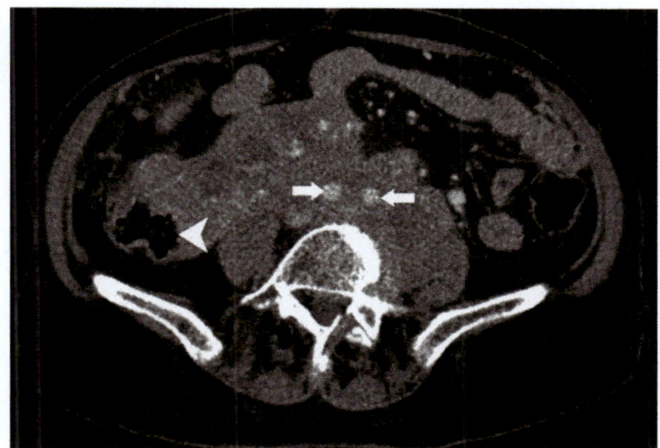

Fig. 4.11.1

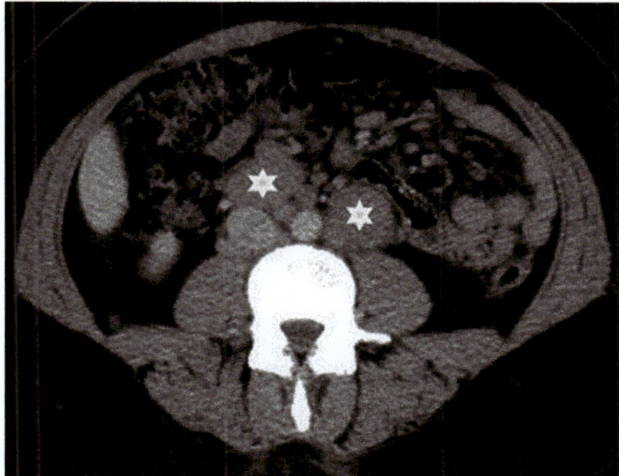

Fig. 4.11.2

Fig. 4.11.3

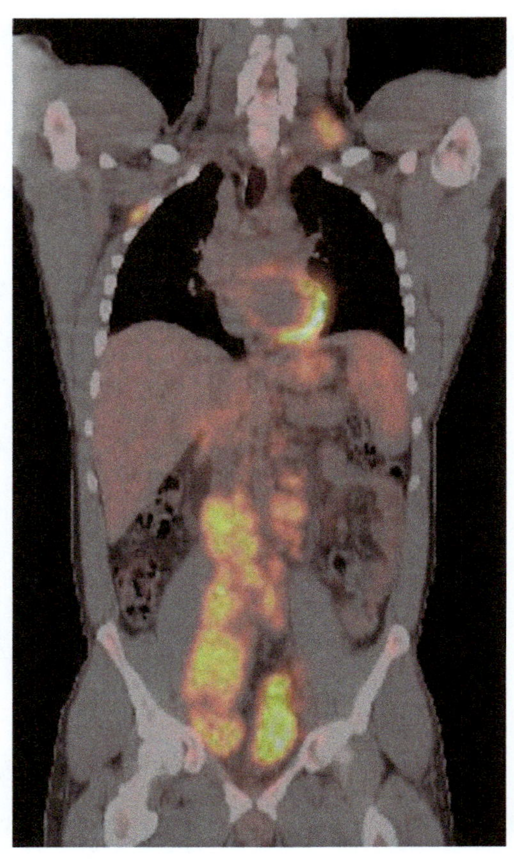

Answers to Case 4.11

1. These are common features of lymphoma on CT with widespread bulky lymphadenopathy and often with hepatosplenomegaly. But virtually any organ can also be involved, including the kidneys or testis. Figure 4.11.1 shows bulky conglomerate retroperitoneal adenopathy encasing the large vessels (arrows) and extending into the small bowel mesentery. There is evidence of direct involvement of the left psoas muscle and the caecum (arrowhead). Figure 4.11.2 shows separate, rounded enlarged lymph nodes in the retroperitoneum (stars) and, to a lesser degree, in the mesentery. Anatomical boundaries are maintained. Figure 4.11.3 is the fused coronal image from an 18-FDG-PET showing FDG-avid disease in the retroperitoneum and pelvis in a patient with follicular lymphoma. Also note additional sites of disease in the right axilla and left supraclavicular fossa.
2. The first patient is more likely to have an aggressive lymphoma as there is extensive evidence of invasion and these are often of the large B cell variety, whereas appearances in the second suggest a more indolent pathology such as chronic lymphocytic leukaemia (CLL) or follicular lymphoma.
3. High-grade lymphomas are treated with curative intent at first presentation, whereas low-grade non-Hodgkin's lymphomas are generally considered incurable.

Further Reading

Matasar MJ, Zelenetz AD. Overview of lymphoma diagnosis and management. *Radiol Clin North Am.* 2008;46(2):175–198.

Case 4.12

1. This 44-year-old female was scanned for right upper quadrant pain. Her only other complaint was of irregular sweats. Describe the salient findings on this axial enhanced CT?
2. What is the differential diagnosis?
3. Histologically this proved to be metastatic disease from a poorly differentiated carcinoma. What is the likely source of origin?

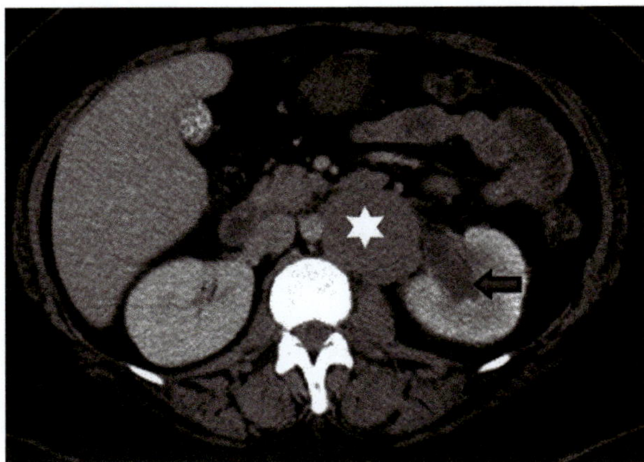

Fig. 4.12.1

Answers to Case 4.12

1. In Fig. 4.12.1 there is a 6 cm retroperitoneal left paraaortic lymph node mass (star) with mild left hydronephrosis (arrow). Multiple gall bladder stones are also noted.
2. The main differential in this case would include lymph node metastasis, lymphoma and neurogenic tumours including schwannoma and paraganglioma.
3. In a female the chief primary sites to be considered include ovarian, gastrointestinal and pancreatic carcinoma; but myriad other malignancies can also present with retroperitoneal lymphadenopathy, including bladder or ureteric TCC. In men the testes and prostate should also be examined as possible primary sites. Biopsy is usually necessary to establish cellular type.

Further Reading

Jerusalem G, Rorive A, Ancion G, Hustinx R, Fillet G. Diagnostic and therapeutic management of carcinoma of unknown primary: radio-imaging investigations. *Ann Oncol*. 2006;17(suppl 10):168–176.

Case 4.13

1. Describe Figs. 4.13.1a,b and 4.13.2. What do they show and what is the diagnosis? Suggest the next diagnostic investigation.
2. Figure 4.13.2 is an H and E section of this condition, describe the typical appearances.
3. What are the commonest aetiological factors causing this condition and how might it develop?
4. What does the post-mortem specimen (Fig. 4.13.3) show and what other complications may arise?

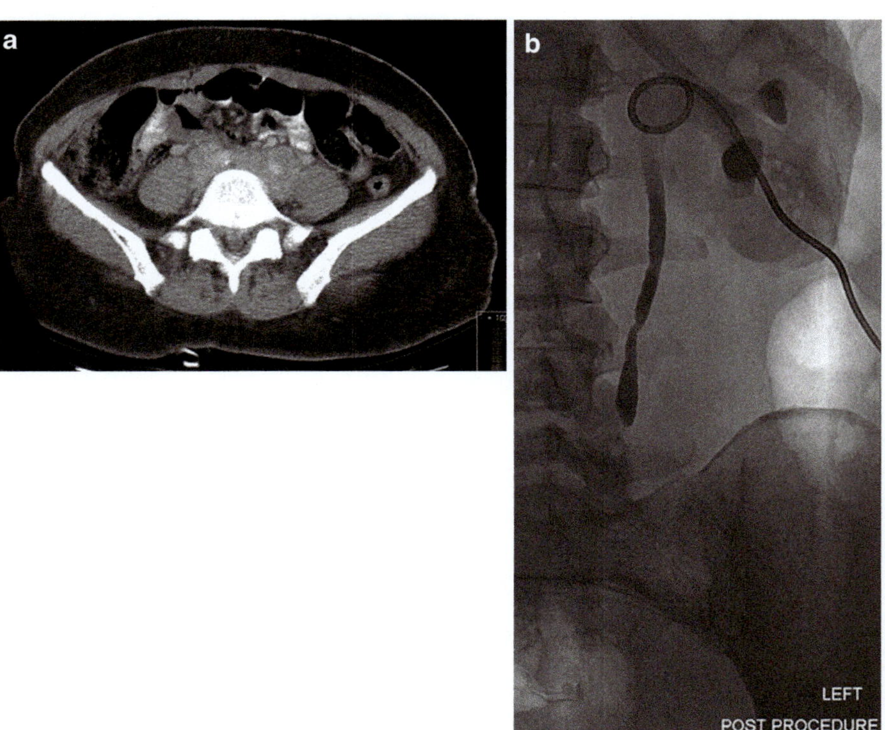

Fig. 4.13.1

Fig. 4.13.2

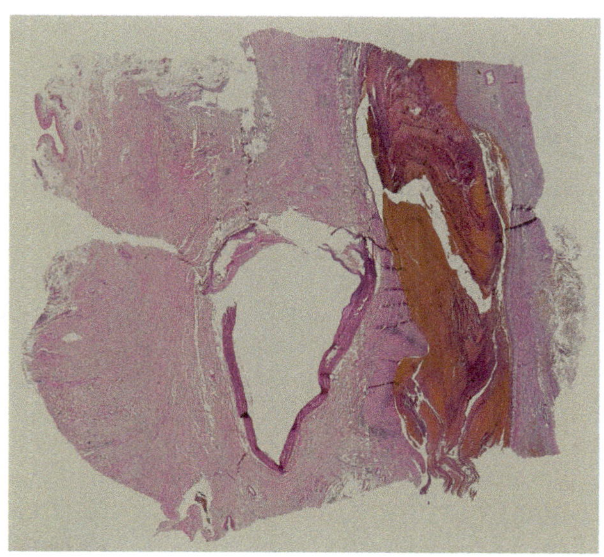

Fig. 4.13.3

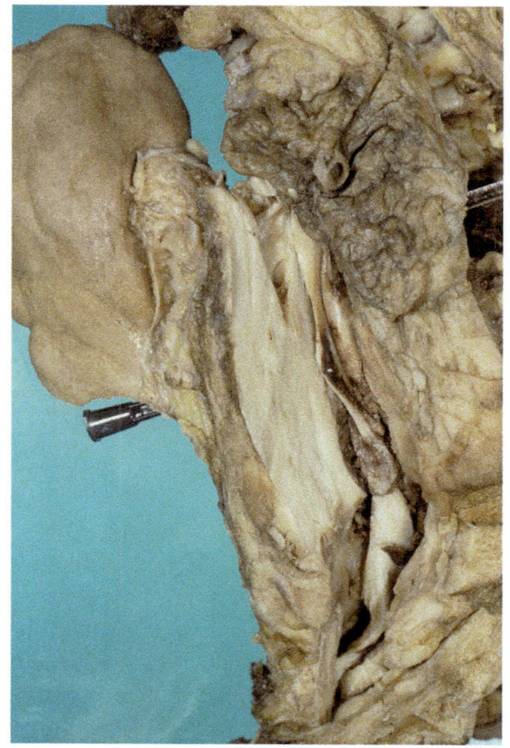

Answers to Case 4.13

1. Figure 4.13.1a, b are an axial CT and nephrostogram image. The CT image is a cut through the upper pelvis showing that both common iliac vessels are encircled by a contiguous enhancing soft tissue mass. The mass is separate from the psoas muscles. In the second image a nephrostomy has been inserted and the ureter is completely obstructed at the level of L4/5 vertebral body. Note the ureter smoothly tapers down to the point of narrowing, a feature of extra-luminal disease constricting the lumen. In the presence of both bilateral disease and the ureteric appearances, retroperitoneal fibrosis is the most likely diagnosis. But alternative possibilities are lymphoma, or extensive and confluent retroperitoneal lymphadenopathy. Retroperitoneal fibrosis is most probable as it is usually centred round L4/5. Computed Tomography guided biopsy is usually necessary for diagnostic confirmation.
2. Figure 4.13.2 is an H and E slide of idiopathic RPF. Idiopathic RPF is characterised by a fibrous tissue reaction of varying density which replaces adipose tissue and encases the inferior vena cava, aorta and ureters. Microscopically a variety of appearances may be seen ranging from a mixed (but predominantly chronic) inflammatory infiltrate with associated fibrosis to dense, virtually acellular collagen fibres which may appear refractile resembling those seen in keloid scars. These tissue reactions infiltrate adipose tissue and extend into nerves, blood vessel and ureteric walls.
3. The aetiology of RPF is idiopathic in 70% of cases. Defined causes include retroperitoneal malignancy either metastatic disease or lymphoma, inflammatory periaortitis, drugs (including methysergide, methyldopa and β-blockers), irradiation and autoimmune conditions. Current theories with respect to the pathogenesis of idiopathic RPF include an immunological response starting at the site of an atherosclerotic plaque. Low-density lipoproteins, for example ceroid, constitute potential antigens as they leak through the diseased aorta. The frequent association of idiopathic RPF with aortic aneurysms and the reported regression of fibrosis following aneurysm repair supports this theory, though other factors including a genetic predisposition and an association with auto-immune connective tissue disorders may also play a role.
4. Figure 4.13.3 is a post-mortem specimen demonstrating an obstructed, encased ureter. Frequent complications of RPF include obstruction of the ureters leading to renal impairment and hypertension. Inferior vena cava obstruction and deep vein thrombosis are less common sequelae and obstruction of lymphatics may give rise to peripheral oedema, ascites and hydrocoele formation.

Further Reading

Brandt AS, et al. Associated findings and complications of retroperitoneal fibrosis in 204 patients: results of urological registry.*J Urol.* 2011;185:526–531.

Swartz RD. Idiopathic Retroperitoneal Fibrosis: a review of the pathogenesis and approaches to treatment. *Am J Kidney Dis.* 2009;54:546–553.

Zen Y, et al. Retroperitoneal Fibrosis a clinicopathologic study with respect to immunoglobulin G 4. *Am J Surg Pathol.* 2009;33:1833–1839.

The Bladder

5

Dan Wood and Miles Walkden

Case 5.1

1. Give a brief description of how the bladder develops.
2. Look at Fig. 5.1.1 and describe the structure of the bladder wall.
3. Describe the normal anatomical relations of the bladder as seen in Fig. 5.1.2a, b.

S. Bott et al. (eds.), *Images in Urology*,
DOI 10.1007/978-0-85729-769-3_5,

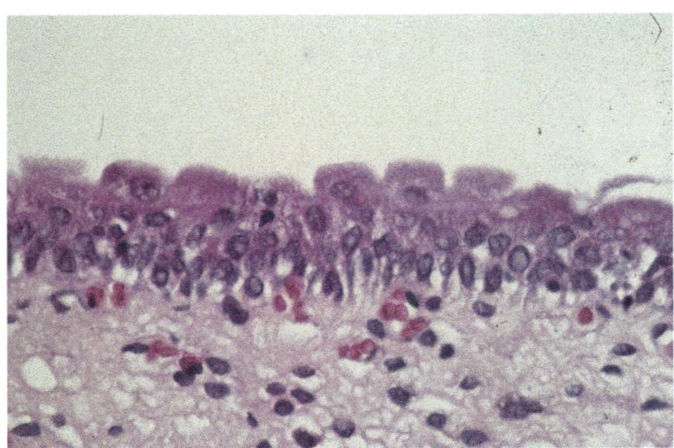

Fig. 5.1.1

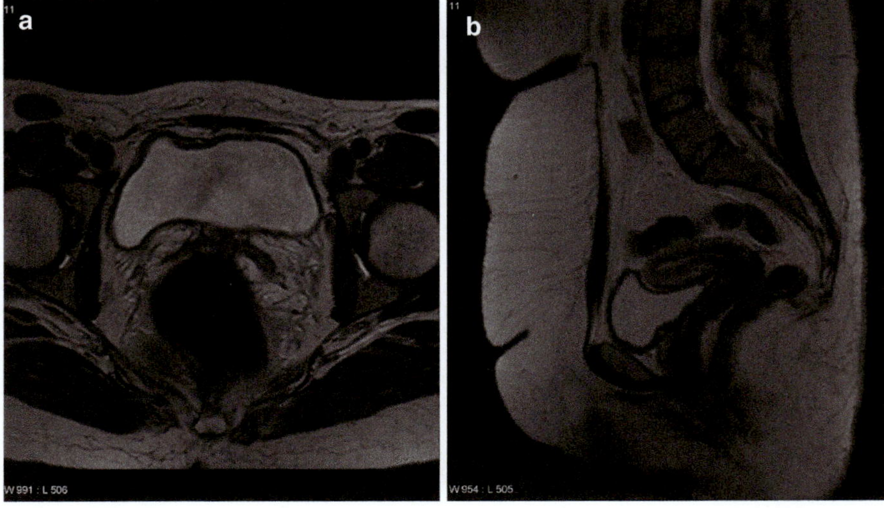

Fig. 5.1.2

Answers to Case 5.1

1. In the 4th to 6th week of gestation, the folds of Rathke grow in from the lateral aspects to divide the cloaca into the urogenital canal anteriorly and an anorectal canal posteriorly. The upper portion of the urogenital canal begins to form the bladder, within which the urothelium induces the surrounding pelvic mesenchyme to differentiate and form the detrusor muscle. The urachus connects the adult bladder to the anterior abdominal wall, and this normally closes in utero, but continued patency may relate to infravesical obstruction.
2. The H and E stained section of the bladder shown in Fig. 5.1.1 demonstrates normal urothelium with a superficial layer of rounded umbrella cells and underlying lamina propria.

   The bladder wall consists of four layers:

   - Urothelium which lines the lumen.
   - The lamina propria, a connective tissue layer directly beneath the urothelium.
   - The muscularis propria or detrusor muscle composed of bundles of smooth muscle. Fibres from the detrusor muscle merge with the prostatic capsule or anterior vagina and pelvic floor muscles.
   - The outer adventitial layer is formed from connective and adipose tissue.

   Note: A thin layer of smooth muscle fibres may be seen in the lamina propria but it is neither uniform nor consistent in the bladder, contrasting with the muscularis mucosae of the intestine.
3. Figure 5.1.2a is an axial T2-weighted image through the bladder in a female patient. The urine is seen as high signal, confirming that this is a T2W sequence. The muscle within the wall forms a low T2 signal rim. The surrounding perivesical fat is also of high T2 signal (fat is of high signal on both T1 and T2W studies, but fluid – or urine – is high on T2W scans only). In bladder tumours disruption of the low T2 signal muscle layer indicates invasive disease. Figure 5.1.2b is a sagittal T2-weighted image in a female patient. This demonstrates the close proximity of the posterior bladder wall to the vagina and explains how vesicovaginal fistula can occur.

   The relations to the bladder are as follows.

   - The superior surface is covered by peritoneum
     i. Anteriorly this is reflected up onto the abdominal wall.
     ii. Posteriorly, in the female the peritoneum continues over the uterus forming the vesicouterine pouch (or pouch of Douglas).
     iii. In males, the peritoneum follows down to the level of the seminal vesicles and meets the peritoneum covering the anterior wall of the rectum.
   - Perivesical fat cushions the bladder from pelvic side walls.
   - The bladder base in the male is related to the seminal vesicles, ampullae of the vasa and distal ureters.
   - In the female the bladder base, bladder neck and urethra are separated from the rectum by the vagina.

Further Reading

Human Embryology. 4th edn. Chapter 15. Larsen: Elsevier Churchill Livingston; 2008.

Case 5.2

1. What is the function of the bladder?
2. Name some common functional abnormalities?
3. How is bladder dysfunction investigated? What investigations are shown in Figs. 5.2.1 and 5.2.2 and what do they demonstrate?

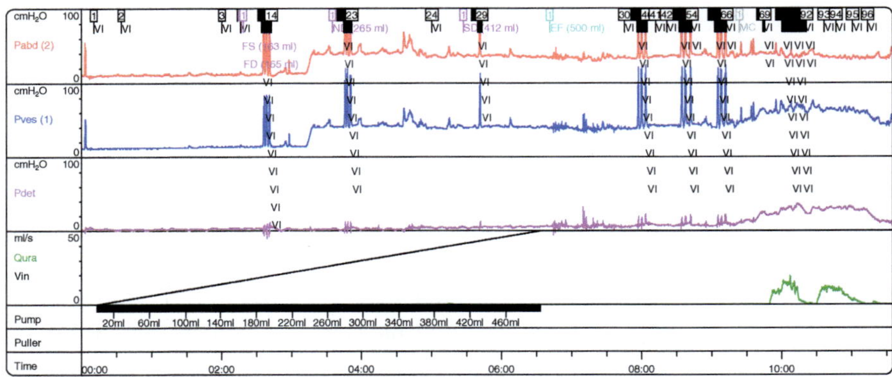

Filling phase results

Infused volume	500 ml
Volume lost through leakage	- ml
Bladder filling	500 ml

Sensation results

Sensation	Bladder filling	Vesical pressure	Detrusor pressure
First sensation	163 ml	14 cmH$_2$O	2 cmH$_2$O
First desire	165 ml	13 cmH$_2$O	1 cmH$_2$O
Normal desire	265 ml	41 cmH$_2$O	2 cmH$_2$O
Strong desire	412 ml	40 cmH$_2$O	5 cmH$_2$O

Voiding phase results

Total bladder capacity	500 ml
Peak flowrate	19 ml/s
Time to peak flow	17 s
Pdet at peak flow	31 cmH$_2$O
Voided volume	542 ml
Flow time	75 s
Voiding time	92 s
Delay time	27 s
Average flowrate	7 ml/s
Computed residual urine	-42 ml
Opening pressure Pdet	22 cmH$_2$O

Fig. 5.2.1

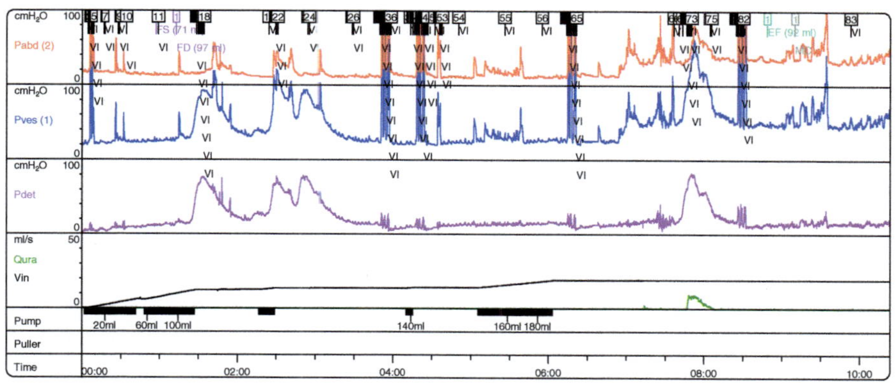

Filling phase results

Infused volume	192 ml
Volume lost through leakage	100 ml
Bladder filling	92 ml

Sensation results

Sensation	Bladder filling	Vesical pressure	Detrusor pressure
First sensation	71 ml	24 cmH_2O	11 cmH_2O
First desire	97 ml	29 cmH_2O	15 cmH_2O

Voiding phase results

Total bladder capacity	92 ml
Peak flowrate	- ml/s
Time to peak flow	0 s
Pdet at peak flow	- cmH_2O
Voided volume	100 ml
Flow time	- s
Voiding time	- s
Delay time	72 s
Average flowrate	- ml/s
Computed residual urine	92 ml
Opening pressure Pdet	- cmH_2O

Fig. 5.2.2

Answers to Case 5.2

1. The bladder has two main functions:
   - Collection and low-pressure storage of urine.
   - Expulsion of urine at the appropriate time in an appropriate place.
2. The commonest functional abnormalities are detrusor overactivity and stress urinary incontinence and either may manifest as lower urinary tract symptoms such as urgency, frequency and/or nocturia. Incontinence occurs when the outlet resistance is less than the pressure within the bladder – resulting in a leak of urine.
3. This depends on the age and sex of the patient as well as the symptoms. Investigations include exclusion of associated pathology (infection, malignancy), frequency volume charts, flow rate, ultrasound and post-void residual measurement (PVR) and invasive urodynamics.

   Figures 5.2.1 and 5.2.2 are traces from urodynamic studies. The detrusor pressure (third row from top) is estimated by the subtraction of rectal pressure (first row) from the total bladder pressure (second row). This removes artefact produced by abdominal straining and provides an accurate detrusor pressure measurement. Figure 5.2.1 shows a normal urodynamic trace. During filling (fourth row, labelled vin) a normal low detrusor pressure is maintained with normal sensation. A normal voiding pressure is seen with a good flow rate. This can be compared with 5.2.2 that shows numerous large phasic detrusor contractions during filling compatible with detrusor overactivity.

Further Reading

Chapple C, MacDiarmid SA, Patel A. *Urodynamics Made Easy*. 3rd edn. Edinburgh: Elsevier; 2009.

Case 5.3

1. Describe the innervation of the bladder.
2. What happens if the nerve supply to the bladder is disrupted and what is shown in Fig. 5.3.1a, b.
3. What is the normal arterial blood supply to the bladder and what is demonstrated in Fig. 5.3.2?

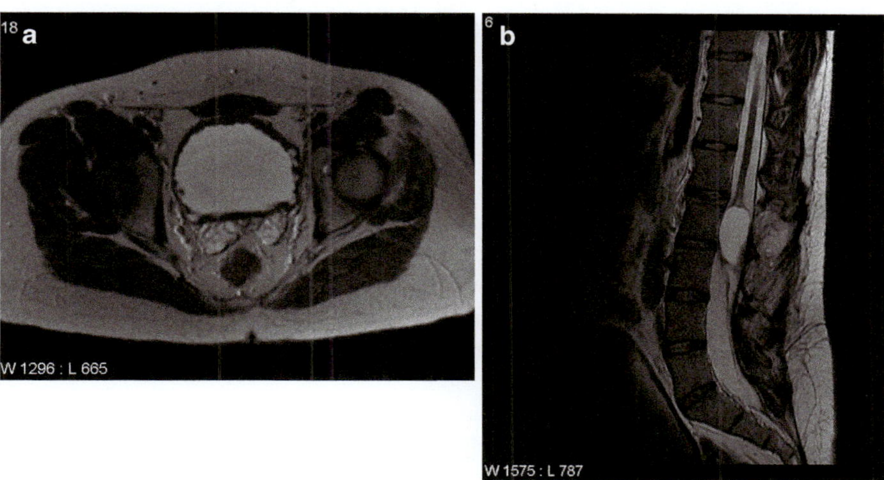

Fig. 5.3.1

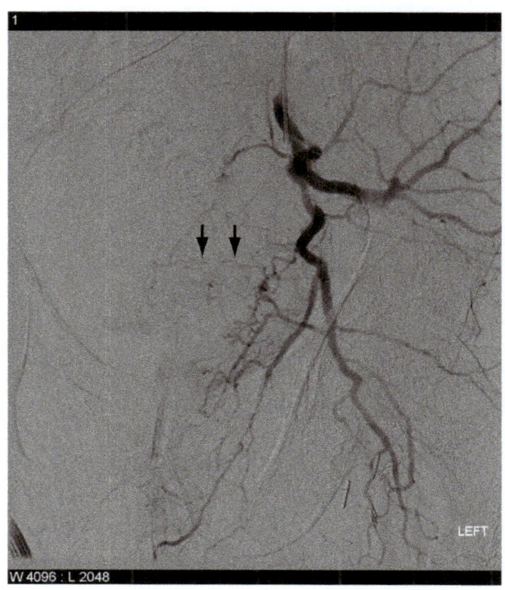

Fig. 5.3.2

Answers to Case 5.3

1. The motor supply to the bladder is parasympathetic via the pelvic plexus nerve roots S 2,3,4. The sympathetic nerves originate in the thoracolumbar spinal cord between T10 and L2 and may mediate bladder relaxation. Sensory nerves via C and Aδ fibres carry afferent information from the bladder and travel with both the parasympathetic and sympathetic nerves.
2. The site of the disruption dictates the effects on the bladder:
   a. Suprapontine – loss of voluntary control but coordination is retained i.e. coordinated relaxation of sphincter with detrusor contraction.
   b. Sub-pontine but Supra-sacral – discoordinated voiding or detrusor sphincter dyssynergia.
   c. Sub-sacral – hypo-contractile detrusor.

   Figure 5.3.1a is an axial T2-weighted MRI in a young male patient showing thickening and trabeculation of the bladder wall with a number of small diverticula. This is typical of a patient with a neuropathic bladder, but similar changes may also be seen with other longstanding causes of outflow obstruction. Figure 5.3.1b is a sagittal T2-weighted MRI of the lumbar spine that shows a large expansible lesion arising from the distal cord compatible with myxopapillary ependymoma of the conus. This is sub-pontine but supra-sacral in location, and accounts for the bladder appearances on the MRI study. This was the cause of the patient's neuropathic bladder.
3. The main arterial supply to the bladder arises from the inferior vesical artery, with some further and variable supply from the superior vesical artery. Both arise from the anterior trunk of the internal iliac artery. Such is the contralateral collateral supply that ligation or embolisation of a whole internal iliac artery is possible with very little risk of ischaemia. Figure 5.3.2 is an AP view from a pelvic angiogram in which the anterior division of the left internal iliac is demonstrated. This was embolised (images not shown) to stop intractable haematuria in a patient with post-radiotherapy telangiectasia, in whom all other treatments had failed. Note the numerous small corkscrew vessels (arrows) compatible with telangiectasia.

Case 5.4

1. What preparation is required for an ultrasound examination of the bladder?
2. What are the normal appearances of the bladder on ultrasound and what do Fig. 5.4.1a–c demonstrate?
3. What pathology is shown in Fig. 5.4.2?

Fig. 5.4.1

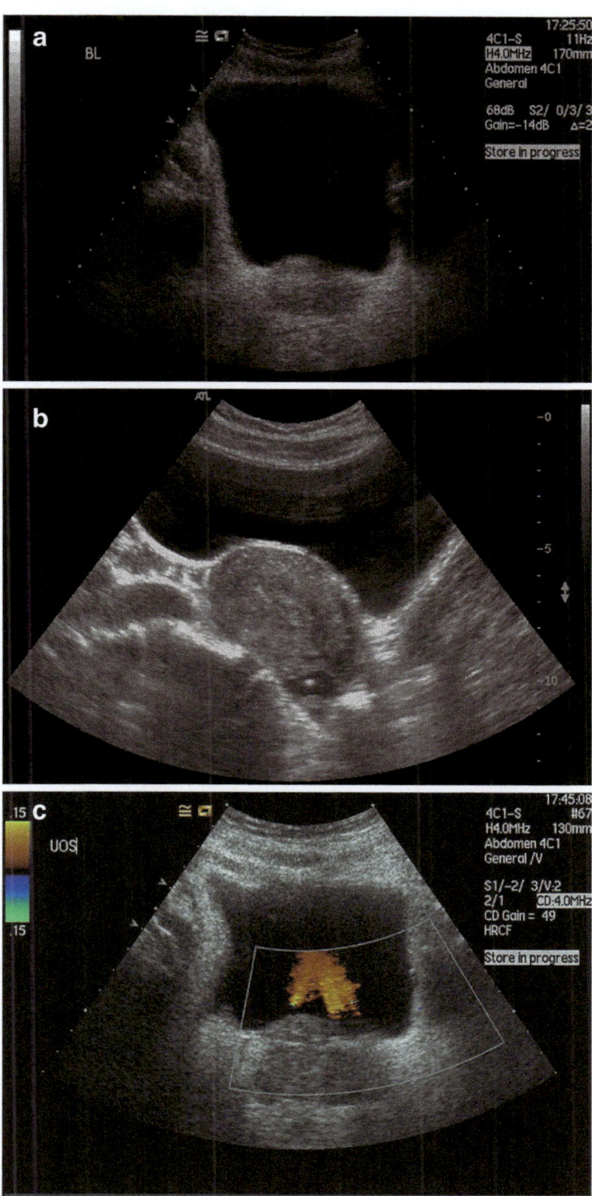

Fig. 5.4.2

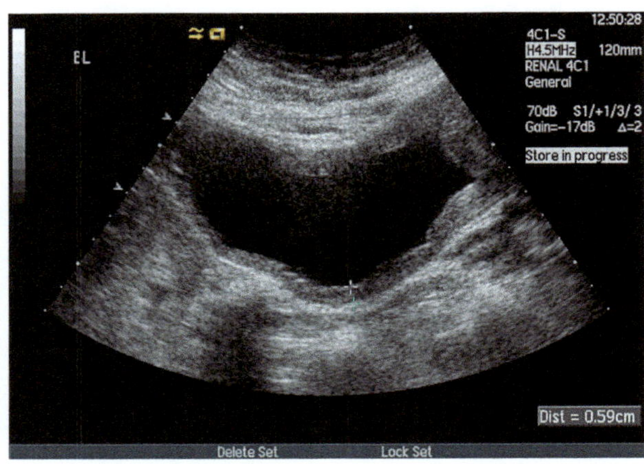

Answers to Case 5.4

1. The patient should have a full bladder (say >350 ml) to allow proper assessment of the bladder wall. If the bladder is not full normal bladder folds make lesion detection difficult. If a patient has a urinary catheter in place, this should be clamped. With good distension the normal bladder wall should be smooth. Ultrasound images are orientated according to standard radiological convention. Thus, on transverse view the left side of the screen represents the right side of the patient; and on a longitudinal or sagittal view the left side of the image represents the cranial aspect of the patient.
2. Figure 5.4.1a is a normal transverse USS of the bladder in a male patient. The prostate can be seen posteriorly indenting the bladder. Figure 5.4.1b shows a normal longitudinal image in a female patient. The uterus can be seen posteriorly. The urine within the bladder appears anechoic (black). Some mixed echoes are seen just beneath the anterior bladder wall, this is an artefact secondary to reverberation echoes, but needs to be differentiated from true pathology such as debris and this can be done by scanning the patient in a lateral position. True debris will move in a dependent fashion. The bladder wall should appear uniformly thin (4 mm maximum) and hyperechoic. Figure 5.4.1c is a transverse colour Doppler image showing bilateral ureteric jets. Note their symmetrical appearance. Unilateral absence of a jet can be taken as a surrogate indicator of a ureteric obstruction, but this is not highly specific.
   The bladder volume and post-void residue can be calculated using the formula: volume = length × width × height × 0.56.
3. Figure 5.4.2 is a transverse USS image of the bladder, showing global wall thickening consistent with bladder outflow obstruction.

Case 5.5

1. What is a CT urogram. Describe the phases shown in Fig. 5.5.1a–d. When should a CT urogram be used?
2. What are the advantages and disadvantages of CT scans?
3. What is MR urography?

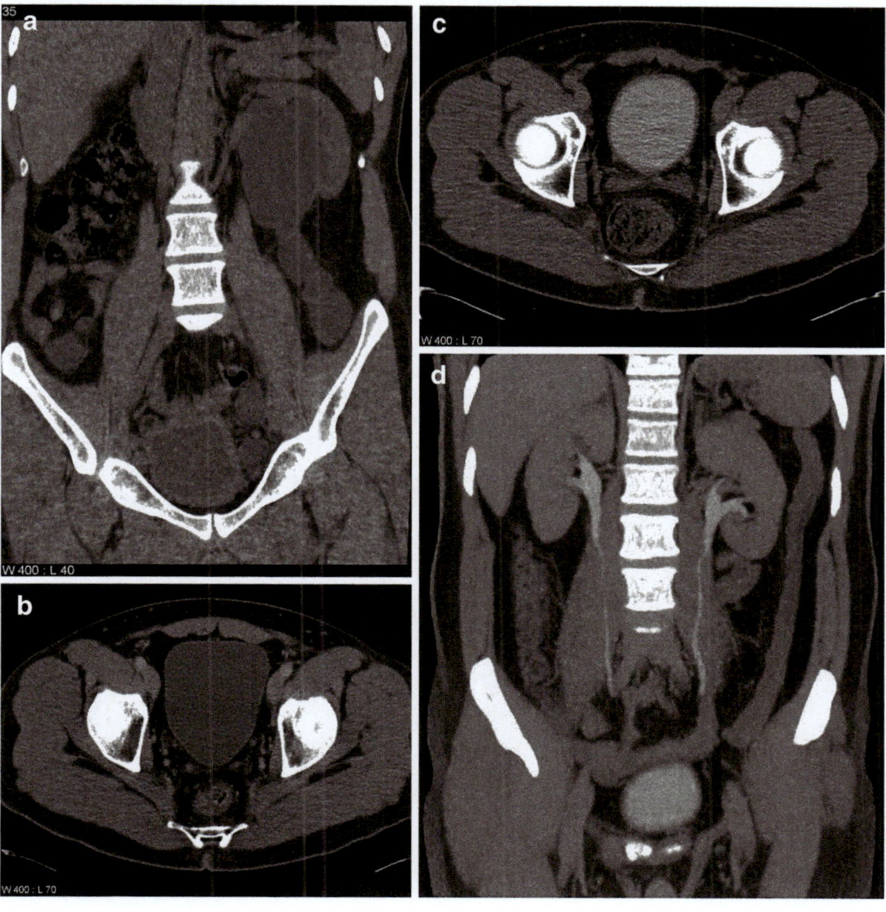

Fig. 5.5.1

Fig. 5.5.2

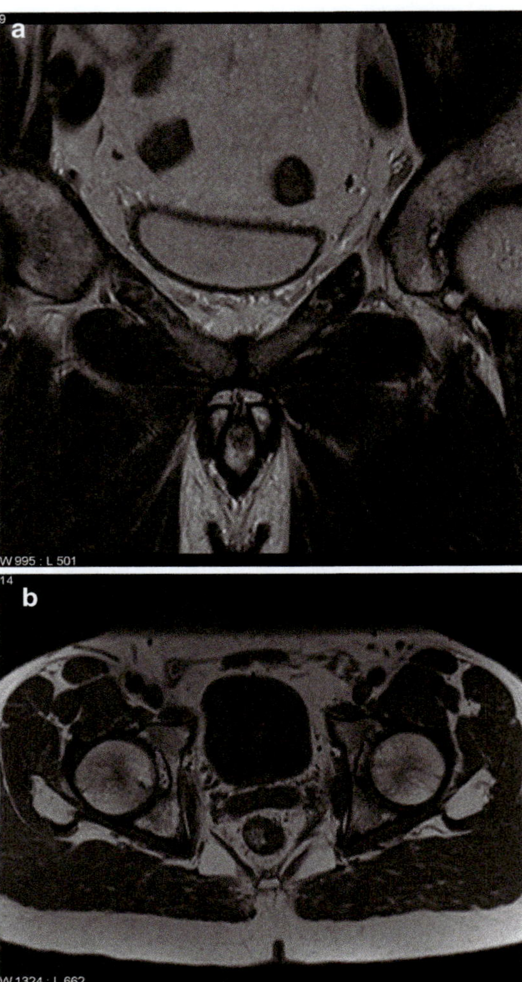

Answers to Case 5.5

1. A CT urogram is a CT scan focused on the kidneys, ureters and bladder, and involves looking at these structures in at least two different phases of contrast excretion. There is still considerable debate as to the best protocol for maximal information, whilst keeping the radiation dose as low as possible. The most thorough protocol is a pre-contrast scan through the entire urinary tract (using CTKUB setting protocol to minimise radiation dose), and further scans at 1 and 10 min after injection of radiographic

contrast medium. The first post-contrast scan will demonstrate the renal parenchyma as optimally opacified whilst the second will demonstrate the collecting system and ureters. There are numerous variations on this theme, designed to either reduce the radiation dose or better visualise the urinary tract. Sometimes a diuretic or a saline load is given to distend the ureters, and the patient mobilised prior to the 10-min scan to better mix the contrast in the bladder. Figure 5.5.1a is a coronal unenhanced study. Figure 5.5.1b is an axial scan through the bladder taken at 90 secs. The urine is of low attenuation. The bladder wall is of uniform thickness and shows subtle and normal enhancement. Figure 5.5.1c is an axial scan taken 10 min after the injection of contrast which has now been excreted by the kidneys and outlines the bladder. Note the homogeneous appearance of the contrast in the bladder, which has been achieved by mobilising/exercising the patient. Any tumour would be seen as a low attenuation filling defect. Figure 5.5.1d is a coronal maximum image projection (MIP) reconstructed image taken 10 min following contrast showing the collecting system, ureters and bladder on one image (please refer to further reading for an explanation of MIP).

2. The advantages of CT are that it is non-invasive (barring the intravenous contrast injection) and is widely available. It has a short acquisition time. In bladder cancer it is able to detect lymph node enlargement and distant metastasis as well as any complications of tumour such as hydronephrosis. It is now also able to provide multi-planar imaging. Disadvantages are mainly those of radiation exposure and the side effects of iodinated contrast media, if used. In bladder cancer it is also not able to reliably distinguish between superficial and deep muscle invasive tumour.
3. MR urography is shown in Fig. 5.5.2a, b. Figure 5.5.2a is a coronal T2-weighted image of the bladder. Opacification of the collecting system, ureter and bladder is achieved with heavily T2-weighted images in which the urine appears of high signal intensity and any lesion is shown as a filling defect within this. The muscle layer is seen as a low T2 signal rim against the high T2 signal urine.

   Figure 5.5.2b is an axial T1-weighted image. The urine is low signal, the bladder wall is intermediate signal and the surrounding perivesical fat is high signal.

   The type of sequence performed can usually be worked out by looking at the bladder (or any area where water or water density is to be expected – e.g. the spinal canal). If the urine (or water) within the bladder appears dark the sequence is T1. If the urine appears bright the sequence is usually T2. *A simple way of remembering the fact that fluid is bright on T2 is that the chemical equation for water is* H_2O *the 2 representing the 2 in T2.*

Further Reading

Walkden M, Patel U. Principles of radiological imaging of the urinary Tract. In: Mundy AR, Fitzpatrick J, Neal D, George NJR, eds. *The Scientific Basis of Urology.* 3rd ed. New York: Informa Healthcare; 2010.

Case 5.6

1. List four urachal anomalies.
2. A 12-year-old boy presented with haematuria and low-grade fever. What is shown in Figs. 5.6.1 and 5.6.2. What type of scan is Fig. 5.6.2 and how else do these anomalies present?
3. What is the likely management of these conditions?

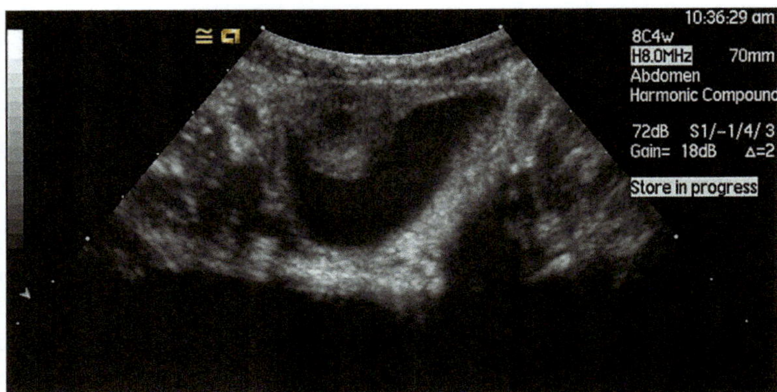

Fig. 5.6.1

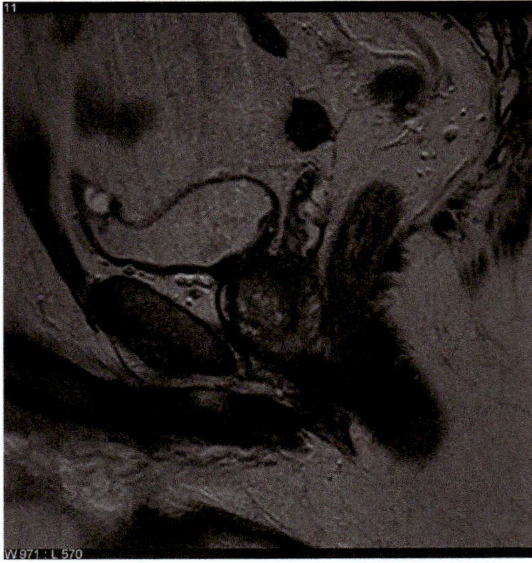

Fig. 5.6.2

Answers to Case 5.6

1. Urachal anomalies include
   - patent urachus (50%).
   - urachal sinus (15%).
   - urachal cyst (30%).
   - urachal diverticulum (5%).
2. Figure 5.6.1 is a transverse ultrasound scan showing a partly cystic/partly solid lesion arising from the dome of the bladder. In this age group the most likely diagnosis is a urachal remnant, or more rarely a tumour. The patient had the lesion excised and it was an infected urachal remnant.

   Urachal anomalies may be asymptomatic or may present with a discharge from the umbilicus, which may indicate bladder outflow obstruction, or if infected, as a painful lower abdominal mass. Adenocarcinoma may also develop in a urachal remnant.

   Figure 5.6.2 is a sagittal T2-weighted image showing a multicystic lesion arising from the wall of the bladder in the position of the urachus consistent with a urachal remnant cyst. It did not demonstrate any enhancing elements. This patient was asymptomatic from this so it was not removed.
3. Imaging with USS, CT or MRI to confirm the diagnosis followed by surgical excision if symptomatic or if malignancy cannot be excluded is the usual management pathway.

Further Reading

Cilento BG Jr, Bauer SB, Retik AB, Peters CA, Atala A. Urachal anomalies: defining the best diagnostic modality. *Urology*. 1998; 52(1):120-122.

Case 5.7

1. What is bladder exstrophy and what is the incidence?
2. What is the embryological failure that occurs in exstrophy?
3. What is shown in Figs. 5.7.1 and 5.7.2 and what are the typical features and associated anomalies of this condition?

Fig. 5.7.1

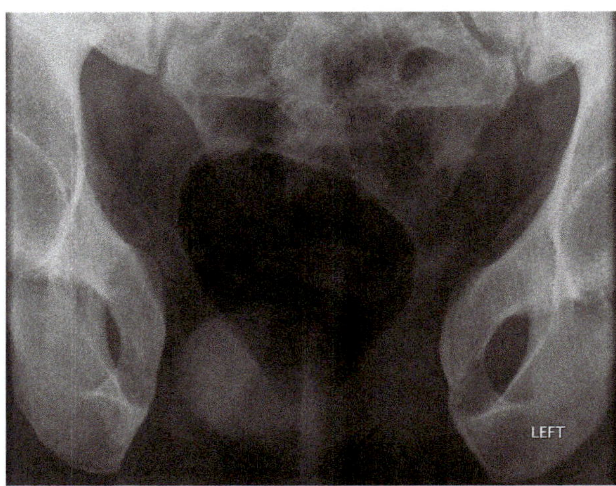

Fig. 5.7.2

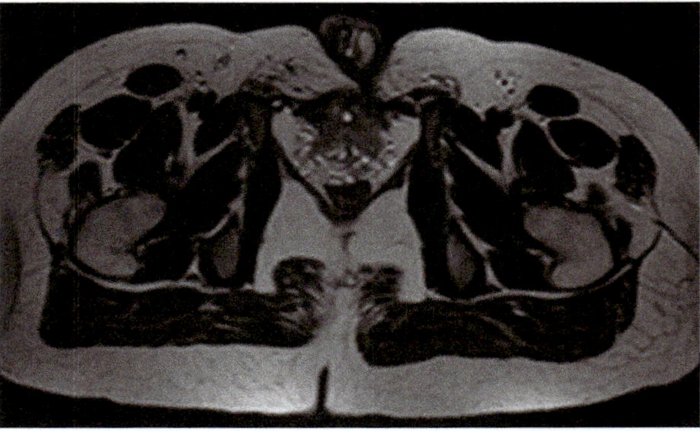

Answers to Case 5.7

1. Bladder exstrophy is a congenital anomaly in which the posterior bladder is turned outward (exstrophy) and located on the anterior abdominal wall. The incidence of bladder exstrophy is between 1/10,000 and 1,50,000. The male to female ratio is 2.3:1, with an estimated incidence in the children of affected adults of 1 in 70.
2. During the first trimester the cloaca separates into the urogenital sinus and the hindgut. Failure of the mesenchyme to migrate between the ectodermal and endodermal layers of the lower abdominal wall leads to premature rupture of the cloacal membrane leading to the exstrophy.
3. Figure 5.7.1 is a plain film of the pelvis showing pubic diastasis consistent with exstrophy. The area of increased density seen lying between the pubic bodies represents the penis. Figure 5.7.2 is a T2 axial MR image of an adult exstrophy patient. Again pubic diastasis is seen. Note also the urethra lies anterior to the prostate.

   Bladder exstrophy is part of a symptom complex, the exstrophy-epispadias complex, involving associated anomalies of the anterior bladder wall, boney pelvis, the urethra and external genitalia. The typical features include

   - Bladder everted through a midline lower abdominal wall defect.
   - Diastasis of the pubic symphysis.
   - Epispadias in males and bifid clitoris in females.
   - Anus and vagina are anteriorly displaced.
   - Undescended testes.
   - Shortened penis due to reduction in corporal size and separation of bases of corpora by attachment to pubic diastasis.

Further Reading

Boyadjiev SA, Dodson JL, Radford CL, Ashrafi GH, Beaty TH, Mathews RI, Broman KW, Gearhart JP. Clinical and molecular characterization of the bladder exstrophy-epispadias complex: analysis of 232 families. *BJUI.* 2004;94: 1337–1343.

Silver R,Yang A, Ben-Chaim J, Robert, Jeffs D, Gearhart JP. Penile length in adulthood after exstrophy reconstruction. *J Urol.* 1997;167:999–1003.

Case 5.8

1. What is shown in Figs. 5.8.1 and 5.8.2 and what are the characteristic features of this condition?
2. What are some of the extra-genitourinary associations?

Fig. 5.8.1

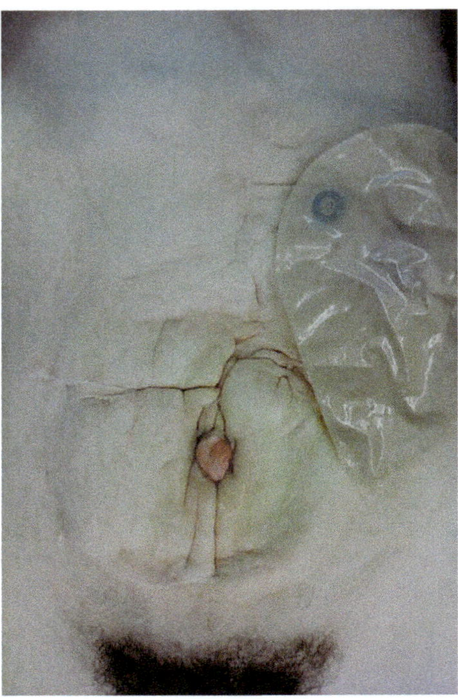

Fig. 5.8.2

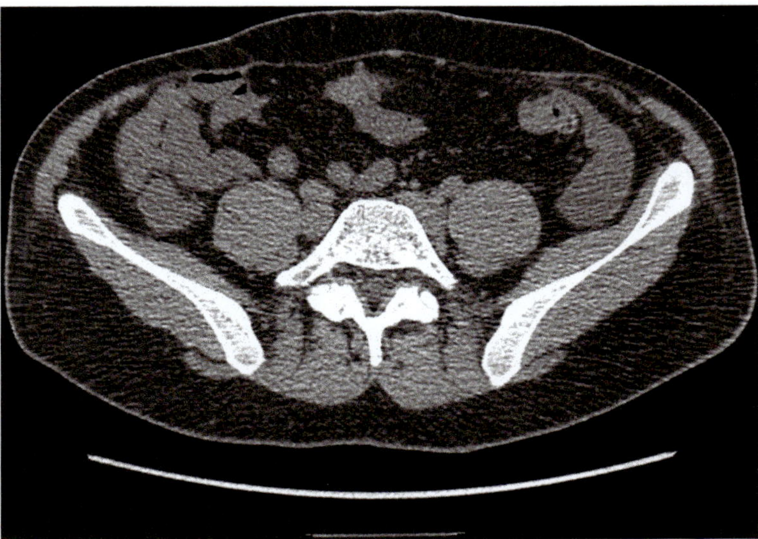

Answers to Case 5.8

1. Figure 5.8.1 shows the anterior abdominal wall of a child with the Prune belly syndrome (PBS). Note the wrinkled skin, colostomy and the herniotomy scars from bilateral orchidopexy for undescended testes. Figure 5.8.2 is an axial CT scan that demonstrates bilateral hydroureters and absence of the anterior abdominal wall musculature.
2. The extra-genitourinary associations are
   - abdominal wall – absence of anterior abdominal wall musculature and wrinkled (prune) like appearance to covering skin.
   - cardiac – patent ductus arteriosus, atrial septal defect, ventricular septal defect, tetralogy of Fallot.
   - pulmonary – pneumothorax/pneumomediastinum, pulmonary hypoplasia, lobar atelectasis.
   - gastrointestinal – Hirschsprung's disease, imperforate anus, intestinal atresia, stenosis, malrotation, omphalocoele, gastroschisis.
   - orthopaedic – congenital dislocation of the hip, genu valgum, talipes equinovares, pectus excavatum, scoliosis, sacral agenesis.

Further Reading

Caldomone AA. Woodard JR. Prune belly syndrome. In: Walsh PC, Retik AB, Vaughan ED. *Campbell's Urology.* 9th edn. Philidelphia: WB Saunders; 2007.

Geary DF, MacLusky IB, Churchill BM, et al. A broader spectrum of abnormalities in the prune belly syndrome. *J Urol.* 1986;135: 324-326.

Manivel JC, Pettinato G, Reinberg Y, et al. Prune belly syndrome: clinicopathologic study of 29 cases. *Pediatr Pathol.* 1989;9: 691-711.

Case 5.9

1. How do posterior urethral valves (PUV) form and what is their incidence?
2. What are the findings on an antenatal ultrasound scan which may indicate (PUVs) and what features suggest a poor prognosis in antenatal scanning?
3. Who described the original valve classification of PUV and what is it?
4. What is shown in Figs. 5.9.1, 5.9.2 and 5.9.3?

Fig. 5.9.1

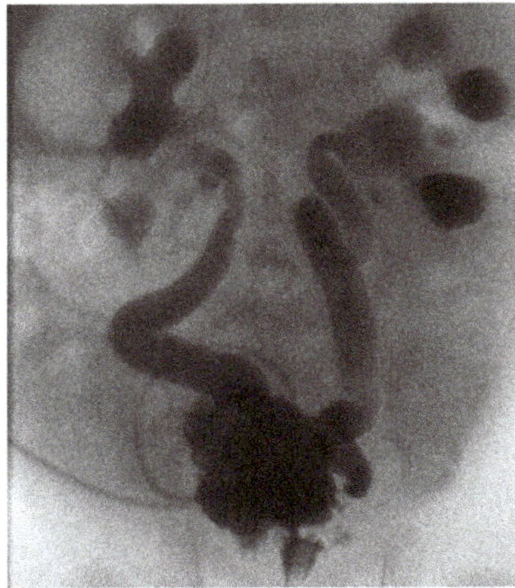

Fig. 5.9.2

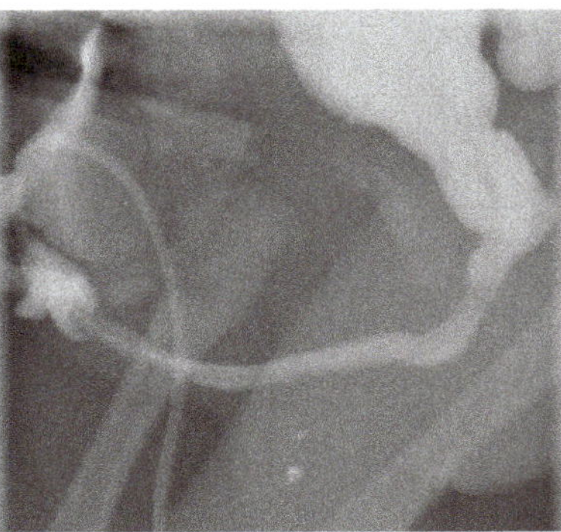

Fig. 5.9.3

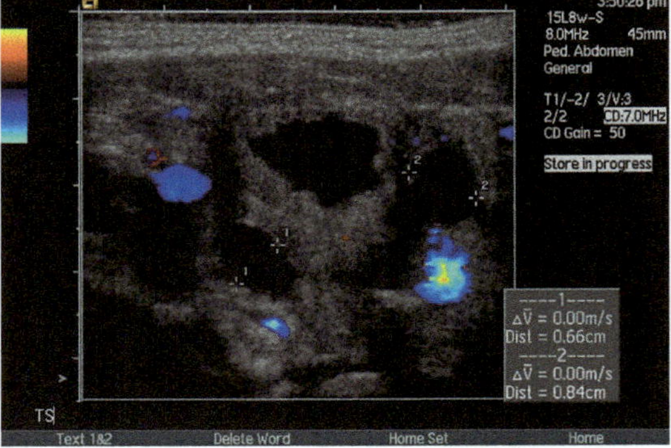

Answers to Case 5.9

1. During the early stages of normal embryogenesis, the most caudal end of the mesonephric duct is absorbed into the primitive cloaca at the site of the future verumontanum. Posterior urethral valves (PUV) are thought to form as the mesonephric duct fuses with the developing cloaca, at approximately 4 weeks gestation. PUV are found in 1/8,000 live births and account for about 10% of antenatal hydronephrosis.
2. Ultrasound findings suggestive of PUV include bilateral hydronephrosis, oligohydramnios, thick-walled bladder and a dilated posterior urethra. The features of poor prognosis, detected on the USS before 24 weeks gestation, are oligohydramnios, thickened bladder wall and renal dysplasia.
3. Hugh Hampton Young made the original PUV classification.
   - Type I (95%) extend anteriorly (upwards and forwards) from the verumontanum.
   - Type II (no longer accepted as valves) extend from the verumontanum along posterior urethral wall towards the bladder neck.
   - Type III (5%) not related to the verumontanum, found at various levels in the urethra and may be circumferentially attached to the urethral wall with a central defect.
4. Figure 5.9.1 is a neonatal micturating cystourethrogram (MCUG) showing gross bilateral vesicoureteric reflux. Also note reflux into the prostatic ducts. Figure 5.9.2 is an image from a MCUG. There is dilatation of the posterior urethra with a change in calibre to the normal anterior urethra. There is a suggestion of a valve seen at this level as a linear filling defect. Figure 5.9.3 is a pelvic ultrasound showing a thick-walled trabeculated bladder and bilateral hydroureters consistent with bladder outflow obstruction secondary to posterior urethral valves.

Further Reading

Desai D, Duffy PG. Posterior urethral valves and other urethral abnormalities. Thomas DFM, Rickwood AMK, Duffy PG. *Essentials of Paediatric Urology*. 2nd edn. London: Informa; 2008.

Young HH, Frontz WA, Baldwin JC. Congenital obstruction of the posterior urethra. *J Urol*. 1919;3:289.

Case 5.10

1. Can you give the eponymous name and describe the classical site of bladder diverticula in young boys, as seen in Fig. 5.10.1.
2. What is the definition of a diverticulum?
3. Give examples of conditions associated with the development of adult bladder diverticula.
4. What complications of a bladder diverticulum are shown in Fig. 5.10.2. What other complications may be occurring in this 61-year-old lady undergoing video-urodynamics, shown in Fig. 5.10.3a, b; and in the cystectomy specimen of a 73-year-old male patient shown in Fig. 5.10.4.

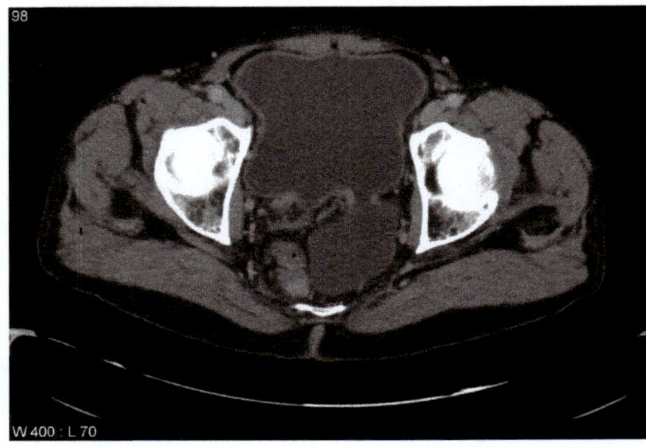

Fig. 5.10.1

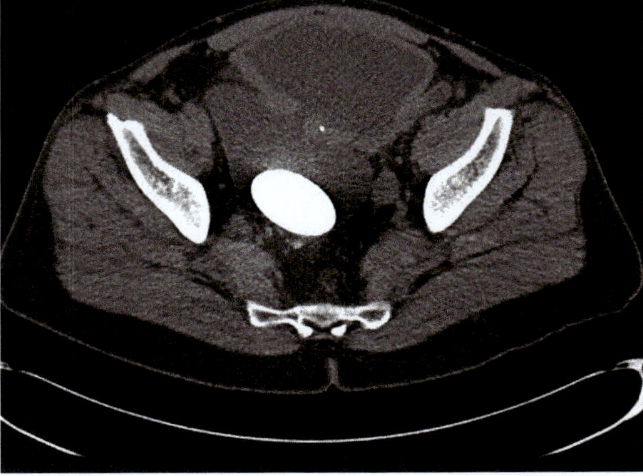
Fig. 5.10.2

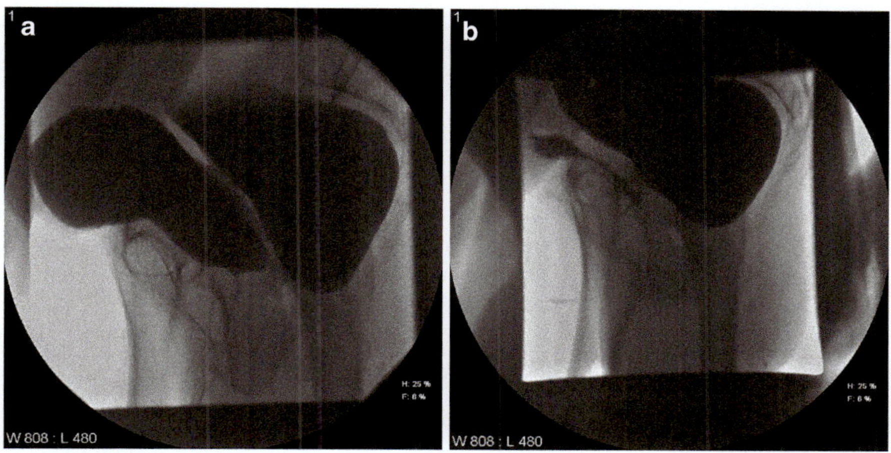

Fig. 5.10.3

Fig. 5.10.4

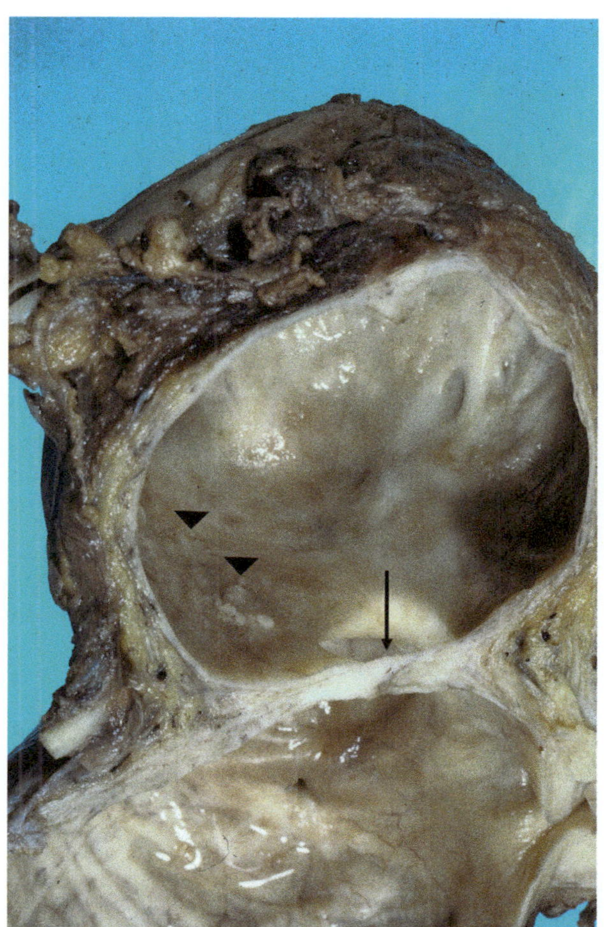

Answers to Case 5.10

1. John Hutch (1961) described primary and secondary paraureteric diverticula, both occur at the ureteric hiatus. Primary are in a smooth walled bladder with no infravesical obstruction, secondary are in trabeculated bladders caused by obstruction. Figure 5.10.1 is an axial CT scan showing a left-sided primary Hutch diverticulum.
2. An out-pouching of the lining of a hollow viscus through its normal external muscle layers.
3. Adult diverticula are found in bladder outlet obstruction and neuropathic bladder dysfunction. These are more common in men than women. If the diverticulum encompasses the ureteric orifice in the context of vesicoureteric reflux and a neuropathic bladder, it is termed a Hutch diverticulum.
4. Diverticula often have a narrow neck which in addition to the limited or absent muscle layer leads to incomplete emptying and stagnant urine. The latter may become infected and stone formation may also occur. Figure 5.10.2 is an axial CT scan showing a large diverticulum arising from the right posterior wall of the bladder that contains a large stone.

   Figure 5.10.3a and b are spot views taken from a video urodynamics study in a lady with incomplete emptying and recurrent urinary infections. Figure 5.10.3a shows the bladder anteriorly and a large diverticulum arising posteriorly. Figure 5.10.3b is a post-micturition image, the bladder has emptied but the diverticulum remains full and on subsequent films slowly re-filled the bladder.

   In addition to infection and stone formation, diverticula are associated with an increased risk of tumour formation, as seen in Fig. 5.10.4. The thin wall and lack of trabeculation of the diverticulum (right) contrasts with that of the bladder. The sessile white tumour (arrowhead) is seen above the narrow neck of the diverticulum (arrow).

Further Reading

Gearhart JP. Exstrophy, epispadias, and other bladder anomalies. In Walsh PC, Retik AB, Vaughan ED Jr, Wein AJ, eds. *Campbell's Urology*. 8th edn. Philadelphia: WB Saunders; 2002:2136-2196.

Hutch JA. Vesico-ureteral reflux in the paraplegic. Cause and correction. *J Urol.* 1952;68:457-467.

Treatment of bladder diverticula, impaired detrusor contractility and low bladder compliance Powell CR, Kreder k. *J Urol Clin N Am.* 2009;36:511–25.

Case 5.11

1. A 25-year-old woman presented with a history of recurrent urinary tract infections and intermittent loin pain. She underwent an ultrasound examination followed by a CT scan. Study images 5.11.1 and 5.11.2a, b. Describe the findings.
2. What is the name of the radiological sign demonstrated in Fig. 5.11.2a?
3. What further radiological investigations may help the management of this condition and why?

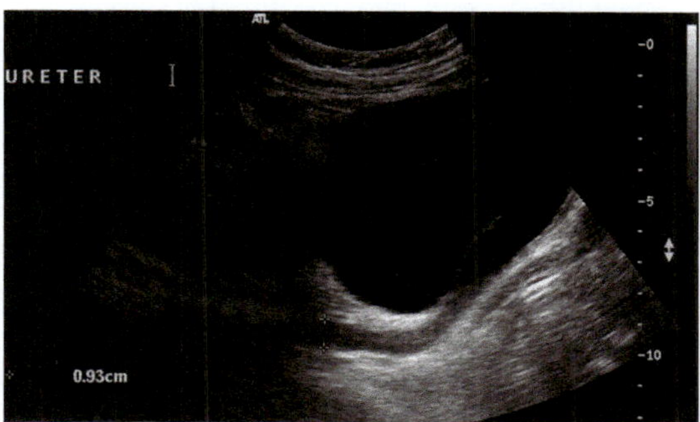

Fig. 5.11.1

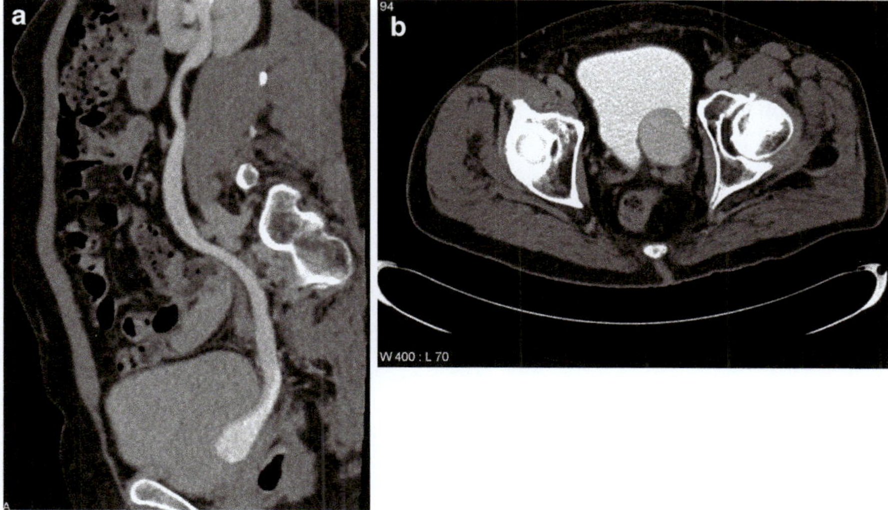

Fig. 5.11.2

Answers to Case 5.11

1. The first image (Fig. 5.11.1) is a sagittal ultrasound scan showing a thin-walled cystic structure. It is transonic and of water density internally, and therefore is not a soft tissue mass. True cysts of the bladder are excessively rare and the most likely diagnosis is an ureterocoele, especially in the context of the history. This was confirmed by a CT urogram study as shown in Fig. 5.11.2a, b. Figure 5.11.2a is a curved re-format study, i.e. the images have been post-processed such that the line of the reconstruction has been curved to follow the orientation of the ureter. The ureter is thus shown as a straightened structure. The ureterocoele is clearly demonstrated protruding into the bladder. Figure 5.11.2b is an axial CT scan image showing a left-sided ureterocoele.
2. Figure 5.11.2a demonstrates the 'Cobra head' sign. The head being the ureterocoele, and the tail is represented by the ureter, which may or may not be dilated.
3. Ureterocoele can either be a solitary finding or part of a duplex system; and the ureterocoele may be causing functional obstruction or not. Thus further radiological studies that may help would be a direct or indirect micturating cystogram to look for reflux. Functional obstruction should be objectively quantified with nuclear scintigraphy, e.g. a Mag3 or DTPA scan; and if the affected kidney is scarred on USS or CT scans, then a nuclear medicine (DMSA) test to document the residual renal function as a poorly functional kidney with a ureterocoele may be better removed than salvaged.

Further Reading

Dyer RB, Chen MY, Zagoria RJ. Classic signs in uroradiology. *Radiographics*. 2004; 24(Suppl 1):S247–S280.

Case 5.12

1. How does bladder cancer present?
2. Examine Fig. 5.12.1 and describe the abnormality seen. How would you further investigate this patient and discuss the other options in assessing a patient with haematuria. Describe the findings seen in Figs. 5.12.2a, b and 5.12.3a,b,c.
3. What does the surgical specimen Fig. 5.12.4 show and how often does this occur?

Fig. 5.12.1

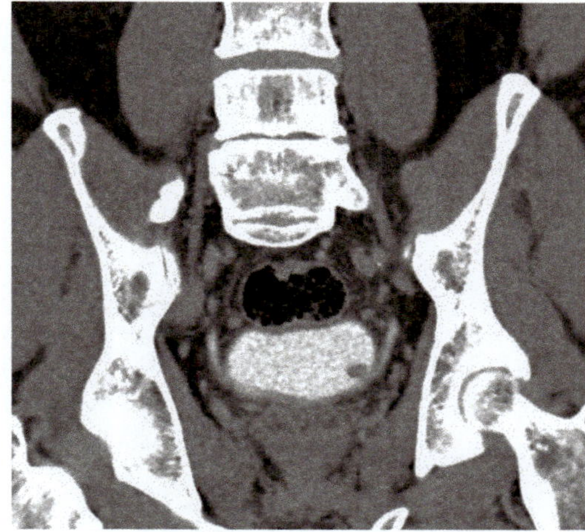

Fig. 5.12.2

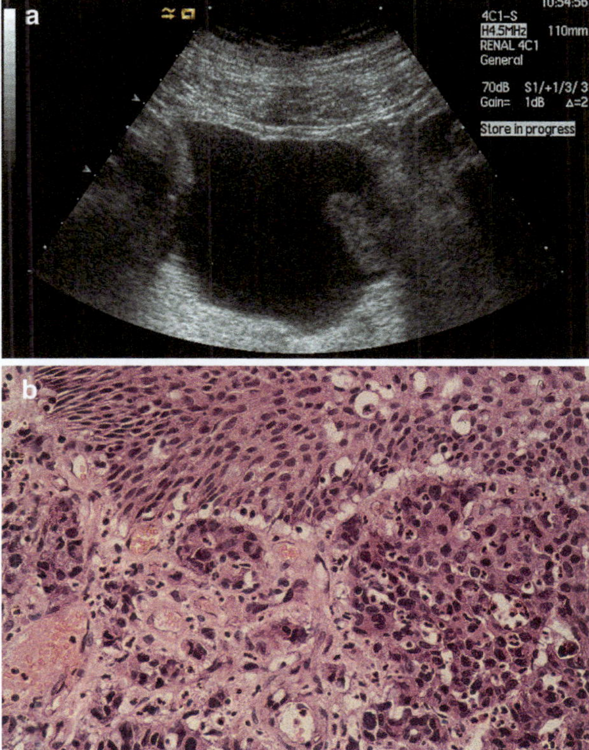

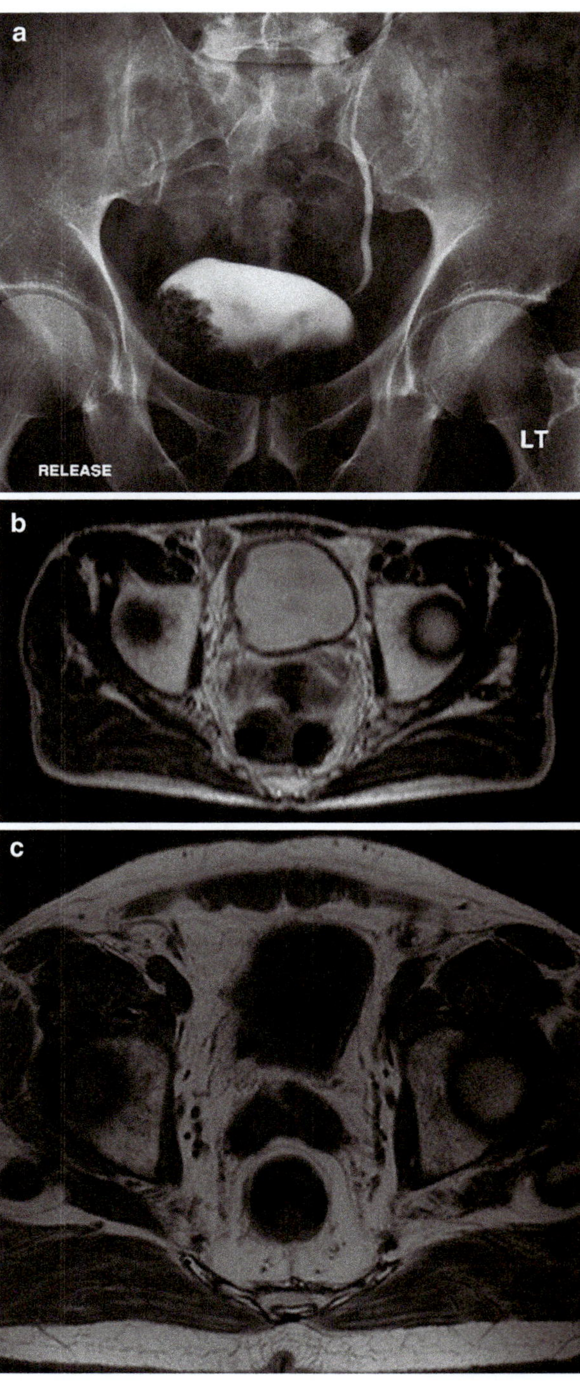

Fig. 5.12.3

Fig. 5.12.4

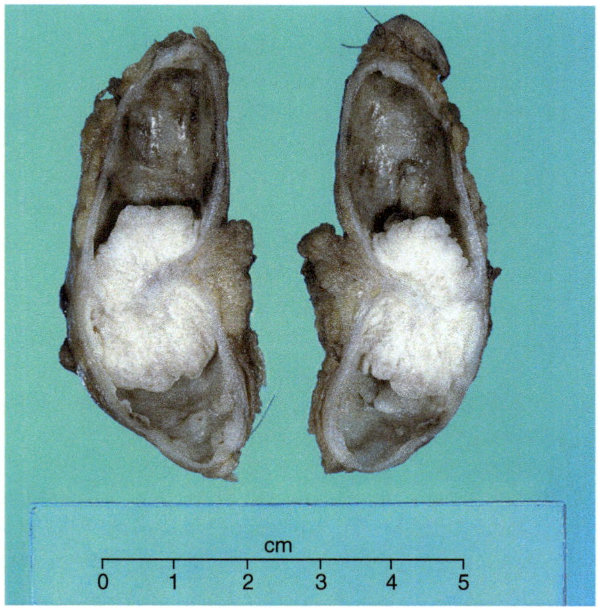

Answers to Case 5.12

1. Transitional Cell (TCC) bladder cancer is the commonest malignancy of the urinary tract, and the 9th most common cancer worldwide. There are 10,000 new cases yearly in the UK with a male to female ratio of 3:1. Approximately 75–85% of patients with bladder cancer present with disease confined to the urothelium (stage Ta, CIS) or lamina propria (stage 1). In patients with non-muscle invasive bladder cancer (Ta and T1), haematuria is the commonest presentation. Patients with carcinoma in situ (CIS) or muscle invasive disease may have storage bladder symptoms, dysuria or bladder pain and in more advanced cases a palpable mass or hydronephrosis.
2. The investigation of haematuria varies from unit to unit. An assessment is made of the upper tracts, in patients with visible haematuria this is usually by means of a CT urogram (CTU), though in some centres and in cases of non-visible haematuria this may be by USS alone and/or IVU. CT has greater accuracy in detecting a primary malignancy and also enables more accurate local and regional staging if tumour is found, but involves administering contrast, a higher dose of radiation and additional cost. Figure 5.12.1 is a coronal image from a CTU showing a small pedunculated filling defect arising from the left wall of the bladder.

Subsequent resection revealed a low-grade pT1 lesion. Figure 5.12.2a is a transverse USS undertaken for haematuria and shows a large solid lesion arising from the left lateral bladder wall. Resection revealed a high-grade pT1 bladder lesion. Figure 5.12.2b shows a TCC of mixed grade. The high-grade component is invading the lamina propria on the left of the figure.

Figure 5.12.3a is part of an IVU series, showing an amorphous right-sided filling defect that proved to be a TCC. MRI may also be used to stage bladder cancer both locally and the regional lymph nodes with similar accuracy to CT, though it is not currently routinely used in the assessment of a patient with haematuria. Figure 5.12.3b is an axial T2-weighted MR showing a T2 bladder cancer on the right lateral wall. Figure 5.12.3c is a T1-weighted MR scan showing thickening along the right lateral and posterior bladder wall, note the irregular outline of the bladder. This was also due to a TCC.

Haematuria investigation may also include urine cytology, which has a high sensitivity for high-grade disease and CIS but a lower sensitivity for lower-grade disease. Cytology has a high specificity, 90%, in experienced hands. Urinary markers including nuclear matrix protein 22 (NMP22) have a higher sensitivity than urine cytology, but at the expense of a lower specificity. Flexible cystoscopy using local anaesthetic is used to assess the bladder, unless imaging or cytology/urinary markers indicate a malignancy when a patient will proceed directly to a rigid cystoscopy under general anaesthetic.

3. Figure 5.12.4 is a segmental excision of the ureter, bisected to show a papillary TCC. Between 1.8% and 5% of patients with bladder TCC will develop an upper tract tumour, increasing to 7.5% in patients with tumours involving the trigone.

Further Reading

Herr HW, Bochner BH, Dalbagni G, et al. Impact of the number of lymph nodes retrieved on outcome in patients with muscle invasive bladder cancer. *J Urol.* 2002;167:1295-1298.

Koch MO, Smith JA Jr. Natural history and surgical management of superficial bladder cancer (stages Ta/T1/Tis). In Vogelzang N, Miles BJ, eds. Comprehensive Textbook of Genitourinary Oncology. Baltimore: Williams and Wilkins; 1996: 405-415.

Skinner DG, Stein JP, Lieskovsky G, et al. 25-year experience in the management of invasive bladder cancer by radical cystectomy. *Eur Urol.* 1998; 33(suppl 4): 25-26.

Sobin LH, Gospodarowicz MK, Wittekind C. Urinary bladder. In: *TNM Classification of Malignant Tumours (Uicc International Union Against Cancer).* New York: Wiley-Liss; 2009.

Case 5.13

1. Study Fig. 5.13.1a–d. What do they show and how is bladder cancer graded?
2. What factors predict recurrence and progression of non-muscle invasive TCC?
3. Figure 5.13.2a-g are non-malignant conditions which may cause papillary or nodular bladder lesions which may be mistaken for TCCs at cystoscopy. List these conditions.

Fig. 5.13.1

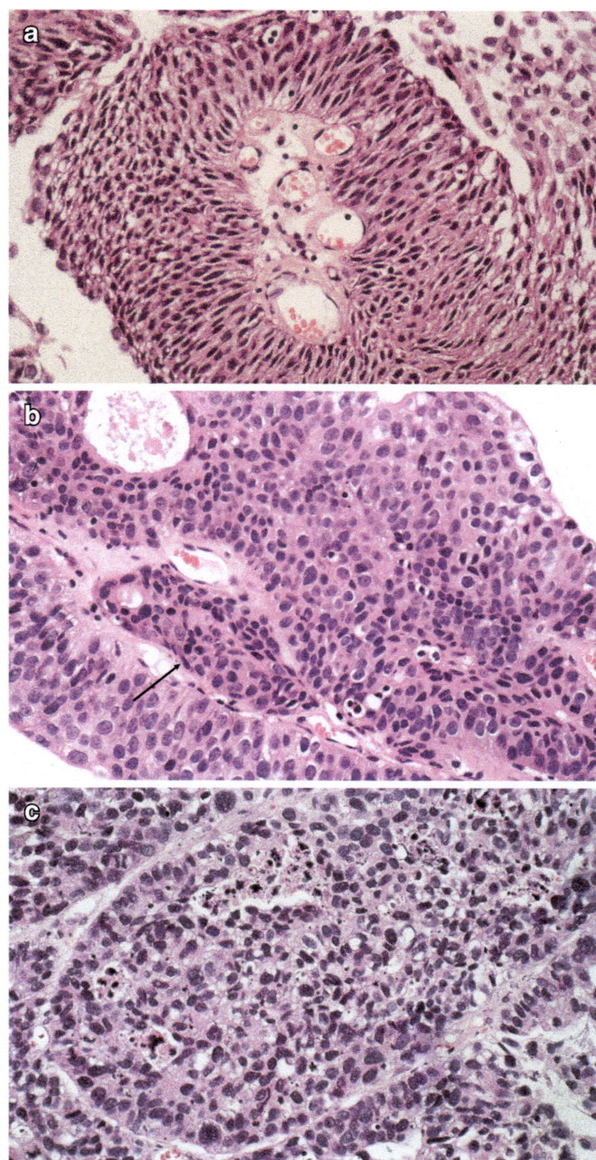

Fig. 5.13.1 (continued)

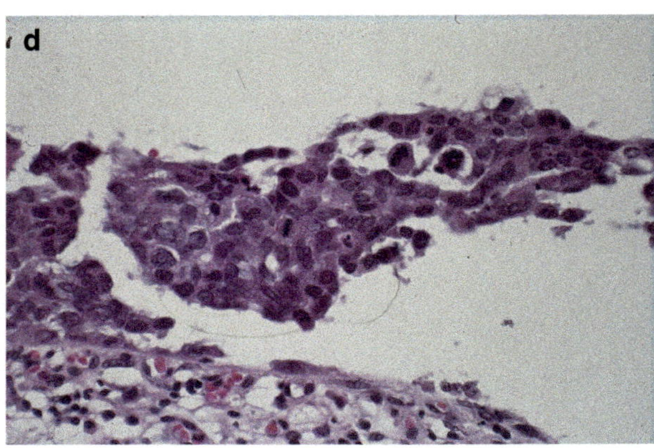

Fig. 5.13.2

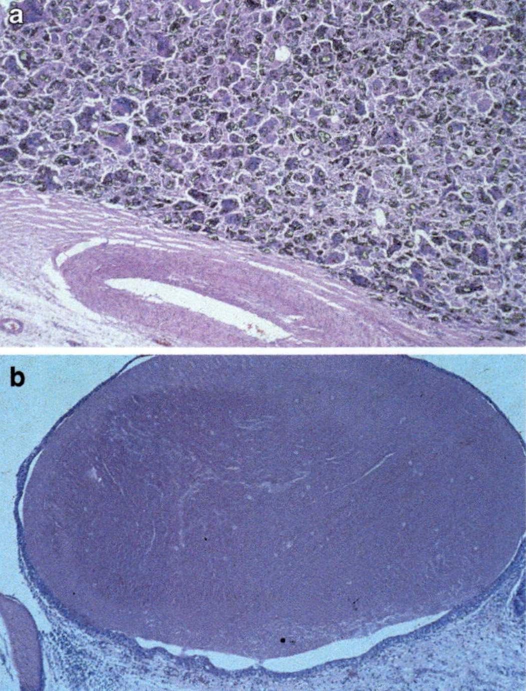

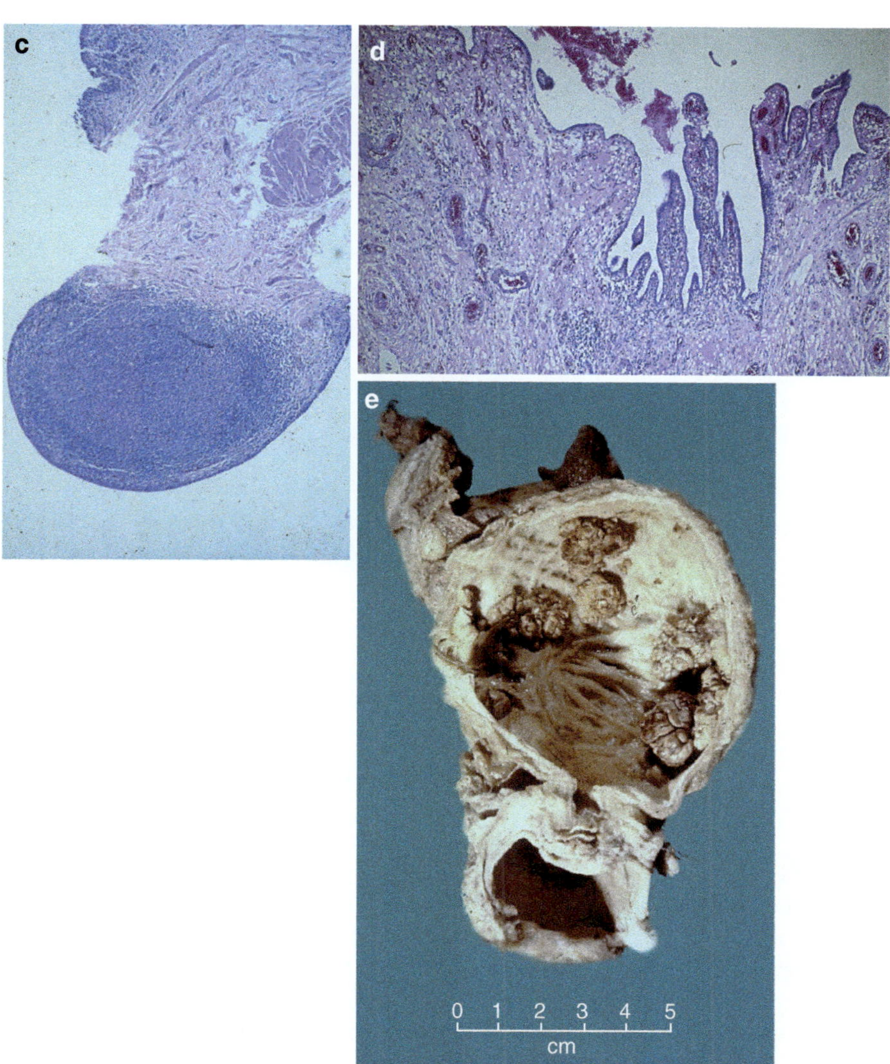

Fig. 5.13.2 (continued)

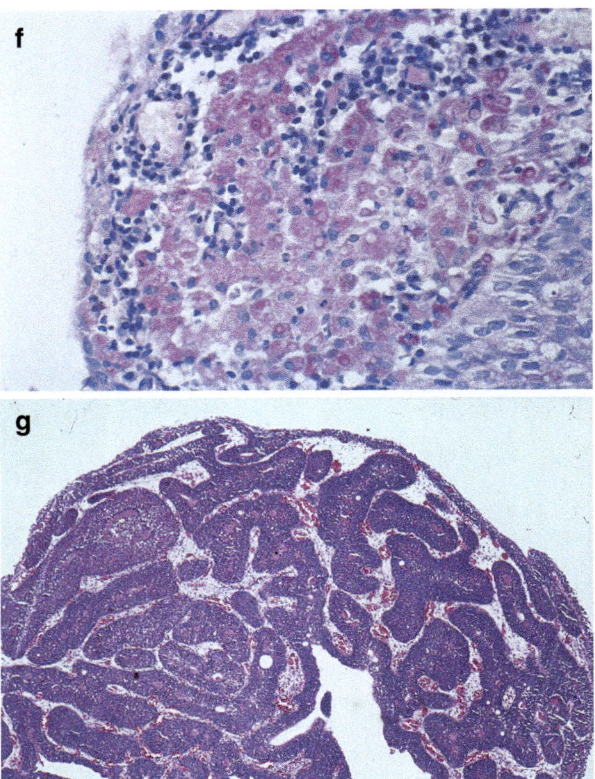

Fig. 5.13.2 (continued)

Answers to Case 5.13

1. Grading categories of urothelial tumours are distinguished by microarchitectural and cytological features resulting in the classification seen in a, b and c.
   a. Papillary Urothelial Neoplasm of Low Malignant Potential (PUNLMP) (Fig. 5.13.1a): fine vascular connective tissue cores are covered by urothelium in which elongated nuclei of similar size and shape with evenly stained chromatin are orientated at right angles to the basement membrane. These features underlie the characteristic orderly appearance of the epithelium.
   b. Papillary urothelial carcinoma, low grade (Fig. 5.13.1b): compared with PUNLMP the nuclei appear more rounded, their polarity is reduced, spacing is irregular with foci of crowding, size, shape and staining are all more variable. These features reduce the orderly microarchitecture. Tumour is invading a papillary core (arrow).
   c. Papillary urothelial carcinoma, high grade (Fig. 5.13.1c): Nuclei have lost polarity and show marked variation in size, shape and staining some being hyperchromatic and including coarse chromatin. Cell borders are indistinct. Mitoses are commonly seen throughout the epithelial thickness and may be atypical. When compared with the previous two grades, the orderly microarchitecture has been lost.

d. Carcinoma in situ (Fig. 5.13.1d): the flat urothelium shows loss of normal nuclear orientation with marked pleomorphism and features resembling high-grade papillary carcinoma. The urothelium lacks cohesion and is frequently shed from biopsies leaving a denuded surface or atypical basal cells. The demarcation between CIS and normal urothelium is commonly abrupt.

2. The risk factors for recurrence and progression are: number of tumours (1, 2–7, >7), tumour diameter (<3 cm, ≥3 cm), recurrence (<1 recurrence per year, >1 recurrence per year), presence of CIS, tumour grade and stage. These factors have been incorporated into low, intermediate and high grade risk tables, derived from European Organization for Research and Treatment of Cancer (EORTC) trials.
3. Lesions that may mimic TCC include:

   Inflammatory polyps: e.g. at a previous biopsy site, associated with an indwelling catheter or adjacent to a fistula, post-operative spindle cell nodule migration of Teflon from a ureterovesical injection site as shown in Fig. 5.13.2a. where numerous multinucleate giant cells incorporate and surround foreign polarisable fragments.

   Cystitis cystica (Fig. 5.13.2b): the term given to cystic change within von Brunn's nests. When such cysts are occasional and microscopic they are considered to be within the range of normality but when large and numerous they produce nodules or polyps which may become visible on cystoscopy. They are usually associated with some form of bladder irritation, e.g. recurrent UTI. Similar cysts are also seen in the upper tracts (ureteritis and pyelitis cystica) and may produce filling defects on IVU (see case 2.6).

   Cystitis follicularis (Fig. 5.13.2c): the lamina propria contains large lymphoid follicles which may cause elevation of the urothelium. This reaction is usually associated with chronic irritation/infection but not invariably so. An identical reaction is also seen in the ureter and pelvis.

   Nephrogenic adenoma: is a form of metaplasia in which the surface transitional epithelium is replaced by benign cuboidal epithelium which also produces numerous tubules in the lamina propria and covers papillary outgrowths (Fig. 5.13.2d). This condition is found throughout the urinary tract and is associated with prior instrumentation and trauma.

   Malakoplakia: a chronic inflammatory response thought to result from the impaired ability of macrophages to phagocytose bacteria. Numerous macrophages with characteristic calcium and iron-rich inclusions give rise to soft yellow plaques seen cystoscopically (Fig. 5.13.2e). Microscopically, malakoplakia is characterised by the presence of granular macrophages with laminated targetoid inclusions seen on the Periodic acid schiff reaction (Fig. 5.13.2f) and known as Michaelis - Gutmann bodies.

   Inverted Papilloma: hyperplastic infoldings of transitional epithelium form cords and islands within the lamina propria with the central layers being composed of umbrella cells. The resulting polyp is covered by benign smooth attenuated transitional epithelium (Fig. 5.13.2g).

Amyloid

Prostatic tissue: Prostatic tissue may prolapse or evert from the ducts to give rise to a papillary lesion at the bladder neck or urethra. Ectopic prostatic tissue may cause a lesion elsewhere in the bladder.

Endometriosis

Specific infection: Polypoid Schistosomiasis.

Further Reading

Grignon DJ. The current classification of urothelial neoplasms *Mod Pathol.* 2009;22:S60–S69.

Lopez-Beltran A, et al. *Tumours of the Urinary system in Pathology and Genetics of Tumours of the Urinary System and Male Genital Organs*. Oxford: IARC Press; 2004.

Sylvester RJ, van der Meijden AP, Oosterlinck W, et al. Predicting recurrence and progression in individual patients with stage TaT1 bladder cancer using EORTC risk tables: a combined analysis of 2,596 patients from seven EORTC trials. *Eur Urol.* 2006;49(3):466-475.

Young RH. Tumor like lesions of the urinary bladder. *Mod Pathol.* 2009;22: S37–S52.

Case 5.14

1. Examine Figs. 5.14.1, 5.14.2, 5.14.3 and 5.14.4. What malignancies other than transitional cell carcinoma (TCC) arise in the bladder?
2. What are the risk factors for these cancers, one example is shown in Fig. 5.14.5.
3. When adenocarcinoma is found in the bladder from which tissues may it have arisen?

Fig. 5.14.1

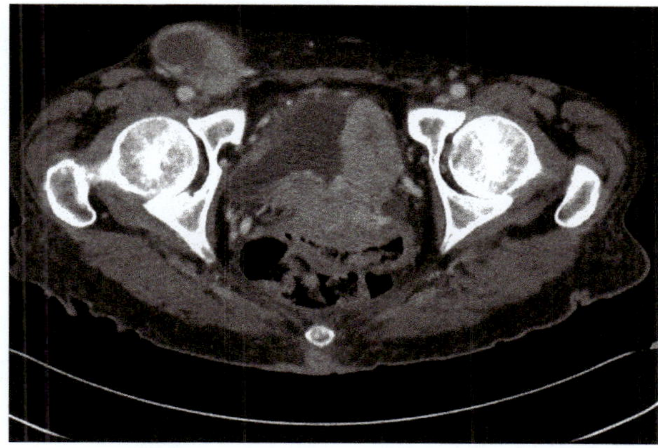

Fig. 5.14.2

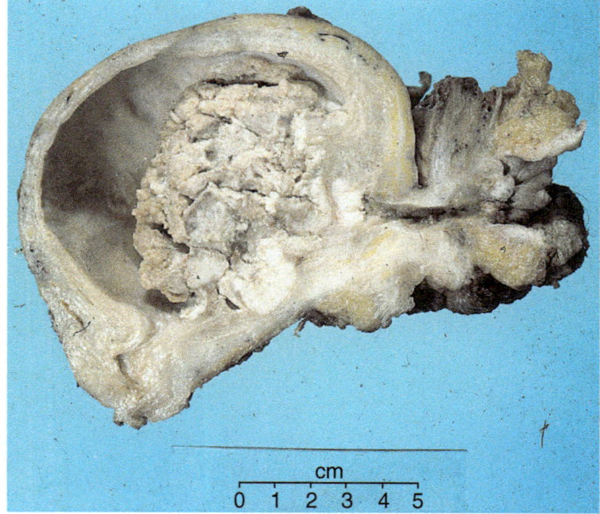

Fig. 5.14.3

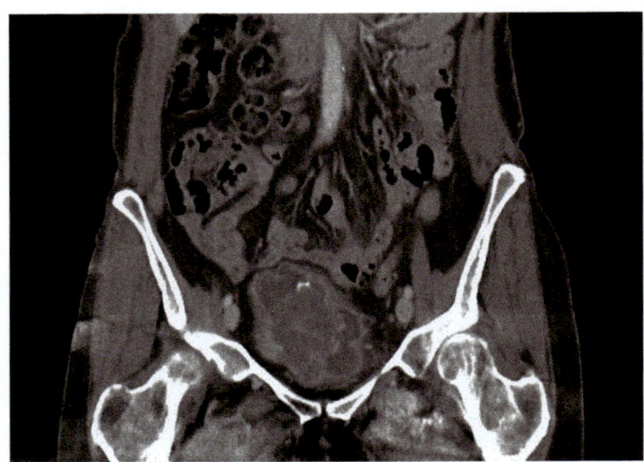

Fig. 5.14.4

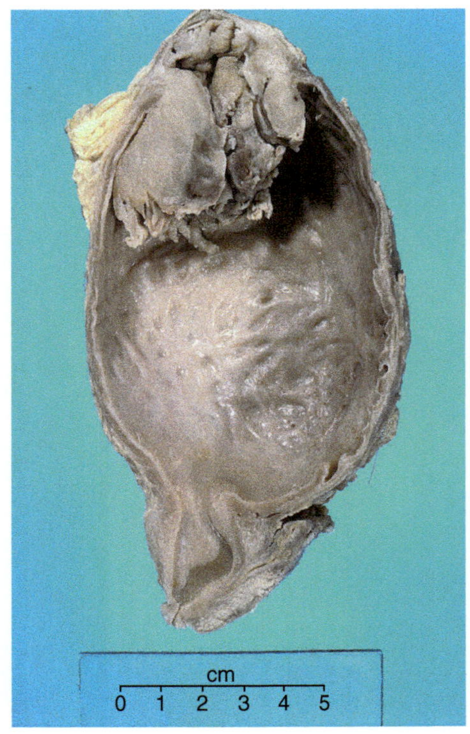

Fig. 5.14.5

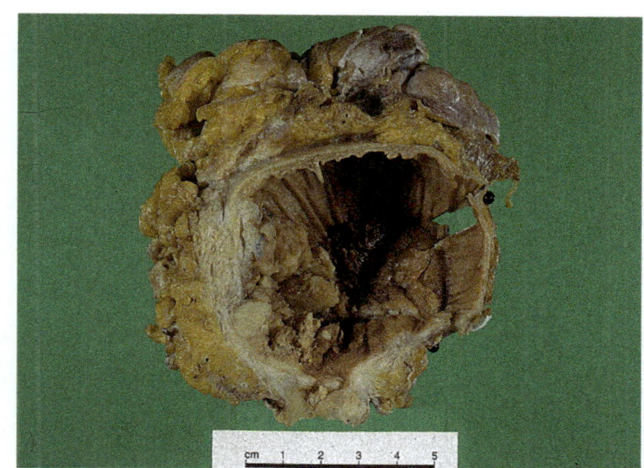

Fig. 5.14.6

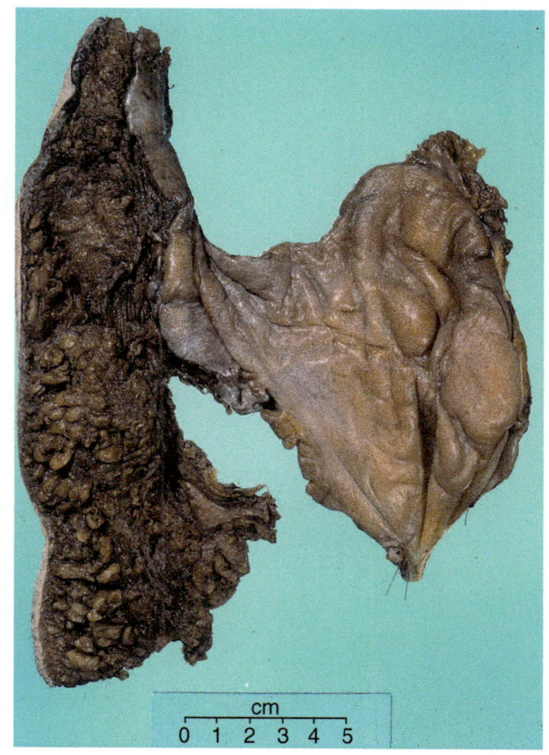

Fig. 5.14.7

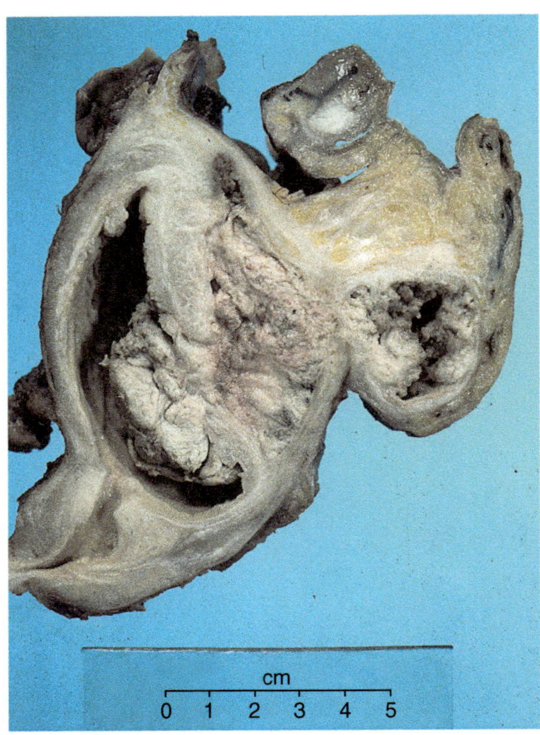

Answers to Case 5.14

1. Transitional cell carcinoma accounts for 90–95% of bladder malignancies. Of the remainder, squamous cell carcinoma (SCC) comprises 1% of bladder tumours in UK, but up to 75% in Egypt. In South Africa there are marked differences between black patients (36% SCC, 41% TCC) and white patients (2% SCC, 94% TCC). The marked regional and racial differences are due to exposure to *Schistosoma haemotobium*. Figure 5.14.1 is an axial CT showing a large solid mass involving the right lateral and posterior wall of the bladder with extravesical extension. Note the large necrotic right inguinal lymph node. Necrotic centres within lymph nodes are more commonly seen with squamous cell carcinoma, although this is not unknown with other tumour types. Figure 5.14.2 is a cystectomy specimen showing a SCC. Figure 5.14.3 is a coronal CT showing a large enhancing mass involving the majority of the bladder. Biopsy showed this to be an adenocarcinoma. Adenocarcinoma of the bladder accounts for 2% of primary bladder cancers.

Less common tumours include neuroendocrine (small cell and carcinoid), mesenchymal (rhabdomyosarcoma (children), leiomyosarcomas (adults)), melanocytic and haemopoietic (lymphoma, plasmacytoma). Figure 5.14.4 is a bisected cystectomy specimen showing a fleshy nodular mass at the dome protruding into the lumen and through the wall. A microscopic diagnosis of leiomyosarcoma was made.

2. Squamous cell carcinoma is usually preceded by squamous metaplasia related to chronic inflammation and smoking, Bilharzia infection, bladder stone, long-term catheterisation, chronic urinary tract infections and bladder diverticula. Adenocarcinoma usually arises from pre-existing intestinal metaplasia, due to non-functioning bladder, obstruction, chronic irritation and in exstrophy. Adenocarcinoma also arises where urine is in contact with bowel mucosa, e.g. uretero-sigmoid anastomoses, Clam ileocystoplasty. Figure 5.14.5 shows an adenocarcinoma arising from an augmented bladder.
3. Adenocarcinomas of the bladder may arise from
   - bladder epithelium – classically seen in the dome or base of the bladder but may occur anywhere. A subtype of primary bladder adenocarcinoma is signet ring, which gives rise to linitis plastica of the bladder.
   - the urachus – usually presenting as a mass deep to the urothelium or within the muscularis. Tumours arising in extra vesical urachal remnants are exceptionally rare. However, the anatomical distribution of urachal vestiges from the dome of the bladder to the umbilicus dictates the surgical approach to the resection of urachal cancer. Figure 5.14.6 is a disc of bladder excised in continuity with the urachus and the umbilicus.
   - direct or metastatic spread from a primary adenocarcinoma elsewhere, e.g. GIT and breast. Figure 5.14.7 is a bisected specimen of bladder and adherent large intestine, on microscopy an adenocarcinoma of the colon was seen to be invading the bladder.

Further Reading

Manunta A, Vincendeau S, Kiriakou G, et al. Non-transitional cell bladder carcinomas. *BJU Int.* 2005;95:497.

Urothelial Tumours of the Bladder. In: Messing EM. *Campbell's Urology*. 9th edn. Philadelphia: WB Saunders; 2007 Eds Walsh PC, Retik AB, Vaughan ED.

Case 5.15

1. Figure 5.15.1a and b are images from the radiographic investigation of a 50-year-old lady who presented with urine leakage per vagina, 1 week after an otherwise uneventful hysterectomy. What do the investigations show?
2. How would you manage this lady and what are the operative principles?
3. List the other causes of this complication, one of which is shown in Fig. 5.15.2.
4. A 73-year-old lady had undergone colectomy and adjuvant radiotherapy 10 years previously for treatment of carcinoma. She presents with recurrent urinary tract infections and pneumaturia. What does Fig. 5.15.3 show and how would you manage this lady?

Fig. 5.15.1

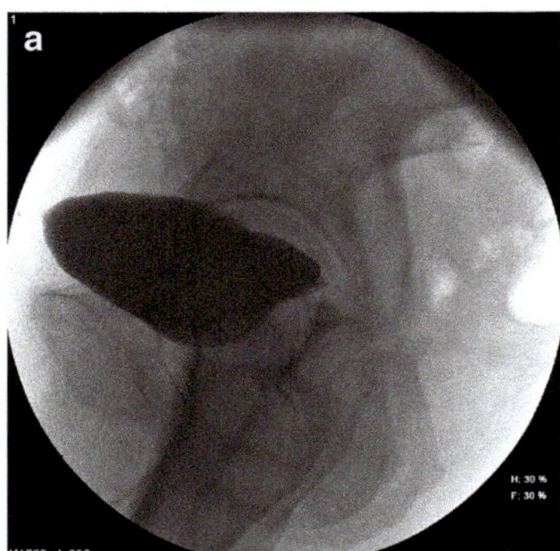

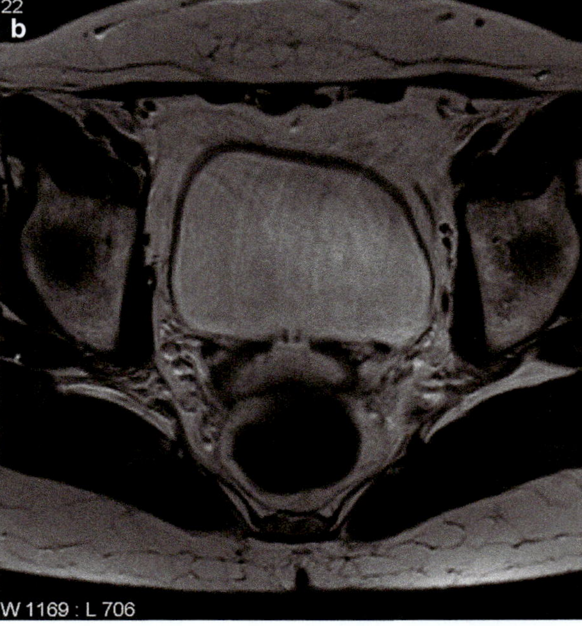

Fig. 5.15.2

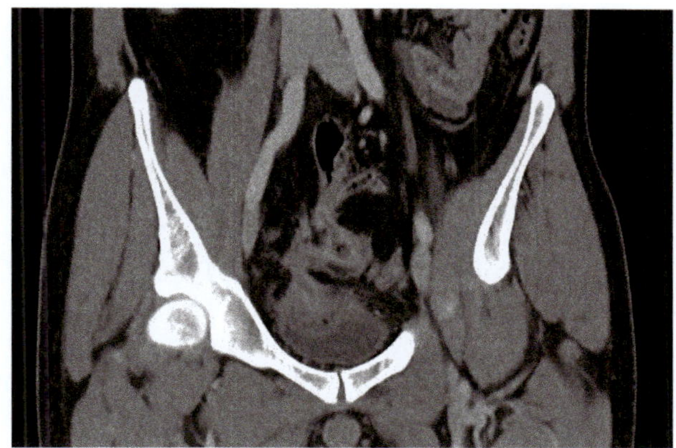

Fig. 5.15.3

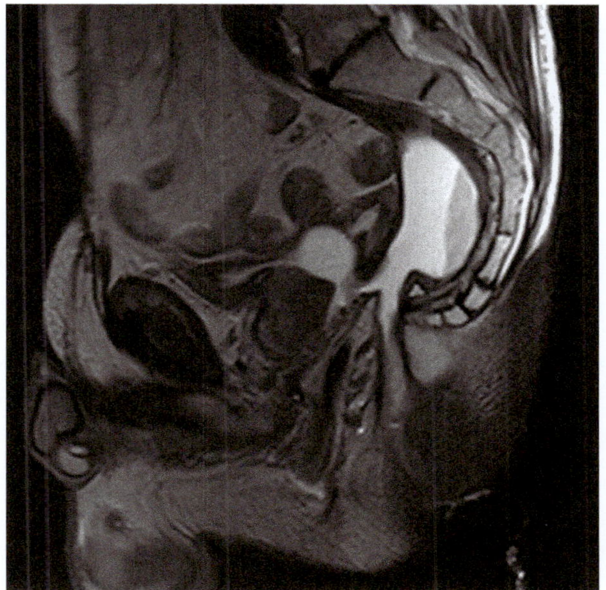

Answers to Case 5.15

1. Figure 5.15.1a is a spot view from a cystogram. It shows a vesicovaginal fistula with the vagina outlined with contrast (note the faint track of contrast outlining the vagina posteriorly). Figure 5.15.1b is an axial T2-weighted MRI in the same patient, and this better demonstrates the exact site of the posteriorly placed vesicovaginal fistula.
2. This lady needs a speculum examination and a bladder catheter to divert the urine away from the fistula. Imaging investigations should include investigation of the upper tracts to exclude a ureteric cause (12% of post-surgical fistulae have a concurrent ureteric injury) by means of a CT urogram or IVU, or cystoscopy and bilateral retrograde pyelograms. If a ureteric fistula is found, a stent may be inserted and the cystoscopy and retrograde pyelogram repeated after 6–12 weeks. If repair is required this should be done early, within 14 days or delayed until after 3 months.

   The operative principles are to ensure accurate localisation of the fistula/injury. Good surgical exposure should be achieved and the fistula mobilised. The tract is excised along with any foreign body and the defect closed with a multiple layer, water-tight, tension-free closure, with suture lines that do not overlap. Where possible, tissue interposition should be undertaken, e.g. omentum or a Martius fat pad. Good post-operative drainage is important to allow healing.
3. The causes of fistula include:
   - Iatrogenic – post-surgical, post-radiotherapy
   - Inflammatory bowel disease
   - Diverticular disease
   - Malignancy
   - Congenital
   - Infection
   - Post-partum – common in the developing world after prolonged labour

   Figure 5.15.2 is a coronal CT showing an enterovesical fistula between the terminal ileum and bladder in a patient with Crohn's disease. Note the central low-density focus within the bladder. This represents air (or more accurately gas). Air within the bladder is a highly specific sign for the presence of a vesicoenteric fistula, in the absence of any other explanation (e.g., recent instrumentation or infection by gas forming organisms).

4. The management is very similar. An MRI is undertaken as shown in Fig. 5.15.3. This is a sagittal view of the pelvis showing a large vesicorectal fistula. A cystoscopy and examination under anaesthetic should be performed to assess the size and position of the fistula, and where necessary a biopsy should be taken. The principles for closure are exactly the same – the literature cites a 95% cure rate for fistulae with good tissue interposition. In a few extreme cases following severe radiation damage urinary diversion may be an option.

Further Reading

Goodwin WE, Scardino PT. Vesicovaginal and ureterovaginal fistulas: a summary of 25 years of experience. *J Urol.* 1980;123:370-374

Wein AJ, Malloy TR, Carpiniello VL, et al. Repair of vesicovaginal fistula by a suprapubic transvesical approach. *Surg Gynecol Obstet.* 1980;150:57-60.

Wein AJ, Malloy TR, Greenberg SH, et al. Omental transposition as an aid in genitourinary reconstructive procedures. *J Trauma.* 1980;20:473-477.

Ockrim J, Greenwell T, Foley C. A tertiary experience of vesico-vaginal and urethro-vaginal fistula repair: factors predicting success. BJU Int.

Case 5.16

1. A 32-year-old motorcyclist hit a stationary care at 30 mph. He was brought into hospital complaining of abdominal pain. He was tender in the suprapubic region and the right hip and had visible haematuria. How would you investigate this man and describe the findings in images 5.16.1a, b. What type of study is Fig. 5.16.2? Has intravenous contrast been given?
2. What alternative imaging modalities may be used for diagnostic evaluation of this patient?
3. Describe a grading system for bladder trauma.

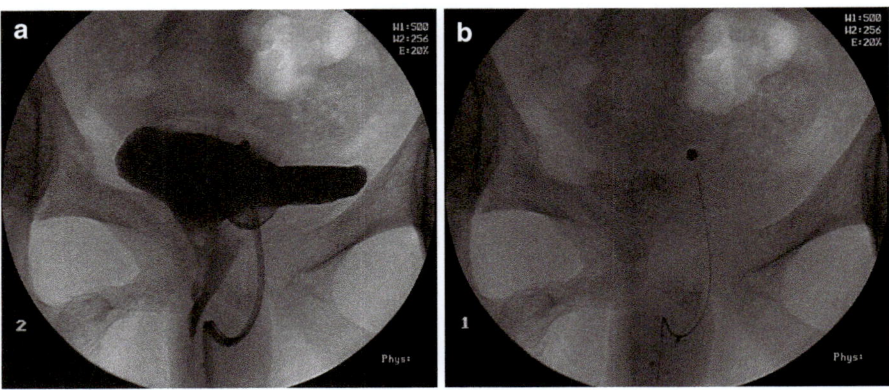

Fig. 5.16.1

Fig. 5.16.2

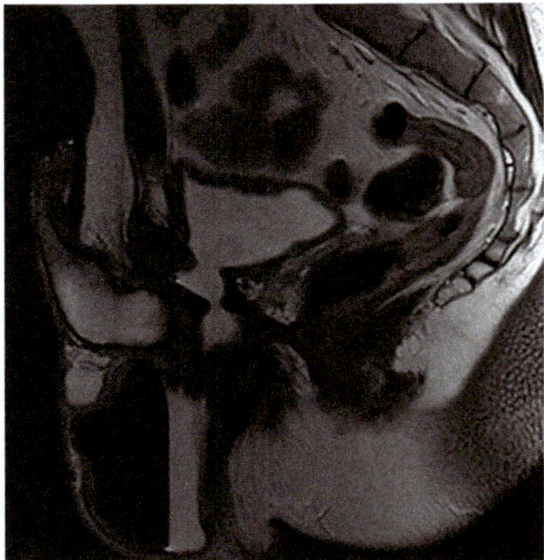

Answers to Case 5.16

1. Figure 5.16.1a is a retrograde cystogram in which contrast can be seen extravasating from the bladder into the pelvis, indicating a bladder rupture. There is also a fracture through the right acetabulum. On subsequent image 5.16.1b, the contrast was seen to remain in the pelvis confirming an extraperitoneal rupture. Figure 5.16.2 is a sagittal T2-weighted MRI study showing extravasated urine in the scrotal sac. There is no intra-peritoneal fluid further confirming that the urine leak was solely extra-peritoneal. No contrast has been given. On T2 MRI studies, the urine (and indeed many body fluids) is of naturally high signal and contrast medium is unnecessary.

   In patients with a ruptured bladder the most common symptoms are gross haematuria (82%) and abdominal tenderness (62%). Other features include the inability to void, bruising and swelling in the perineum and scrotum. Bladder rupture is usually found in patients with pelvic fractures, and though possible, the absence of visible haematuria and pelvic fracture virtually excludes traumatic bladder rupture. Conversely, the presence of pelvic fracture and visible haematuria necessitates an urgent retrograde cystogram.

   Retrograde cystography is the modality of choice for excluding bladder rupture. Conventionally this has been done using either plain film or fluoroscopy and has an accuracy of 85–100%. A minimum of 300–350 ml of contrast must be instilled to ensure adequate distension and prevent false-negative studies. A minimum of three films, pre-contrast, maximum fill and post-drainage must be taken. The post-drainage film is to exclude a posterior wall injury that may be obscured by contrast on the full bladder film.
2. Alternative diagnostic imaging includes CT cystography. This is becoming more popular as it has been shown to have similar sensitivity and specificity (95% and 100%, respectively), as conventional cystography. It does not require post-drainage imaging and the vast majority of patients with traumatic bladder injury will be undergoing CT scanning of the abdomen and pelvis anyway. The contrast protocol is the same as for retrograde cystography. An abdominal CT without cystography is inadequate as it is unable to distinguish abdominal fluid as urine or ascites.
3. There are two main grading systems:

   The AAST-OIS scale which gives five grades
   a. Contusion, intramural haematoma and partial thickness laceration
   b. Extraperitoneal wall lacerations <2 cm
   c. Extraperitoneal lacerations >2 cm or intraperitoneal lacerations <2 cm
   d. Intraperitoneal lacerations >2 cm
   e. Intraperitoneal or extraperitoneal lacerations that extend into the bladder neck or trigone.

   The consensus panel of the Societe Internationale D'Urologie gives 4 grades and is perhaps more commonly used in clinical practice.

a. Bladder contusion
b. Intraperitoneal rupture
c. Extraperitoneal rupture
d. Combined injury

These classifications dictate treatment. Blunt trauma resulting in intraperitoneal bladder perforation requires significant forces and so is often associated with large bladder lacerations as well as injury to other abdominal viscera. Urgent surgical repair and drainage is therefore required in intraperitoneal as well as all penetrating injuries to the bladder. Extraperitoneal injuries can be managed with catheter drainage alone unless there is bladder neck involvement or a bone fragment is embedded in the bladder wall.

Further Reading

Gomez RG, Ceballos L, Coburn M et al. Consensus statement on bladder injuries *BJU Int*. 2004;94:27-32.

Moore EE, Cogbill TH, Jurkovich GJ et al. Organ injury scaling III: Chest wall, abdominal vasculature, ureter, bladder and urethra. *J Trauma*. 1992;33:337-339.

Schneider RE. Genitourinary trauma. *Emerg Med Clin North Am*. 1993;11:137-145.

Case 5.17

1. A 65-year-old man presents and haematuria and dysuria. To investigate this he had a CT scan. What is seen in Fig. 5.17.1 and what is the aetiology?
2. What two abnormalities can you see on the KUB X-ray in Fig. 5.17.2?
3. How is this condition diagnosed on ultrasound? What are the key sonographic findings? What are the sonographic features of uric acid stones?

Fig. 5.17.1

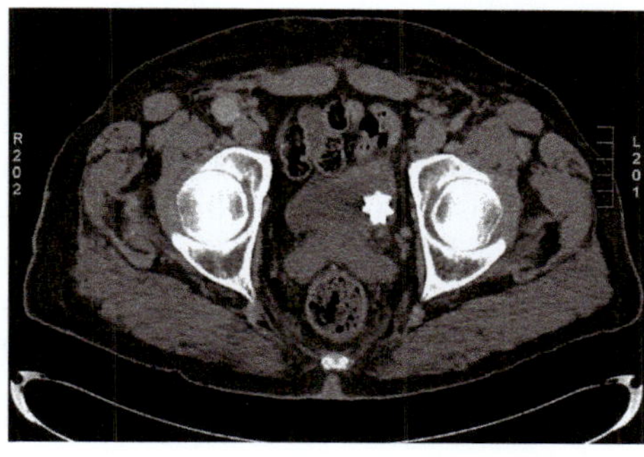

Fig. 5.17.2

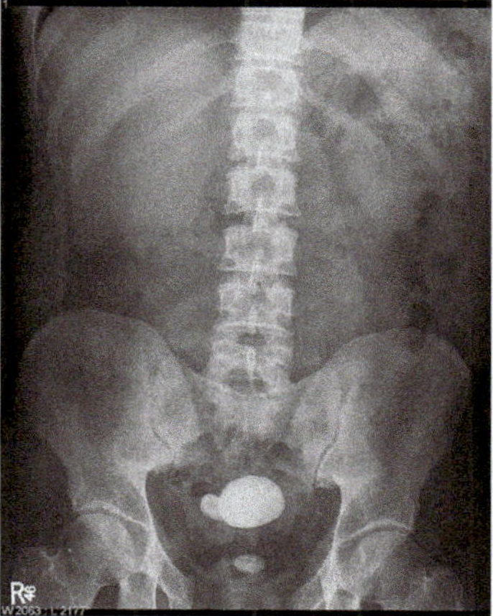

Fig. 5.17.3

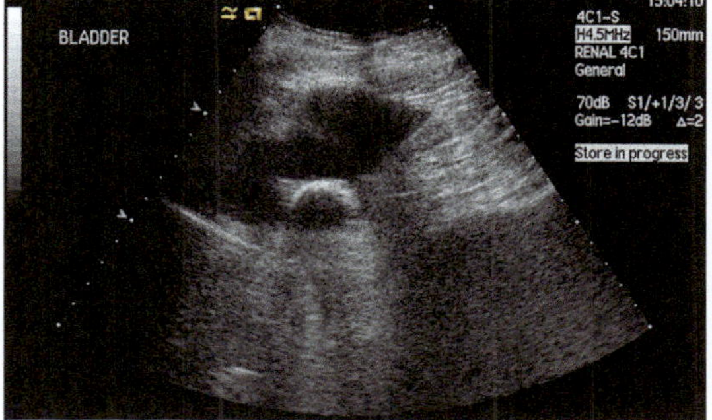

Answers to Case 5.17

1. Figure 5.17.1 is a transverse CT scan showing a left-sided bladder calculus. Bladder stones occur in approximately 0.5% of men with bladder outflow obstruction (BOO). Incomplete bladder emptying is believed to be the underlying cause. Following standard evaluation for BOO the stones are removed either endoscopically or if large or numerous through an open cystolithotomy. Relief of the obstruction by TURP or laser outflow surgery may be performed either at the same sitting or as a staged procedure.
2. Figure 5.17.2 is a KUB radiograph showing a patient with bladder exstrophy with at least three bladder stones; and widened pubic symphysis (diastasis).
3. On USS, bladder stones are typically hyperechoic, cast an acoustic shadow and mobile, as shown in Fig. 5.17.3. The latter is the most important finding as it distinguishes a calculus from a fixed calcified mass in the bladder wall, e.g. a calcified TCC.

   The sonographic features of all calculi, whether uric acid or calcium/magnesium containing, are similar. It is not possible to distinguish stone content on ultrasound. However, on CT uric acid stones (and also cyteine and struvite stones) are of lower density than calcium and magnesium containing calculi. Pure uric acid stones are not visible on plain X-ray. The only stones that are invisible on all imaging modalities are certain drug-related calculi, e.g. Indinavir-related stones.

Further Reading

Hamid R, Robertson WG, Woodhouse CRJ. Comparison of biochemistry and diet in patients with enterocystoplasty who do and do not form stones. *BJUI.* 2008;101:1427-1432.

Wasson JH, Reda DJ, Bruskewitz RC, et al. A comparison of transurethral surgery with watchful waiting for moderate symptoms of benign prostatic hyperplasia. The Veterans Affairs Cooperative Study Group on Transurethral Resection of the Prostate. *N Engl J Med.* 1995; 332:75-79.

Case 5.18

1. What is the difference between a complicated and uncomplicated urinary tract infection (UTI) and what are the most common causative organisms?
2. A 82-year-old diabetic lady presented with symptoms of a UTI and a temperature of 38.4°C. What is shown in Fig. 5.18.1? Which organism can cause this?
3. What does the cystogram show in Fig. 5.18.2 and with what organism might this occur?
4. A 64-year aid worker presented with frequency, dysuria and terminal haematuria. What does the CT (Fig. 5.18.3) demonstrate?
5. What are the typical cystoscopic appearance of this condition and what does the biopsy (Fig. 5.18.4) show?

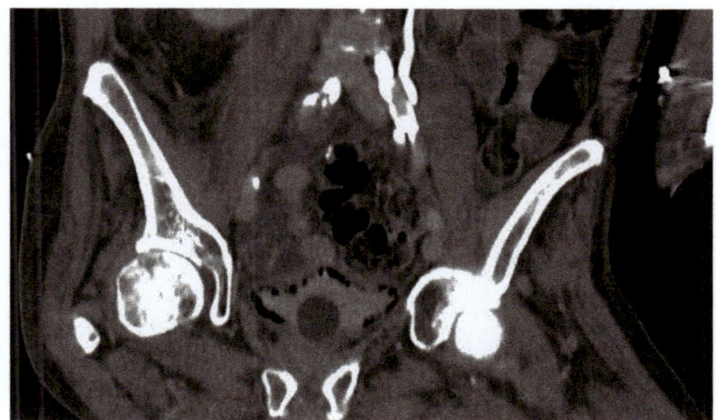

Fig. 5.18.1

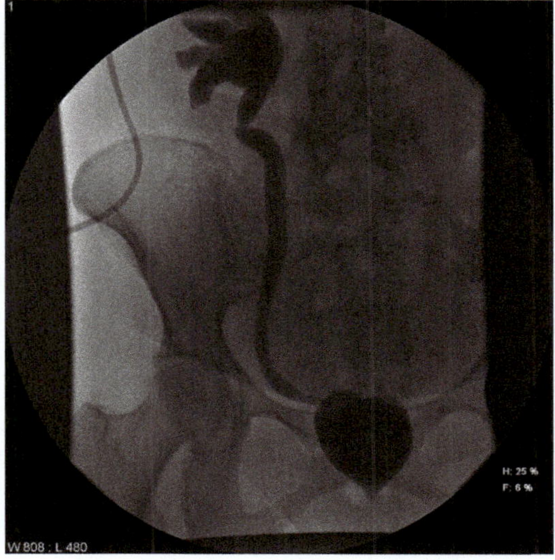

Fig. 5.18.2

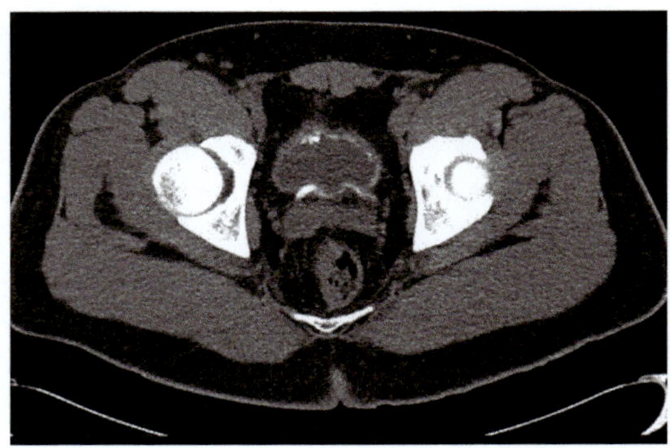

Fig. 5.18.3

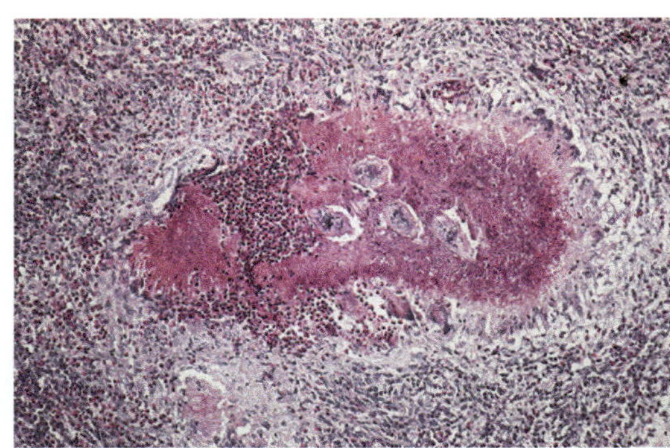

Fig. 5.18.4

Answers to Case 5.18

1. An uncomplicated UTI occurs in a healthy patient with a structurally and functionally normal urinary tract. A complicated UTI is associated with host factors making infection more likely to occur or more difficult to eradicate, e.g. an anatomical abnormality of the urinary tract, male gender, pregnancy, immunosuppression, indwelling catheter, stones, diabetes mellitus, renal insufficiency, surgery. In addition, the pathogen may have increased virulence or antimicrobial resistance.
   a. Uncomplicated UTI – *Escherichia coli* (80%), *Staphylococcus saprophyticus* (5–15%), *Klebsiella* spp. (4%), *Enterococcus faecalis* (6%), *Proteus mirabilis* (5–10%).
   b. Complicated UTI – *Escherichia coli* (55%), *Klebsiella* spp. (17%), *Enterobacter cloacae, Seratia marascens, Proteus mirabilis* (14%), *Pseudomonas aeruginosa* (5%), *Enterococcus faecalis* (4%), *Group B streptococci, candida species.*

2. Figure 5.18.1 is a coronal delayed phase CT scan showing air within the bladder wall compatible with emphysematous cystitis, there is also a catheter balloon in the bladder. These are generally synergistic infections and classically affect patients with chronic disease such as diabetes mellitus. The most common organism is *E. coli*, but other organisms reported to produce emphysematous cystitis include *Enterobacter aerogenes, Klebsiella pneumonia, Proteus mirabilis, Staphylococcus aureus, streptococci, Clostridium perfringens and Candida albicans.*
3. Figure 5.18.2 is a spot image from a cystogram showing a small capacity bladder with severe right-sided reflux. Any small volume, high-pressure bladder can result in similar radiographic appearances, and an infective cause is tuberculosis.
4. Figure 5.18.3 is an axial CT scan in the same patient confirming the presence of bladder wall calcification with no evidence of any other renal tract calcification. Urinalysis confirmed the presence of schistosomiasis. Bladder wall calcification is also seen in TB, bladder cancer, amyloidosis and rarely cyclophosphamide-induced cystitis.
5. At cystoscopy the bladder is usually inflamed with classic 'sandy patches'. A biopsy taken during the active phase is shown in Fig. 5.18.4. This biopsy (H and E stain) contains schistosome ova surrounded by a dense inflammatory infiltrate, including eosinophils and a granulomatous element. When inactive the eggs calcify leading to both the formation of fibrous polyps and ulceration.

Further Reading

Neal DE Jr. Complicated urinary tract infections. *Urol Clin North Am.* 2008;35(1):13–22.

Nicolle L.E. Uncomplicated urinary tract infection in adults including uncomplicated pyelonephritis. *Urol Clin North Am.* 2008;35(1):1–12.

Case 5.19

1. Figure 5.19.1a is from an IVU and Fig. 5.19.1b a CT of a 27-year-old man who presents with haematuria, frequency, nocturia and urgency. He admits to recreational drug taking. He underwent a cystoscopy and biopsy (Fig. 5.19.1c). What does the IVU and the biopsy show and what is the likely diagnosis? How is this managed?
2. What are the other causes of non-infective cystitis?
3. What are the diagnostic criteria for interstitial cystitis? What treatment modalities have been suggested in interstitial cystitis?

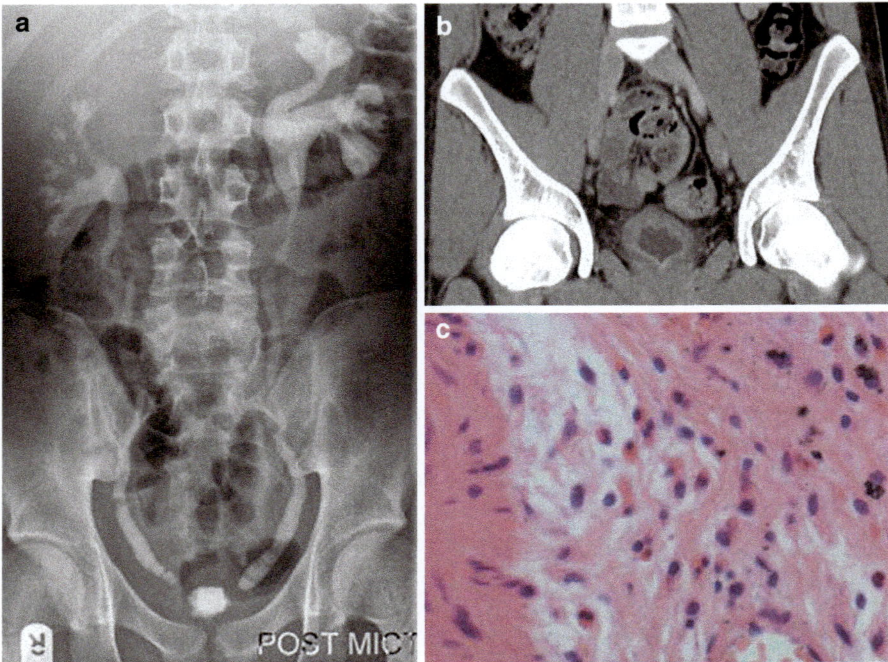

Fig. 5.19.1

Answers to Case 5.19

1. Figure 5.19.1a is a post-micturition IVU film and 5.19.1b is a coronal CT image of a patient with ketamine cystitis showing a small volume bladder. The ureters are dilated down to the thick-walled bladder. The histopathological findings on biopsy are similar to those of interstitial cystitis, including ulceration and pan mural inflammation followed by fibrosis. Scattered eosinophils are found in the inflammatory infiltrate, as seen with their characteristic bi-lobed nuclei in Fig. 5.19.1c. However, eosinophils may be present in the bladder wall in a variety of conditions including post-biopsy, as part of 'catheter reaction', associated with invasive carcinoma, schistosomiasis, in allergic responses involving the respiratory and gastrointestinal tract and other forms of drug induced including cyclophosphamide.

   The management includes full urinary tract evaluation, cessation of ketamine and reassessment for reversible symptoms. In cases where symptoms fail to resolve or consequences such as upper tract obstruction occur, cystectomy and urinary diversion may be necessary.
2. Non-infective causes of cystitis include radiation, systemic lupus erythematosis (SLE), Sjögrens syndrome, chemical cystitis (e.g. cyclophosphamide, ketamine) and interstitial cystitis.
3. The presence of any one of the criteria below excludes interstitial cystitis:
   - Bladder capacity of greater than 350 mL whilst awake
   - Absence of an intense urge to void with the bladder filled to 150 ml using a fill rate of 30–100 ml/min
   - The demonstration of phasic involuntary bladder contractions on cystometry
   - Duration of symptoms less than 9 months
   - Absence of nocturia
   - Symptoms relieved by antimicrobial agents, urinary antiseptic agents, anticholinergic agents, or antispasmodic agents
   - Daytime frequency of urination of less than 8 times/day
   - A diagnosis of bacterial cystitis or prostatitis within the last 3 months
   - Bladder or ureteral calculi
   - Active genital herpes
   - Uterine, cervical, vaginal or urethral cancer
   - Urethral diverticulum
   - Cyclophosphamide or any type of chemical cystitis
   - Tuberculous cystitis
   - Radiation cystitis
   - Benign or malignant bladder tumours
   - Vaginitis
   - Age younger than 18 years

Dietary modification including avoidence of spicy food, caffeine, alcohol, fruit juices helps about half of sufferers. Oral medical therapies including antibiotics (doxycycline), antihitamines, anticholinergics, amitriptyline, sodium pentosan polysulphate, calcium channel blockers have all been proposed as treatments for interstitial cystitis, with varying degrees of success.

Further Reading

Chu P, Ma W, Wong SC et al. The destruction of the lower urinary tract by ketamine abuse: a new syndrome?. *BJU Int*. 2008;102(11):1616–1622.

Hanno P. Keay S. Moldwin R. Van Ophoven A. International Consultation on IC - Rome, September 2004/Forging an International Consensus: progress in painful bladder syndrome/interstitial cystitis. Report and abstracts. *Int Urogynecol J*. 2005;16(Suppl 1):S2–S34.

The Prostate

6

Kevin Lessey and Susan Heenan

Case 6.1

1. Study Fig. 6.1.1a–d and name structures labelled a–g.
2. Name and describe the terminology applied to the zones of the prostate.
3. Why is MRI preferred to CT for imaging of the prostate?

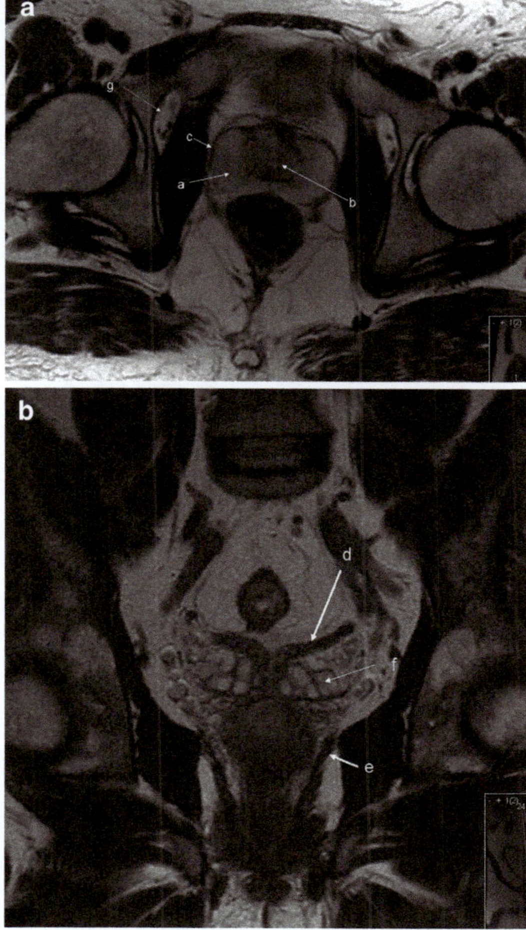

Fig. 6.1.1

S. Bott et al. (eds.), *Images in Urology*,
DOI 10.1007/978-0-85729-769-3_6, © Springer-Verlag London Limited 2012

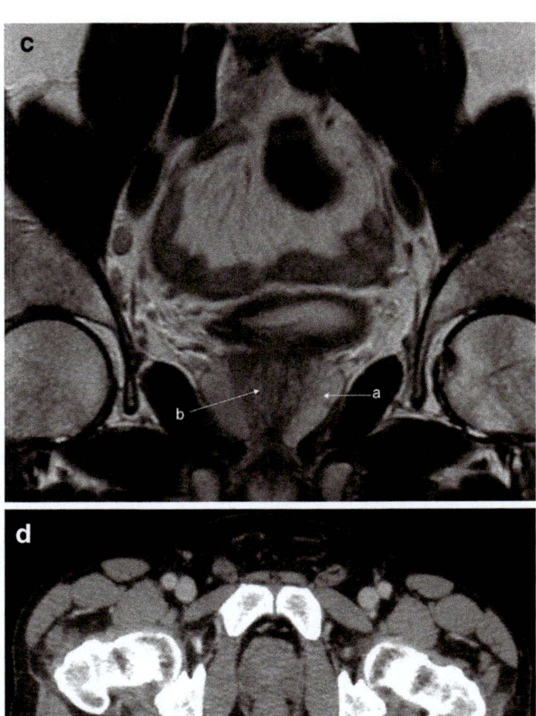

Fig. 6.1.1 (continued)

Answers to Case 6.1

1. Figure 6.1.1a–c are axial and coronal high-resolution T2-weighted images through the prostate and seminal vesicles (SVs). Figure 6.1.1d is an axial CT image.
   (a) Peripheral zone (PZ) also note the fine fibromuscular bands traversing the PZ which should not be confused with malignancy.
   (b) Central gland, it is generally impossible to distinguish the central and transition zones as separate regions on radiological imaging.
   (c) 'Capsule'.
   (d) Vas deferens.
   (e) Levator ani.
   (f) Seminal vesicle.
   (g) Obturator canal.
2. The zones of the prostate were described as peripheral, central and transition zones (PZ, CZ and TZ) by John McNeal in 1968, distinguished by microanatomical boundaries, duct drainage and acinar morphology. The PZ forms the bulk of the normal

gland, enveloping the posterior, lateral and apical aspects and forming the entire apical region. The CZ is wedge shaped; surrounding the ejaculatory ducts with its base at the bladder neck and its apex at the veru. The TZ extends from the base to the veru encircling the proximal urethra. Anteriorly a variable amount of fibromuscular stroma unites the anterior lateral horns of the PZ. McNeal demonstrated that the majority of carcinomas (75–85%) arise in the PZ and 15–25% in the TZ; with multifocal disease seen in more than 85% of cases. The TZ is the usual site of benign prostatic hyperplasia (BPH) and infarction. Prostatitis and atrophy are thought to be most common in the PZ as a consequence of the longer length of the drainage ducts. The prostatic 'capsule' is composed of fibrous connective tissue and smooth muscle with a variable striated muscle component in the apical region. Both the internal and external limits of the capsule are ill-defined as it blends with prostatic stroma and pelvic connective tissue, respectively. The 'capsule' is often indistinct or absent at the apex and base, so the prostate does not have a complete distinct capsule like the kidney, for example.

3. Magnetic resonance imaging (MRI) is the most appropriate modality for imaging the prostate, given its better soft tissue resolution. On T2-weighted sequences, the PZ demonstrates a homogeneous high signal against the lower signal inner gland; the CZ and TZ cannot be differentiated on MRI and are usually of mixed signal because of BPH. The addition of functional imaging techniques, such as diffusion weighted sequences and spectroscopy, may increase diagnostic accuracy. CT cannot delineate prostatic zonal anatomy (Fig. 6.1.1d) but may be required for local staging if contraindications to MRI, such as a pacemaker, exist. CT may be used to assess lymph nodes and disease burden elsewhere within the abdomen and pelvis, but cannot accurately define the local tumour T stage.

Further Reading

McNeal JE. Regional morphology and pathology of the prostate. *Am J Surg Pathol.* 1968;49:347–357.

McNeal JE, Redwine EA, Freiha FS, Stamey TA. Zonal distribution of adenocarcinoma. Correlation with histologic pattern and direction of spread. *Am J Surg Pathol.* 1988;12(12):897–906.

Case 6.2

1. Study the ultrasound images in Fig. 6.2.1. What type of probe would be used and with which frequency range. Describe the orientation of the images and what is being measured – describe the formula being used. What is the most accurate method for volume measurement of the prostate gland?
2. What are the indications for performing a transrectal ultrasound (TRUS) guided prostate biopsy?
3. Explain the features (arrowed) on the MRI images (Fig. 6.2.2a, b) seen soon after prostate biopsy.
4. When should MRI staging be performed?
5. Explain the features seen along the right side of the prostate gland in Fig. 6.2.3.

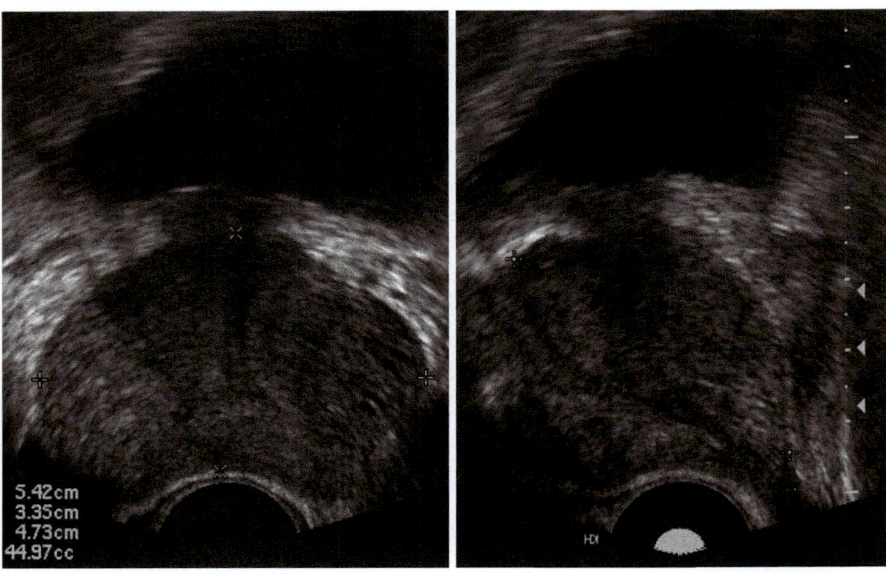

Fig. 6.2.1

Fig. 6.2.2

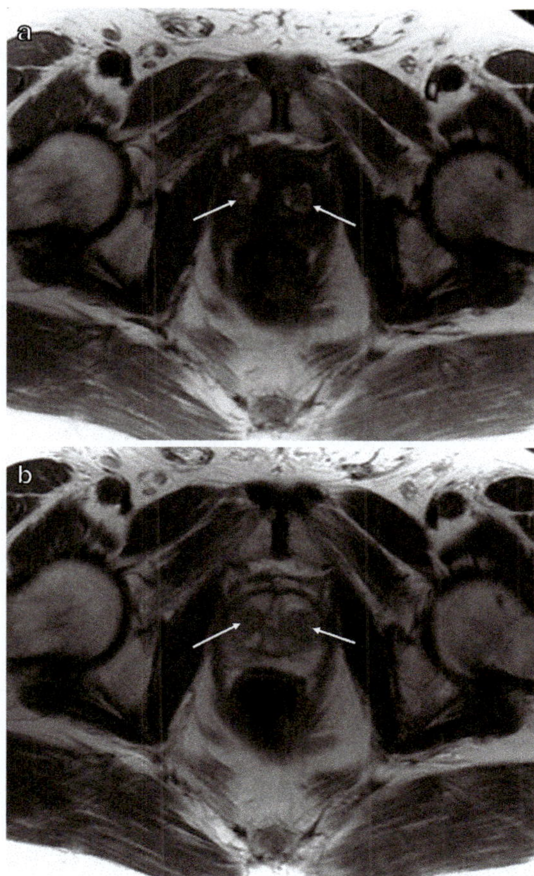

Fig. 6.2.3

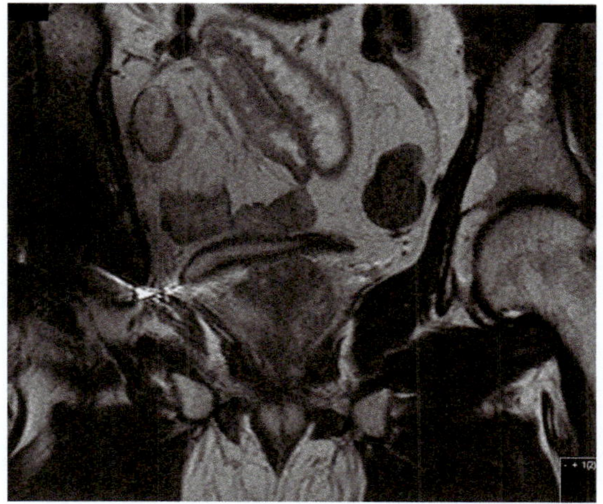

Answers to Case 6.2

1. Figure 6.2.1 shows a normal axial (left image) and sagittal (right image) ultrasound image taken with a transrectal probe using a frequency range of 6-9MHz. The volume is being measured and the formula used is: height (apex to base) × width × antero-posterior length × 0.52, this assumes the prostate is a prolate ellipsoid. In larger glands the prostate is more spherical in shape and so the formula becomes inaccurate. When more accurate volume measurement is required, for example in brachytherapy planning, step planimetry is used.
2. A TRUS biopsy should be offered to men with suspected prostate cancer. Suspicion may be raised by an elevated serum prostate specific antigen (PSA) and/or an abnormal digital rectal examination (DRE). Other indications are in men with a strong family history or suspected metastatic disease, even if the PSA level is normal (as a small minority of prostate cancers do not secrete PSA).
3. In Fig. 6.2.2a, b, two foci of high signal are demonstrated within the central gland on T1-weighted images indicative of post-biopsy haemorrhage. Normally the prostate gland is of homogenous low signal on T1-weighted studies. High T1 signal is seen with fat (other causes include blood products, melanin, protein, colloid or gadolinium based contrast agents). In comparison, high T2 signal is seen with fluid such as water or urine, i.e. those fluids with high hydrogen ion content. In this case high T1 signal is due to blood products, commonly seen for up to 3-6 months after prostate biopsies. However, on T2 weighted images blood products are seen as low signal foci (arrows) mimicking multifocal malignant disease. This can limit diagnostic evaluation of MRI after a biopsy. Most of such artefacts will have resolved by 6 weeks, but can take up to 6 months.
4. MRI staging should be performed in men with intermediate or high-risk disease (e.g. tumours with a Gleason score ≥7, clinical stage≥T2b, extensive tumour involvement in biopsy cores or PSA>10 ng/l) for whom radical treatment is intended.
5. Figure 6.2.3 shows a right hip replacement is causing susceptibility artefact distorting the right side of the prostate, which can lead to problems with interpretation of both intraprostatic cancer extent and evaluation of potential extraprostic extension.

Further Reading

National Institute for Health and Clinical Excellence. *Prostate Cancer; Diagnosis and Treatment.* London: National Institute for Health and Clinical Excellence. Available at: http://guidance.nice.org.uk/CG58. Accessed October 2010.

Case 6.3

1. Name the components arrowed in Fig. 6.3.1a, b.
2. Describe the normal microscopic features of the prostate.
3. How may immunohistochemistry be diagnostically useful in prostatic pathology?

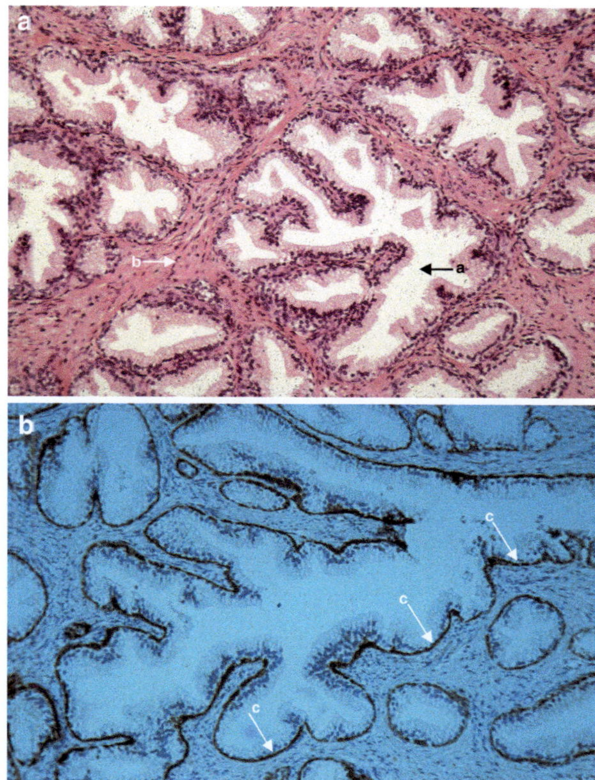

Fig. 6.3.1

Fig. 6.3.2

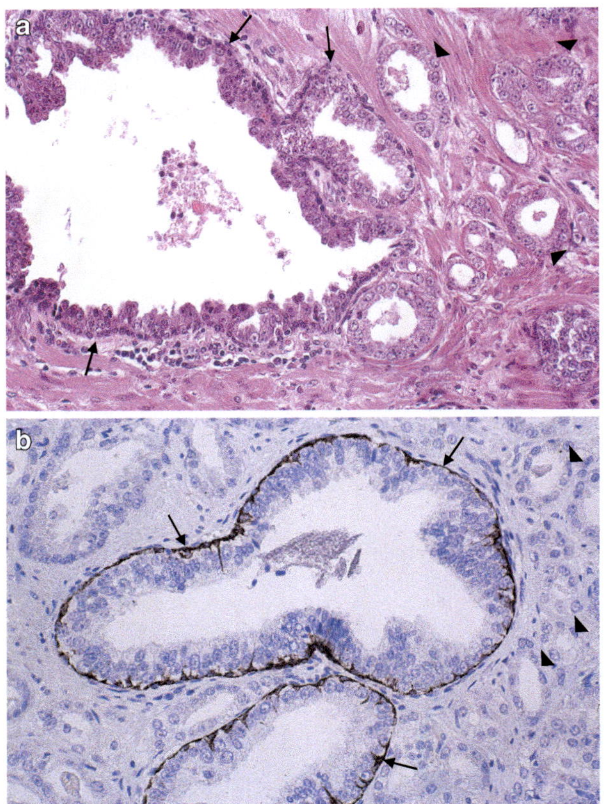

Answers to Case 6.3

1. Components labelled in Fig. 6.3.1a, b
   a. Prostatic acinus
   b. Prostatic stroma
   c. Basal cells of acini defined by immunohistochemistry (IH).
2. The prostate is composed of a fibromuscular stroma which surrounds epithelial elements. The latter have a tubulo-acinar architecture continuous with a series of ducts which lead into the large primary ducts lined by urothelium for a variable distance before opening into the urethra. The epithelial lining of the acini and small ducts is similar, being composed of inner/luminal, tall, secretory cells (in which prostatic acid phosphatase and PSA can be demonstrated), outer basal regenerative cells which are much smaller with dark nuclei and scant cytoplasm (sometimes difficult to see on H and E sections) and rare scattered neuro-endocrine cells.

   Basal cells may be distinguished from secretory cells immunohistochemically by the detection of a variety of antigens absent from the luminal cells and stroma. The antibodies most commonly used are those against cytokeratins, singly or in groups, which produce cytoplasmic staining (e.g. CK 5 and 6, LP34, 34BE12) and an antibody against p63 which provides nuclear staining.
3. Basal cells in either a complete or intermittent distribution around acini showing marked atypia support a diagnosis of high-grade prostatic intra-epithelial neoplasia (HGPIN) in contrast to invasive carcinoma. This distinction is seen in Fig. 6.3.2a, b in which H and E and IH preparations from the same tissue show HGPIN on the left (arrows) and invasive carcinoma on the right (arrowheads).

   Similarly a diagnosis of atypical adenosis, in contrast to well-differentiated carcinoma, would be confirmed by the presence of basal cells (see Case 6.7). The demonstration of cytoplasmic alpha-methylacyl coenzyme A racemase is used as an adjunct to the diagnosis of carcinoma in association with appropriate morphological and other IH findings.

   The presence of IH staining of PSA in a poorly differentiated pelvic tumour or a metastasis will indicate a prostatic origin. A variety of other antibodies may also be useful in the identification of rare tumours, e.g. neuro-endocrine neoplasia, lymphomas, sarcomas and metastases to the prostate.

Further Reading

Paner GP, Luthringer DJ, Amin MB. Best practice in diagnostic immunohistochemistry: prostate carcinoma and its mimics in needle core biopsies. *Arch Pathol Lab Med*. 2008;132(9):1388–1396.

Case 6.4

1. Describe the abnormality demonstrated on these MRI (Fig. 6.4.1a,b) and TRUS (Fig. 6.4.2) images.
2. How may it present and describe any potential complications?
3. What is the differential diagnosis?

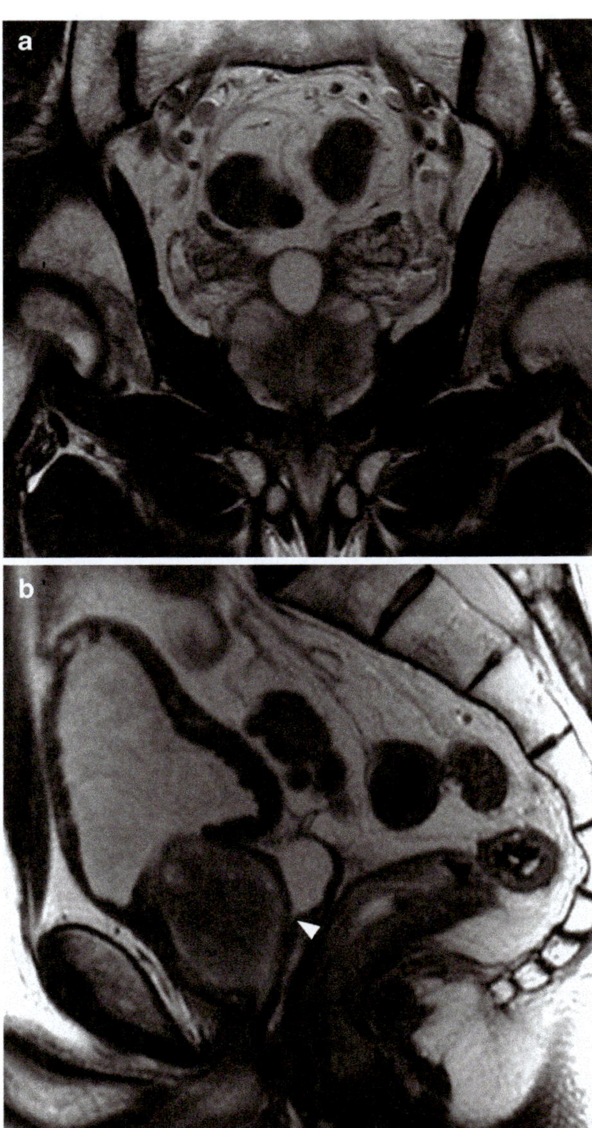

Fig. 6.4.1

Fig. 6.4.2

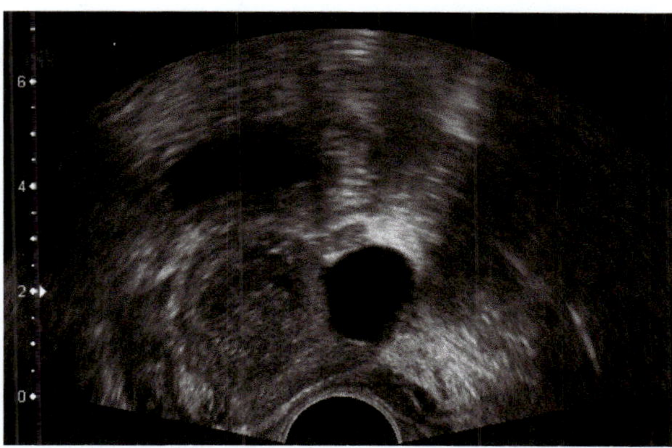

Answers to Case 6.4

1. These T2-weighted MR (Fig. 6.4.1a, b) and TRUS (Fig. 6.4.2) images show a well-defined thin-walled simple cyst arising within the midline of the prostate with a communication with the urethra (Fig. 6.4.1b arrowhead) consistent with a prostatic utricle cyst. Note the especially high T2 signal consistent with fluid content. The prostatic utricle is a Müllerian vestige (paramesonephric duct) and these cysts often communicate with the urethra.
2. Prostatic utricle cysts may present with obstructive urinary symptoms, pelvic pain and haematuria as well as reduced ejaculatory volume as a result of duct obstruction. They may cause post-void dribbling due to their urethral communication. Utricle cysts may contain pus or haemorrhage leading to difficulties in interpretation as appearances may overlap with those of an abscess or cystic tumour.
3. The differential diagnosis of a utricle cyst includes other cysts within the region: cysts within prostatic hyperplasia, cystic dilatation of the ejaculatory duct or cysts within a phyllodes tumour. These are all said to originate laterally (in contrast to utricle cysts), but resulting gland distortion can make this distinction difficult. Very rarely pelvic cysts outside the prostate, arising from peritoneum or lymphatics, may cause diagnostic problems.

Further Reading

Coppens L, Bonnet P, Andrianne R, Leval J. Adult müllerian duct or utricle cyst: clinical significance and therapeutic management in 65 cases. *J Urol.* 2002;176:1740–1747.

Curran S, Akin O, Agildare AM, et al. Endorectal MRI of prostatic and periprostatic cystic lesions and their mimics. *AJR.* 2007;188:1373–1379.

Case 6.5

1. Describe the findings featured in Fig. 6.5.1a–c. How common is this condition?
2. What is the surgical resection specimen seen in Fig. 6.5.2?
3. What do the H and E stained sections of prostate in Fig. 6.5.3a–c show?

Fig. 6.5.1

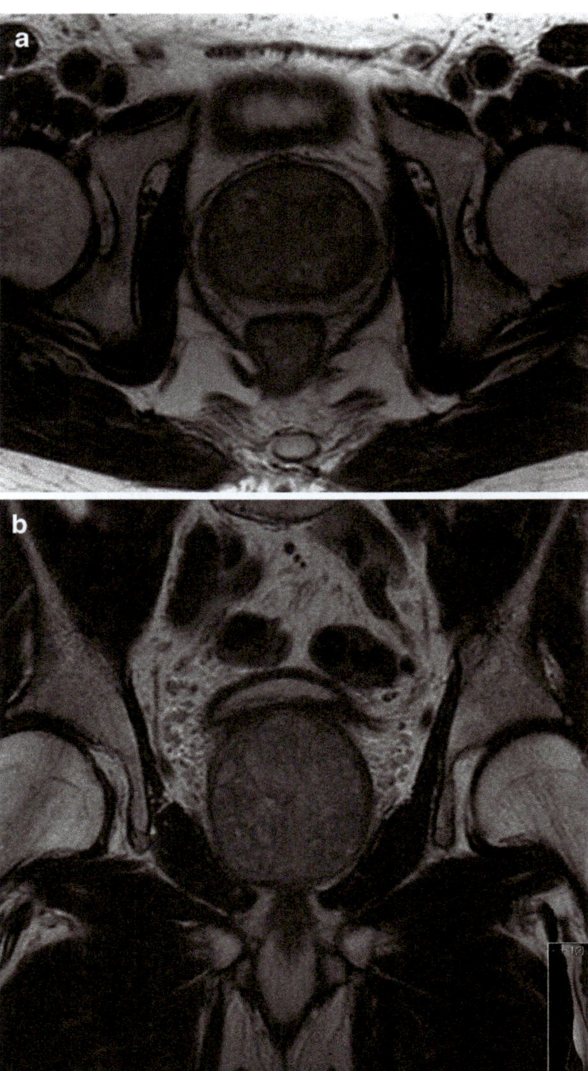

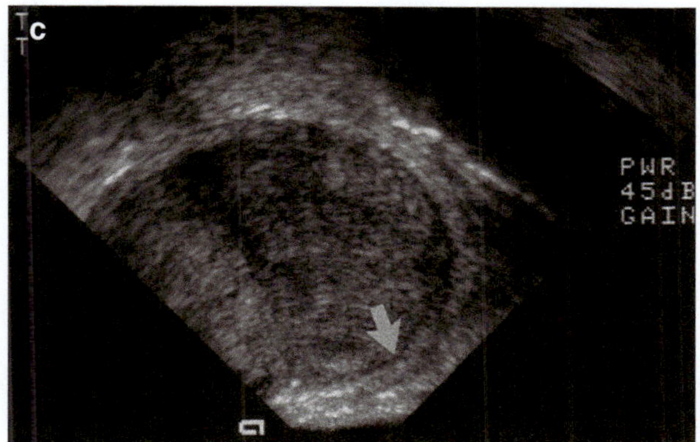

Fig. 6.5.1 (continued)

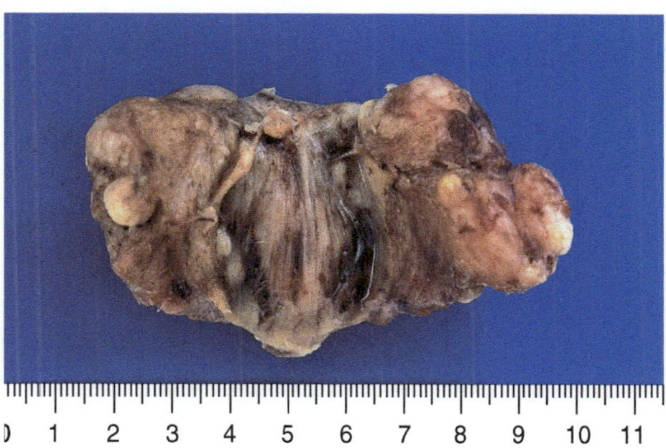

Fig. 6.5.2

Fig. 6.5.3

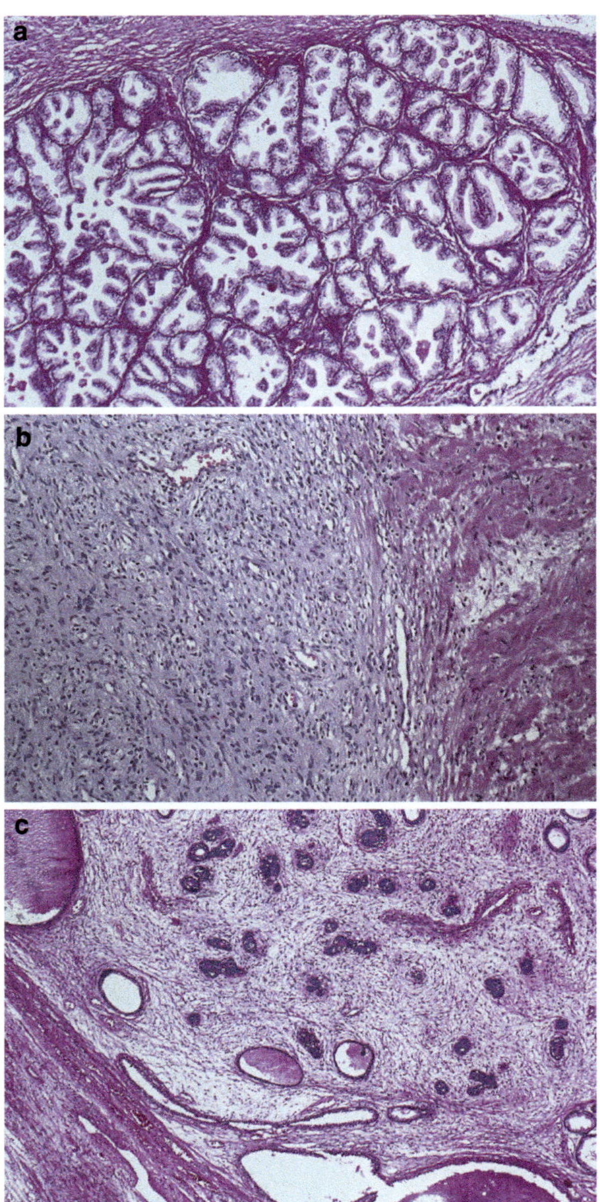

Answers to Case 6.5

1. The axial and coronal T2-weighted MR image (Fig. 6.5.1a, b) shows benign enlargement of the central gland (TZ) which is of heterogeneous signal, compressing the PZ. A very large central gland can cause significant thinning of the PZ and even reduce the normally high T2 signal intensity of the PZ, but usually not to the same extent as malignancy. Similar changes are seen on TRUS (Fig. 6.5.1c), with a thinned PZ (arrow) and heterogeneous inner gland. The PZ may retain its normally hyperechoic quality or may be of intermediate echogenicity.

   In a sample of men in Olmstead County (USA), aged 40–79 years, moderate to severe symptoms relating to BPH were present in 13% of men aged 40–49 years and among 28% of those older than 70 years. The frequency of histological BPH in all age groups is higher than in clinical studies. Pathology studies report BPH is not present before 30 years but rises to 88% by the age of 90.
2. The resection specimen (Fig. 6.5.2) is from an open retropubic enucleation of the prostate. Although this form of surgery is now rarely preformed, the illustration demonstrates the potential size of hyperplastic enlargement, its nodularity and the manner in which it can be shelled out from the compressed PZ. Hyperplasia is also seen in Fig. 6.6.1 (next case) where the cystic hyperplastic nodules compress the urethra to a slit. Hyperplasia commonly involves the TZ, nodules are rarely seen in the PZ. As ductal and glandular architecture become distorted by nodule formation, cystic dilatation occurs associated with atrophy of the epithelium, inspissation of secretions, inflammation and the development of corpora amylacea and calcification. Infarction may also be a feature.
3. Figure 6.5.3a–c shows the three morphological forms of prostatic hyperplasia: epithelial, stromal and mixed, respectively. Stromal nodules commonly occur just deep to the urethral urothelium and are thought by some authorities to represent the first form of nodule into which epithelium extends.

Further Reading

Chute CG, Panser LA, Girman CJ, Oesterling JE, Guess HA, Jacobsen SJ, Lieber MM. The prevalence of prostatism: a population based survey of urinary symptoms. *J Urol.* 1993;150(1):85–89.

Petersen RO, Sesterhenn IA, Davis CJ. *Prostate in Urologic Pathology*. 3rd ed. Philadelphia: Lippincott Williams and Wilkins; 2009.

Case 6.6

1. Figure 6.6.1 is a transverse section of a prostate gland removed at autopsy. What abnormalities does it show?
2. What is the clinical significance of this condition?
3. Figure 6.6.2 is an H and E stained section from the lesion seen in Fig. 6.6.1. What does it show?

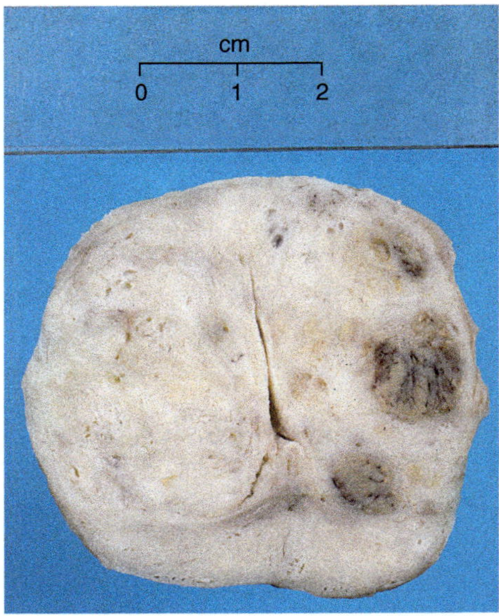

Fig. 6.6.1

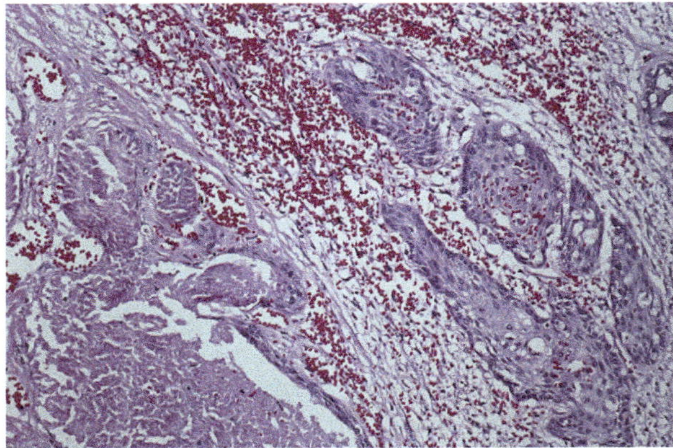
Fig. 6.6.2

Answers to Case 6.6

1. Figure 6.6.1 shows nodular hyperplasia of the prostate gland, with compression of the urethra to a slit. In the right side of the gland, within the hyperplastic area there are three haemorrhagic foci suggesting recent infarction. Infarcts are found in up to 25% of hyperplastic glands.
2. Prostatic infarcts are usually asymptomatic but rarely may trigger acute urinary retention, secondary to oedema with a sudden rise in serum PSA. The aetiology of all infarcts is not known but infarction has followed cardiac surgery (thought to be associated with hypotension), infection and trauma.
3. This section (Fig. 6.6.2) shows an area of necrosis (left side of image) in which cell boundaries and nuclei have been lost. Adjacent ducts/acini show squamous metaplasia. Scattered erythrocytes are present in the viable tissue. In addition to infarction, necrosis and adjacent squamous metaplasia may be seen in the prostate at the site of a biopsy track, bordering a TUR cavity or following cryotherapy. Squamous metaplasia is also common after oestrogen treatment and radiotherapy.

Further Reading

Male reproductive system. In: Rosai J, ed. *Rosai and Ackerman's Surgical Pathology*. 9th ed. London: Mosby; 2004.

Milord RA, Kahane H, Epstein JI. Infarct of the prostate gland: experience on needle biopsy specimens. *Am J Surg Pathol.* 2000;24:1378–1384.

Case 6.7

1. Compare Fig. 6.7.1, an H and E section of the prostate, with that of the normal gland (e.g. Fig. 6.3.1a). Describe the abnormalities in the former and give the diagnosis.
2. What is the pathological and clinical significance of this condition?
3. Describe the lesion seen in H and E and IH preparations of prostate in Fig. 6.7.2a, b and give the diagnosis.

Fig. 6.7.1

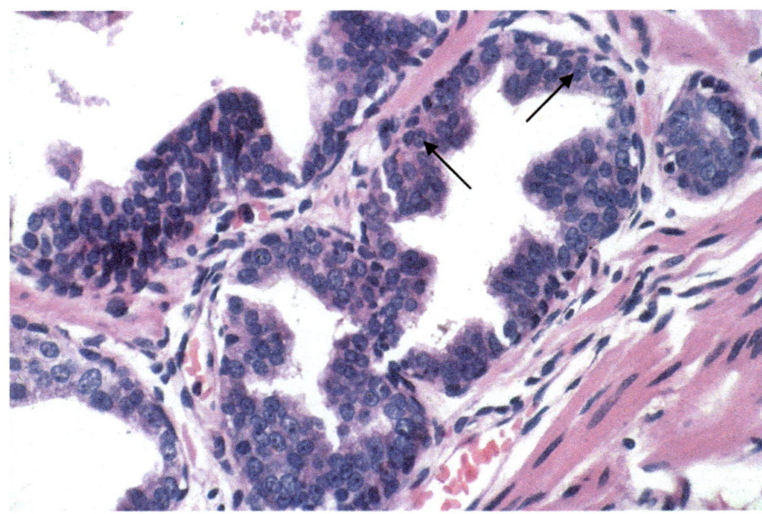

Fig. 6.7.2

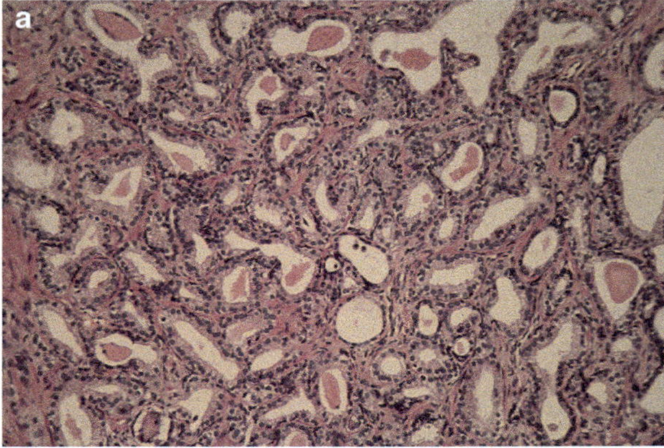

Fig. 6.7.2 (continued)

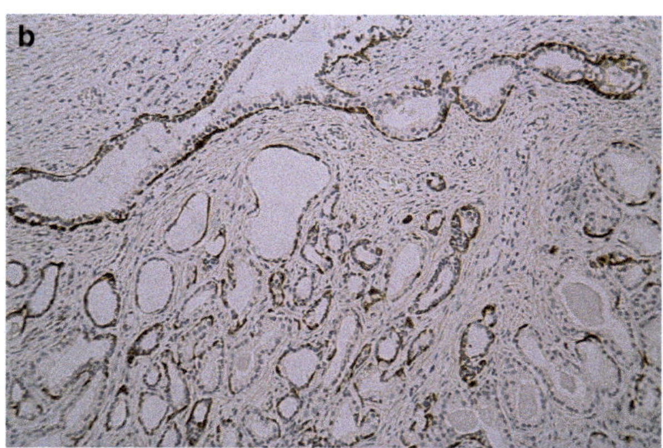

Answers to Case 6.7

1. The following features in Fig. 6.7.1 are in marked contrast to those of the normal glandular epithelium seen in Fig. 6.3.1a. The secretory cells are crowded and stratified with nuclei at varying levels, thus the clear column of cytoplasm with basal nuclei seen in the normal secretory layer has been lost and the lesion appears basophilic at low power. The nuclei of the secretory cells are larger, darker (hyperchromatic) and more variable in shape and size; nucleoli (arrowed) are prominent and often multiple. Intermittent basal cells are represented by small dark nuclei. The diagnosis is high grade PIN (HGPIN).
2. McNeal described PIN (under the term intraductal dysplasia) in 1965. Its premalignant nature was supported by its morphological similarity to and microanatomical association with invasive carcinoma in the PZ, being less common in the CZ and TZ and its peak incidence in post-mortem studies preceding that of invasive carcinoma. More recent studies have shown that adenocarcinoma and HGPIN share certain biomarkers. Following a consensus statement in 1989 two types of PIN were described – high grade and low grade. More recently, the reporting of low-grade PIN has largely been abandoned due to poor interobserver reproducibility and a relatively low risk of cancer following re-biopsy. Over recent years, with the advent of more extensive biopsy regimes, the association of HGPIN with concomitant invasive cancer has been called into question. The incidence of invasive cancer found if the prostate is re-biopsied is the same if the first biopsy was benign or showed a single core of HGPIN (~10%). If multifocal (≥2 biopsy cores) HGPIN is present, the cancer detection rate on subsequent biopsy is 30%.
3. In Fig. 6.7.2a small acini are crowded together suggesting a diagnosis of well-differentiated carcinoma. However, the atypical cytological features of malignancy are not apparent and as an intermittent basal cell layer is defined on IH in Fig. 6.7.2b, the diagnosis is atypical adenomatous hyperplasia (AAH). The major significance of AAH, in the absence of IH, is the possibility of a misdiagnosis of well-differentiated adenocarcinoma. It is seen more commonly in the TZ than the PZ, thereby presenting a diagnostic problem in TUR specimens.

Its pre-malignant status has been investigated but remains controversial. Currently no clinical response to this lesion is required.

In contrast, the term atypical small acinar proliferation (ASAP) arose as a 'working diagnosis' to describe the quandary when a small number of acini are 'suspicious of cancer but not diagnostic'. Such foci are often so small that they disappear on the deeper levels precluding the additional help given by IH. It is acknowledged that on biopsy a restricted sample of a variety of entities can prompt a diagnosis of ASAP. Nevertheless, the average risk of cancer following a diagnosis of ASAP is 40%. Currently, early re-biopsy is recommended when ASAP is identified.

Further Reading

Epstein JI. Precursor lesions to prostatic adenocarcinoma. *Virchows Arch.* 2009;454:1–16.

McNeal JE, Bostwick DG. Intraductal dysplasia: a premalignant lesion of the prostate. *Human Pathol.* 1986;17:64–71.

Merrimen JL, Jones G, Srigley JR. Is high grade prostatic intraepithelial neoplasia still a risk factor for adenocarcinoma in the era of extended biopsy sampling? *Pathology*. June 2010;42(4):325–329.

Case 6.8

A 62-year-old man presented with a PSA of 6.7 ng/ml and clinically he was staged T2a. Part of one prostate biopsy core is shown below. He underwent an MRI study, and after considering his options he elected to have a radical prostatectomy.

1. What is seen on the H and E of the biopsy core at low and high power field (Fig. 6.8.1a, b).
2. Describe the features in MR image (Fig. 6.8.2)? The rest of the study was normal. What is the radiological staging?
3. Figure 6.8.3a shows three transverse macroscopic sections of a radical prostatectomy (RP) specimen and the equivalent H and E from the upper slice in the illustration (and Fig. 6.8.3b). What do these specimens show?

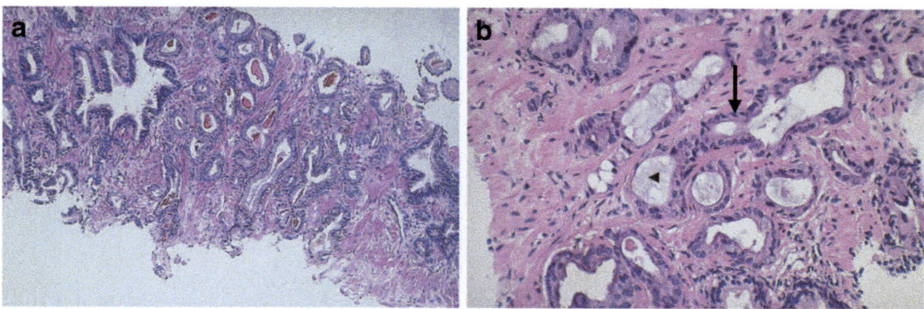

Fig. 6.8.1

Fig. 6.8.2

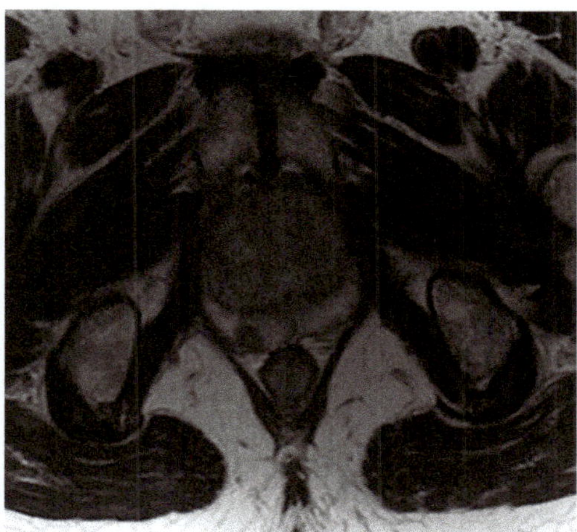

Fig. 6.8.3

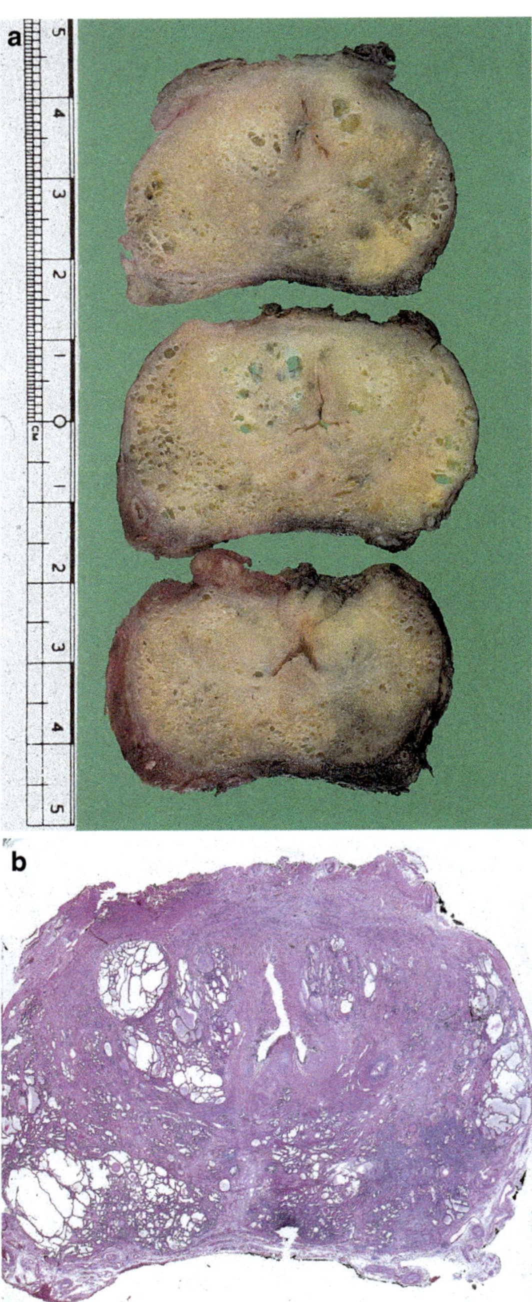

Answers to Case 6.8

1. Figure 6.8.1a is an H and E of the core biopsy in which malignant acini of varying size invade between the benign acini seen at both limits of the field. This is Gleason score 3+3=6. On the high-power image (Fig. 6.8.1b), nucleoli (arrow) and intraacinar mucin (arrowhead) can be seen in the carcinoma.
2. Figure 6.8.1 is a T2-weighted axial MRI image showing a single focal area of low signal within the right posterior PZ (left side of the image). It abuts the edge of the gland ('capsule') but the contour remains smooth; thus using MRI criteria there is no extracapsular spread. In the rest of the study (images not shown), the seminal vesicles were morphologically normal, there was no nodal enlargement and no focal marrow abnormality. As the tumour occupies less than one half of the right lobe with no nodal involvement, this represents T2a N0 disease.
3. In Fig. 6.8.2a, the upper and middle slices of the gland show a solid yellow/cream coloured area in the right side of the image posteriorly, typical of cancer in both appearance and site (and corresponds to the MRI findings). Hyperplastic nodules are also present in the TZ. The H and E of the upper slice (Fig. 6.8.2b) shows a basophilic area equivalent to the macroscopic yellow focus and confirmed on higher power to be invasive cancer (Please note that radiological convention assumes that the reader is viewing images of a patient lying supine on a bed in front of them and therefore these appear inverted when compared to the pathological images).

Case 6.9

1. Describe the abnormalities on the TRUS (Fig. 6.9.1a) and MR images (Fig. 6.9.1b, c).
2. Figure 6.9.2 is an H and E section of prostate invaded by cancer, what is the Gleason sum score?
3. Describe the Gleason grading system, how it is scored and its recent modification.

Fig. 6.9.1

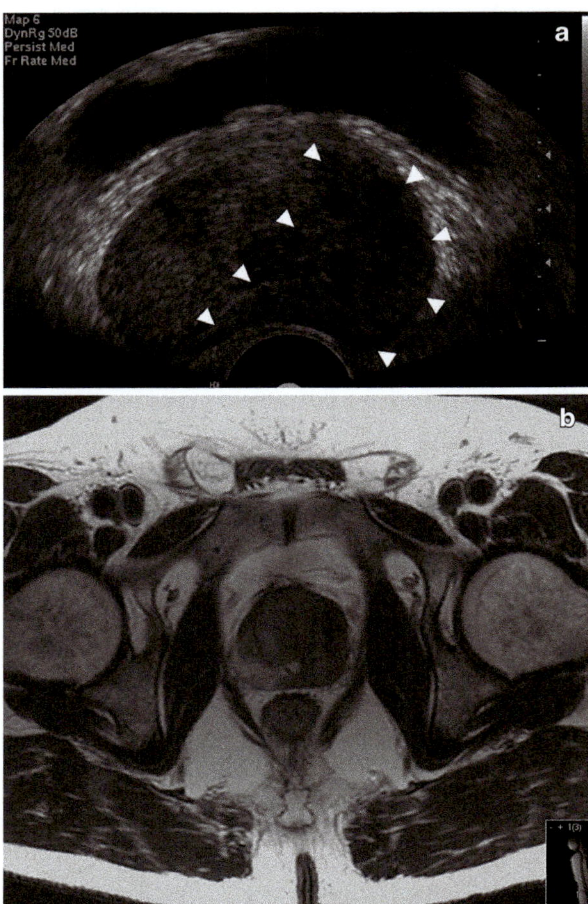

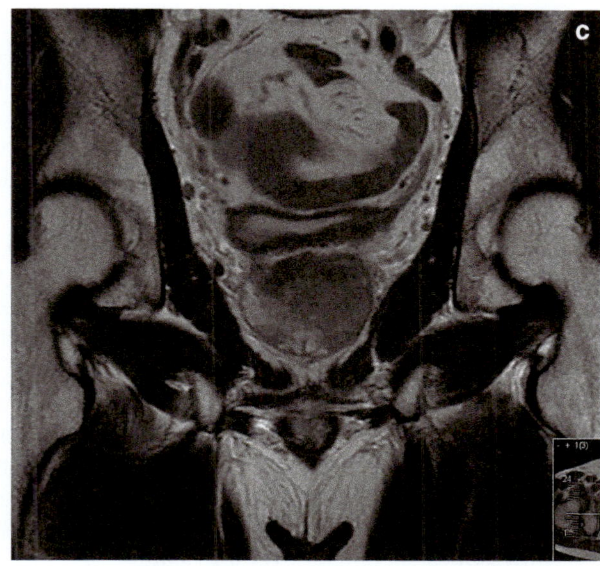

Fig. 6.9.1 (continued)

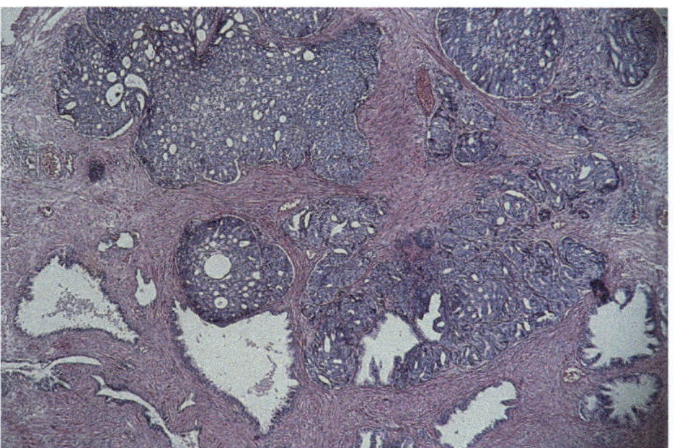

Fig. 6.9.2

Answers to Case 6.9

1. Figure 6.9.1a is an axial TRUS image illustrating a region of decreased echogenicity (arrowheads) within the left peripheral zone extending into the central gland. The axial T2-weighted MRI (Fig. 6.9.1b) confirms a large area of low signal in the left PZ, that crosses the midline as well as a further area of low signal in the right apex, as seen on the T2-weighted coronal image (Fig. 6.9.1c). The capsule of the gland has a smooth intact contour. This therefore represents T2c prostate cancer as it involves both lobes, but does not extend through the capsule.
2. Figure 6.9.2 shows large irregular cribriform tumour conforming to Gleason 4+4=8. Benign distended ducts/acini are present at the lower edge.
3. In 1966 Donald Gleason described a grading system with prognostic significance derived from the histopathological assessment of specimens (biopsies, TURs and RPs), later validated in a larger number of patients. The Gleason system is based on the glandular micro-architecture (patterns) at low power (in contrast to cancer diagnosis and other grading systems which incorporate high-power cytological features). The five grades range from 1 and 2 which include uniform, compact glands forming nodules with a smooth edge, through 3 in which glands of more variable size and shape infiltrate between benign acini to 4 characterised by fusion of glands often into large irregular tumour masses and 5 in which sheets, cords and single tumour cells are seen.

   Multiple Gleason patterns within a tumour are common. Adenocarcinoma is assigned a Gleason sum score according to the two predominant patterns by area. The most extensive pattern being the primary grade followed by the secondary grade, e.g. 3+4=sum score 7. If only one pattern is present, the number is doubled, e.g. 4+4=8. This system gives a potential sum scores 2–10.

   In 2005, an international consensus meeting agreed modifications to the Gleason classification which were extended in 2010. The major changes with respect to needle biopsies were: sum score 2–4 should be rarely used with respect to needle biopsies; certain morphological changes to the definition of grade 3 resulting in upgrading of a proportion of pattern 3 to pattern 4; definition of the grading of the adenocarcinoma variants; in biopsies a third (tertiary) grade should be given if a smaller area than the two most predominant patterns is seen which is of higher grade (e.g. Gleason score 3+4+5); the sum score of a biopsy series was to be summarised as the highest score and not as an average. Similar changes were specified for Gleason scoring of RP specimens.

   These changes have implications for the comparison of database information and the use of nomograms.

Further Reading

Epstein JI. An update of the Gleason grading system. *J Urol.* 2010;183:433–440.

Gleason DF, Mellinger GT. The Veterans Administration Cooperative Urological Research Group. Prediction of prognosis for prostatic adenocarcinoma by combined histological grading and clinical staging. *J Urol.* 1974;111:58–64.

Case 6.10

1. Describe the radiological features seen in Fig. 6.10.1a, b.
2. What are the most common sites for extraprostatic extension and how does this occur?
3. Examine Fig. 6.10.2a, b. What is a positive surgical margin, where do they commonly occur and what is their significance?
4. Figure 6.10.3a, b are images from another patient. What types of studies are these and describe the abnormalities seen?

Fig. 6.10.1

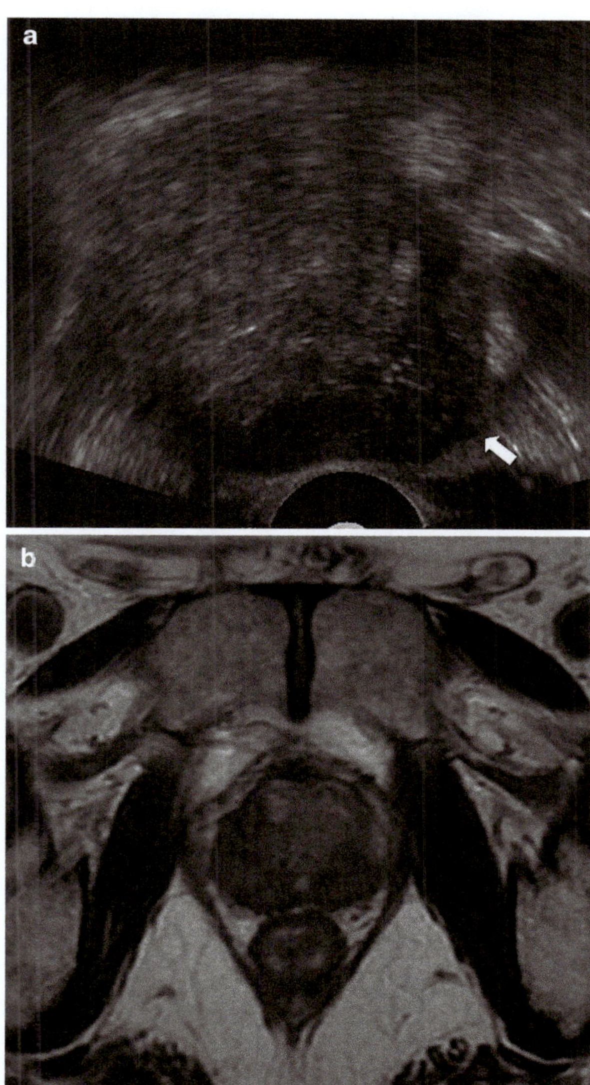

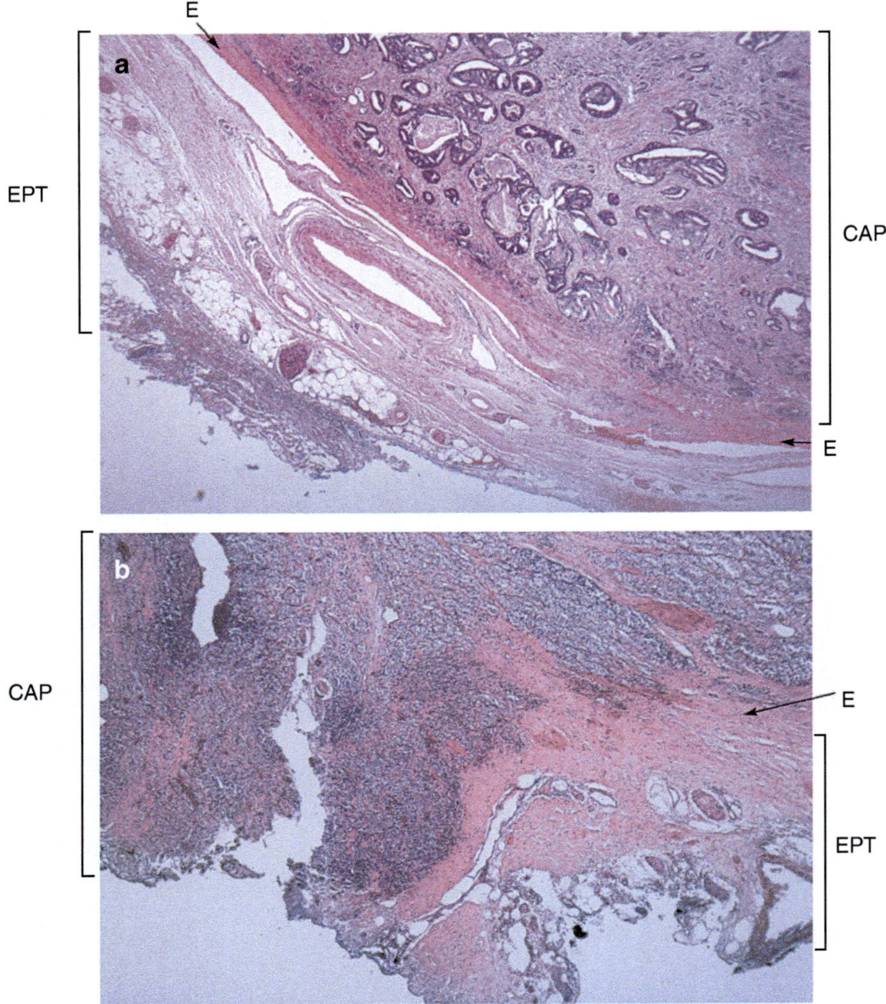

Fig. 6.10.2

Fig. 6.10.3

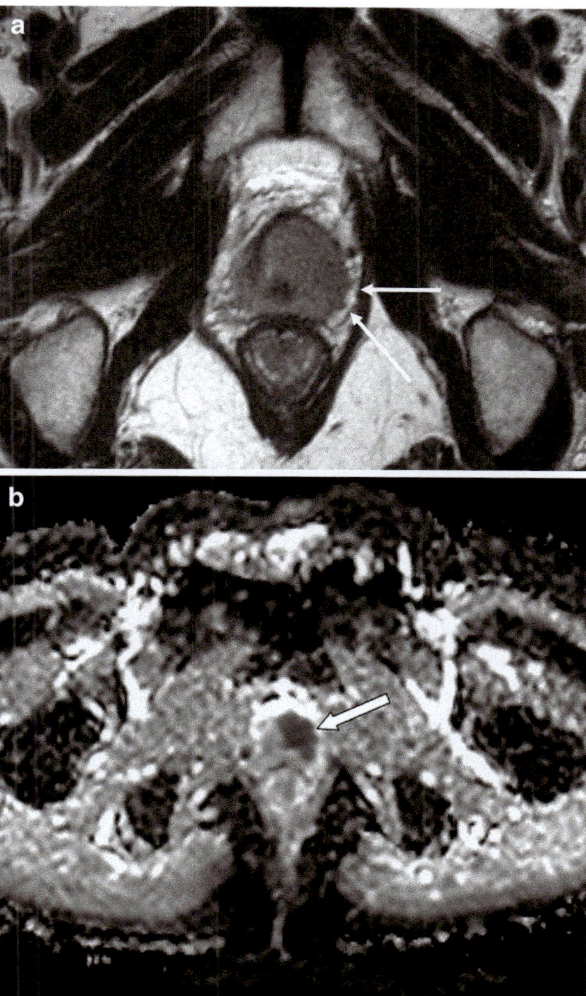

Answers to Case 6.10

1. In Fig. 6.10.1a (axial TRUS image) there is reduced echogenicity seen in the PZ bilaterally with some irregularity to the capsule on the left (arrow). The corresponding axial T2-weighted MRI image in Fig. 6.10.1b confirms low signal throughout the PZ, abutting and extending outside the prostate causing irregularity of the gland contour laterally and posteriorly. The appearances are of locally advanced prostate cancer, at least T3a on the evidence from these images.
2. Extraprostatic spread occurs when tumours invade along nerves posterolaterally or directly into extraprostatic soft tissue. On MRI, the rectoprostatic angles should be examined carefully and the presence of low-signal tissue within this normally fat-filled area is highly suggestive of extraprostatic spread. Other features of T3a disease include thickening, retraction or distortion of the capsule. Alternatively tumour may invade superiorly into the bladder neck and seminal vesicles, or inferiorly at the apex where the capsule is deficient. This is best appreciated on the coronal and sagittal images, as an absence of a fat plane between the tumour and the relevant structure. However, other pathologies such as infarction, inflammation and biopsy-related haemorrhage may also cause low T2 signal within the peripheral zone. The National Comprehensive Network guidelines, published in 2003, have suggested that men with T3a or T3b disease can be considered for either radical prostatectomy or curative radiotherapy as long as their life expectancy is over 5 years.
3. To facilitate surgical margin assessment whilst fixing (see Chap. 1) the external surface of a radical prostatectomy specimen is painted with ink, frequently using two different colours to indicate laterality. Following division into tissue blocks and embedding in paraffin, sections are taken for microscopic examination.

   In Fig. 6.10.2a carcinoma of the prostate (CAP) is separated from the extraprostatic tissue (EPT) by a fibromuscular layer (E) ('the capsule'), the tumour is organ confined. Ink is not in contact with the tumour so the margins at this site are negative. In Fig. 6.10.2b tumour (CAP) is seen invading through the fibromuscular layer (E) and is in contact with the ink the tumour is described as having a positive surgical margin.

   Two types of positive margins occur – where tumour has extended beyond the confines of the prostate and has been cut across by the surgeon (pT3a R1), as shown in Fig. 6.10.2b, or inadvertent intraprostatic incision into a tumour which is otherwise confined within the gland (pT2+ or pT2X). The margin is negative if tumour cells are very close to the inked surface of the margin but not touching or when the tumour cells are at the surface of the tissue but lacking any ink. The most common sites for intraprostatic positive margins (pT2X) include the apex when the open retropubic approach is used, the bladder neck for the perineal approach and postero-lateral for the laparoscopic and robotic technique.

   Patients with positive surgical margins have a significantly increased risk of biochemical progression compared with those with negative margins (biochemical progression-free survival 58–64% R1 vs. 81–83% R0, at 5 years). Multifocal and extensive positive margins confer an increased risk of progression. Several studies suggest the site of positive margins also impact on risk of progression – apical positive margins have a lower rate of failure than bladder neck positive margins.

4. Figure 6.10.3a, b are T2 and diffusion weighted MR images (DWI) respectively from the same patient. The latter is a functional MR sequence that demonstrates areas of restricted diffusion within malignant tissue as a result of its increased cellularity; areas of cancerous tissue are seen as areas of low signal. Malignant disease is confirmed on the DWI study as an area of significantly reduced low signal compared to the rest of the gland (large arrow). The diagnostic value of this study, as well as the use of dynamic contrast enhanced MRI studies, is the subject of active research.

Further Reading

Claus FG, Hricak H, Hattery RR. Pretreatment evaluation of prostate cancer: role of MR imaging and 1H MR spectroscopy. *Radiographics*. 2004;24:S167-S180.

Choi YJ, Kim JK, Kim N, Kim KW, Choi EK, Cho K.S. Functional MRI of prostate cancer. *Radiographics*. 2007;27:63–75.

Scher D, Swindle PW, Scardino PT. National Comprehensive Cancer Network guidelines for the management of prostate cancer. *Urology* 2003;61:14–24.

Tan PH et al. International Society of Urological Pathology (ISUP) consensus conference on handling and staging of radical prostatectomy specimens. Working group 5: surgical margins. *Mod Path*. 2011;24:48–57.

Case 6.11

1. What tumour stage do Figs. 6.11.1 and 6.11.2a, b demonstrate?
2. What is the differential diagnosis of these appearances, one example is shown in Fig. 6.11.3?

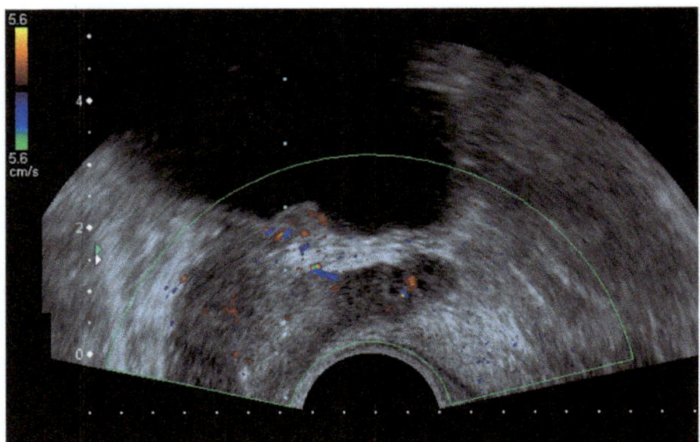

Fig. 6.11.1

Fig. 6.11.2

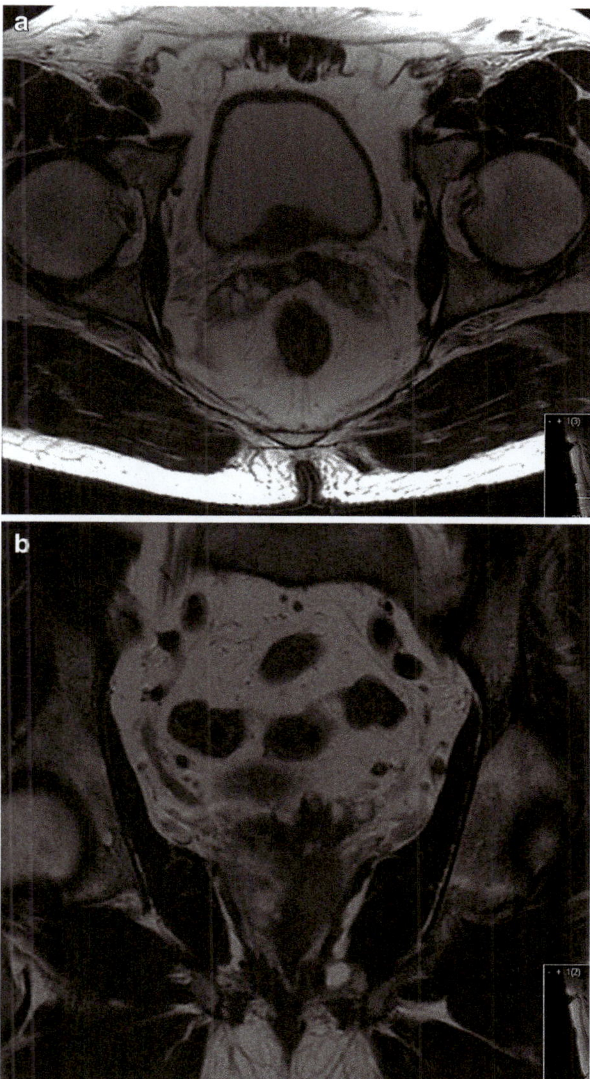

Fig. 6.11.3

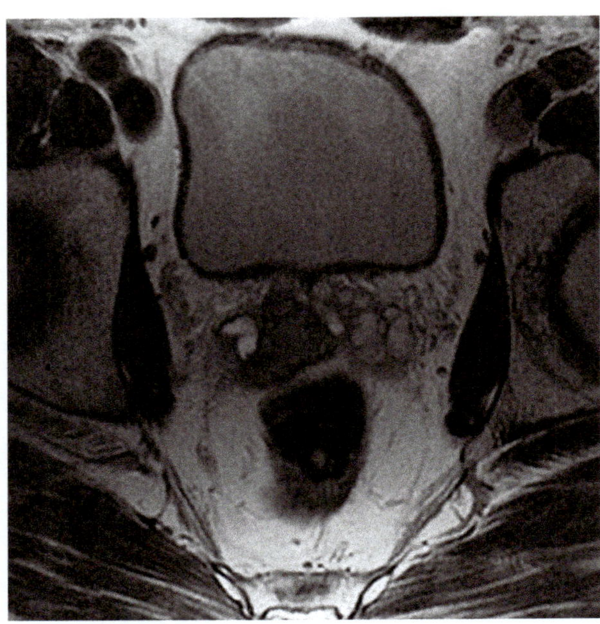

Answers to Case 6.11

1. Figure 6.11.1 is a sagittal TRUS image showing decreased echogenicity within the seminal vesicle (SV), with marginally increased vascularity on colour Doppler scans. Figures 6.11.2a, b are T2W MR images, and show the tumour to have an abnormally low signal intensity, well demonstrated against the typical high T2 signal returned from normal seminal vesicles and consistent with SV invasion. This feature is important to recognise, as tumours with SV invasion have a higher rate of treatment failure. Invasion is defined as tumour infiltrating the muscular coat of the extraprostatic SV. Asymmetrical changes within the SV should be viewed with suspicion.
2. In older men SV atrophy may result in loss of the normal high signal and differentiation between tumour and benign atrophic changes can present a diagnostic difficulty. Post-biopsy haemorrhage is a common mimic of apparent SV invasion. This mistake can be avoided by comparing with the T1-weighted studies. True tumour will have a low signal on both T1 and T2 studies, but haemorrhage will be of high signal on the T1 studies. Significant amyloid deposition is a rarer mimic of tumour involvement. Similarly metastatic disease from elsewhere can cause problems with interpretation.

   Figure 6.11.3 shows an abnormal mass of low signal within the right SV in a 30 year old man. The prostate gland appeared normal and at biopsy this proved to be metastatic melanoma.

Further Reading

Berney DM et al. International Society of Urological Pathology (ISUP) consensus conference on handling and staging of radical prostatectomy specimens. Working group 4: seminal vesicles and lymph nodes. *Mod Path.* 2011;24:39–47.

Hull GW, Abbani F, Abbas F, Wheeler TM, Kattan MW, Scardino PT. Cancer control with radical prostatectomy alone in 1000 consecutive patients. *J Urol.* 2002;167:528–534.

Case 6.12

1. Describe the radiological features seen on the images below.
2. What is the explanation for the appearances of the hips?
3. What type of study is shown in Fig. 6.12.1d and what does it show?
4. What clinical stage is this?

Fig. 6.12.1

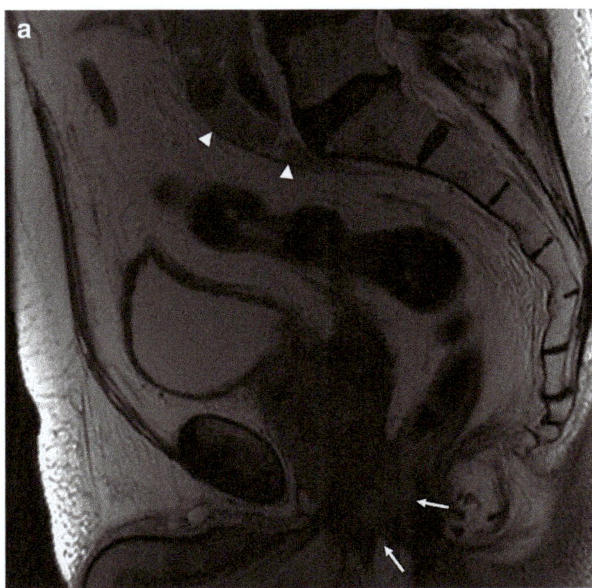

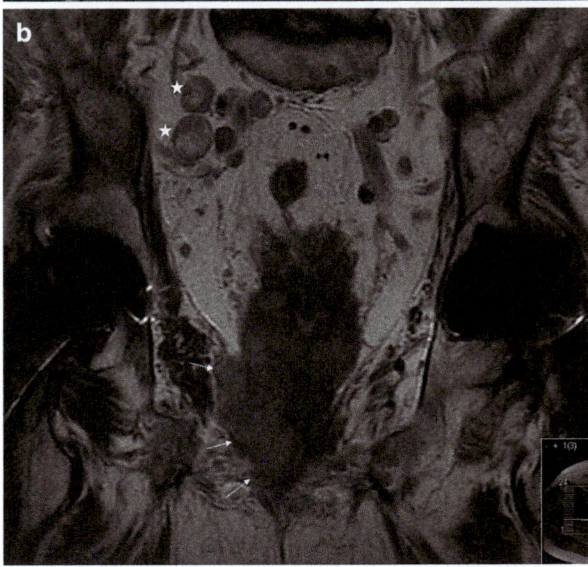

Fig. 6.12.1 (continued)

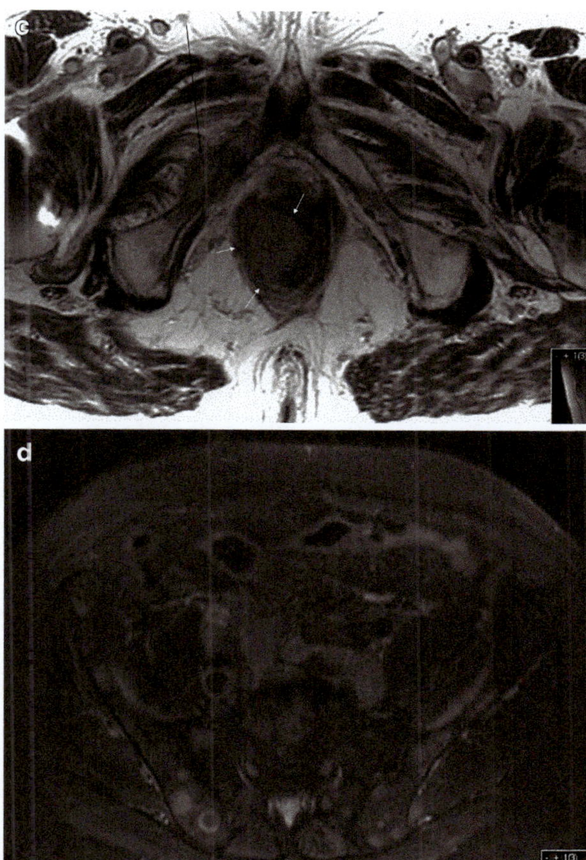

Answers to Case 6.12

1. Figure 6.12.1a–c are sagittal, coronal and axial T2W MRI studies illustrating loss of normal zonal anatomy and almost complete replacement of the prostate by tumour (seen as low T2 signal) which is invading the lower rectum, anal canal and pelvic floor (arrows; Fig. 6.12.1a). Other features include enlarged pathological left external iliac lymph nodes (stars), presacral lymphadenopathy (arrowheads) and a pathological fracture through the right inferior pubic ramus (black arrow, Fig. 6.12.1c).
2. Low signal in the region of both hips represents bilateral hip replacements.
3. Figure 6.12.1d is a T2W image with fat suppression allowing better visualisation of significant pathology within bone marrow. This image shows multiple round bone metastases and lymphadenopathy within the retroperitoneum.
4. This is Stage T4N1M1b prostate cancer.

Case 6.13

These are images taken from a man who presented with severe lower urinary tract symptoms and a PSA level of 854 ng/ml.

1. Describe the abnormal radiological findings on these MR images.
2. How was Fig. 6.13.1b acquired? What does it show and what are the diagnostic possibilities?
3. What is the clinical stage?

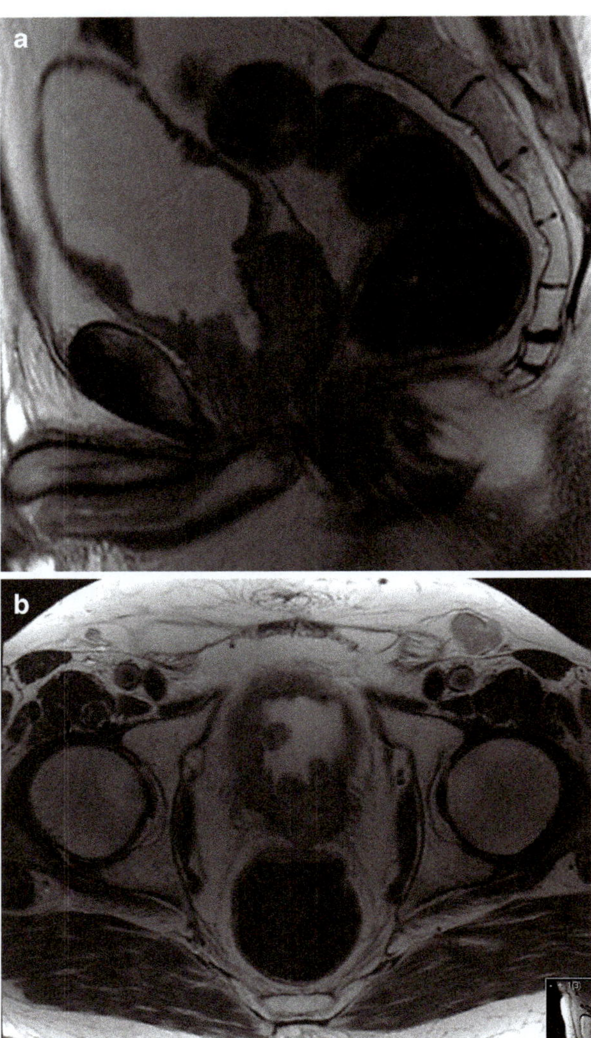

Fig. 6.13.1

Fig. 6.13.1 (continued)

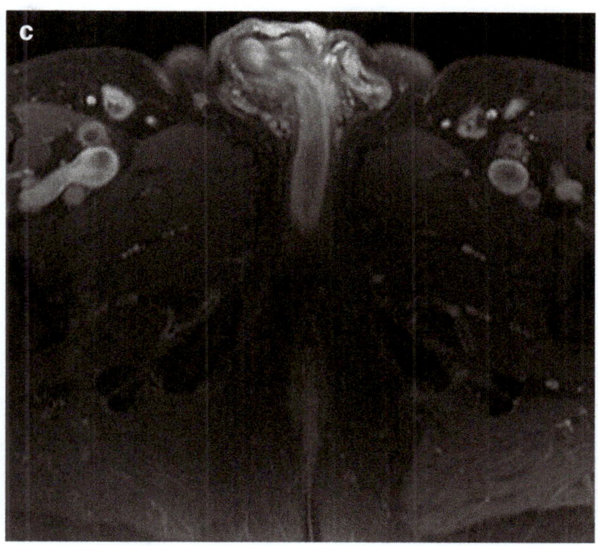

Answers to Case 6.13

1. Figure 6.13.1a, b (sagittal and axial T2W MRIs respectively) show a centrally lying TUR defect (note the wide bladder neck), while the rest of the gland is enlarged and infiltrated by low-signal tumour. The SVs have been engulfed and there is direct invasion of the bladder base. The tumour also extends posteriorly to abut, but probably does not invade, the anterior wall of rectum. Irregularity of the bulbar urethral signal is demonstrated on the sagittal image (Fig. 6.13.1a) and an enlarged left inguinal node is also present.
2. Figure 6.13.1c is a fat-suppressed T1 weighted image post-contrast and this confirms an irregular, nodular urethra that does not enhance as intensely as adjacent corpus spongiosum. The differential diagnosis includes both a primary urethral cancer and metastatic prostate cancer. The latter was proven at biopsy.
3. This is stage T4N1M1c prostate cancer.

Case 6.14

1. What is a bone scintigram, how is it carried out, what agent is used? What are the indications?
2. Describe the findings in Fig. 6.14.1.
3. Describe the findings in Fig. 6.14.2a, b.
4. Figure 6.14.3 is a postmortem coronal section of vertebral bodies of a patient with the same condition. Figure 6.14.4a, b show microscopic sections of bone. What staining technique is used in each and what are they likely to demonstrate?

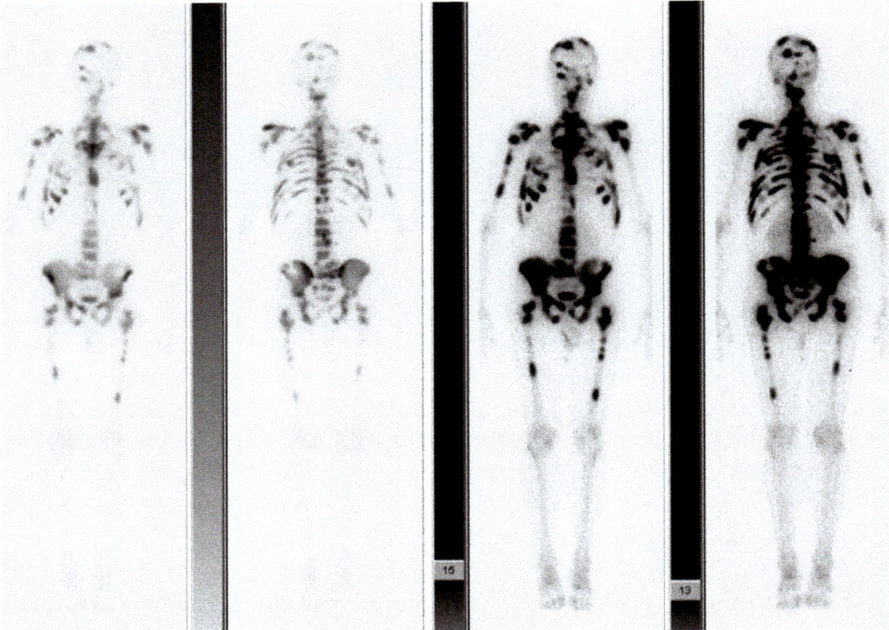

Fig. 6.14.1

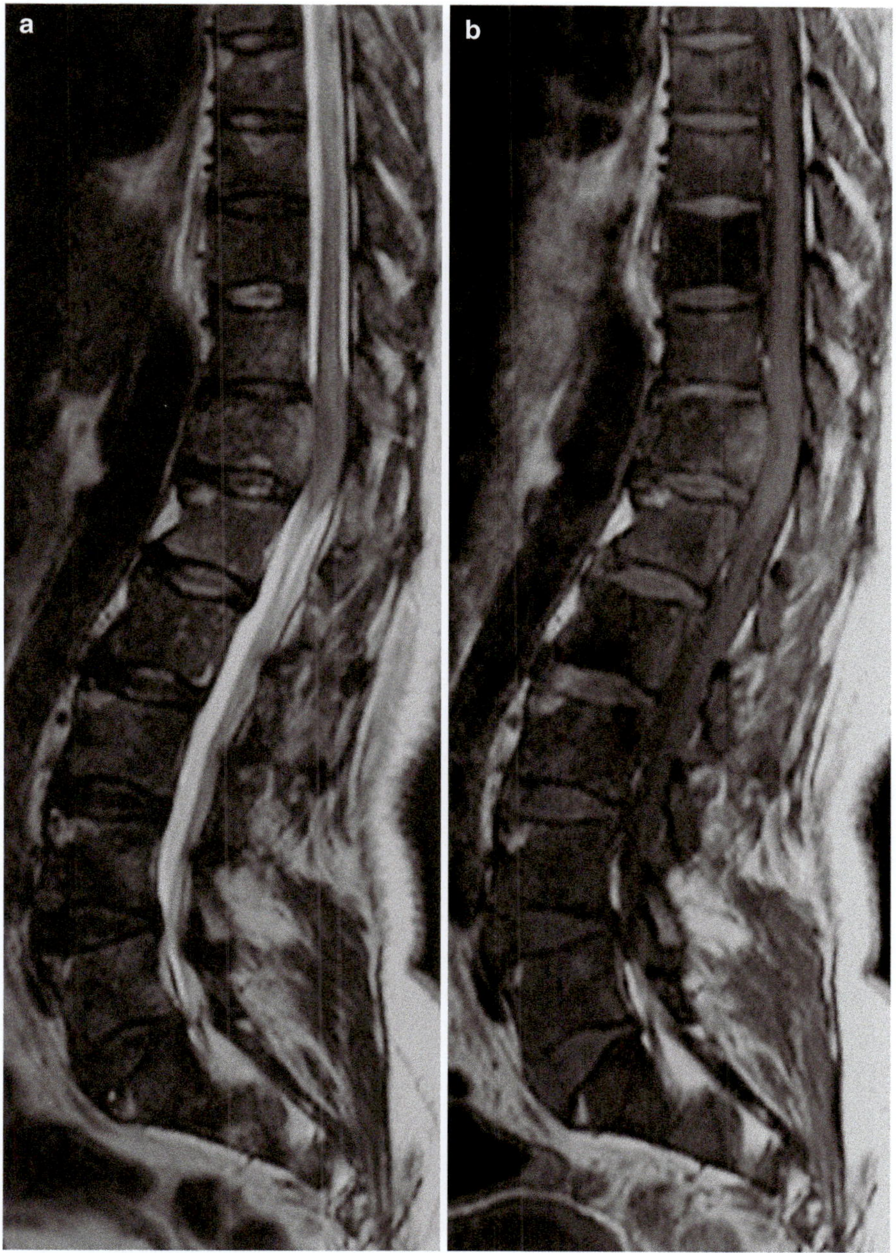

Fig. 6.14.2

Fig. 6.14.3

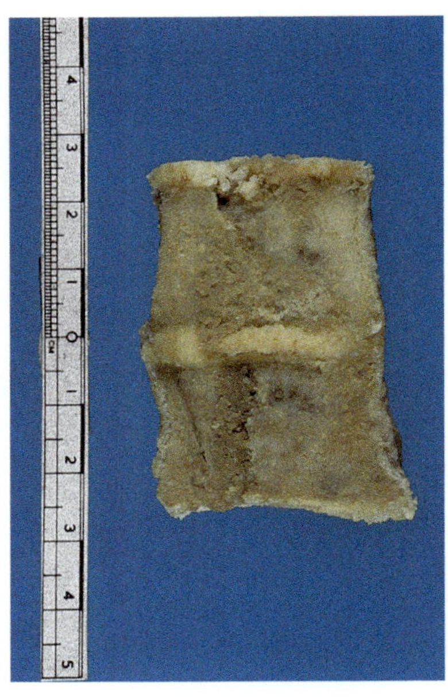

Fig. 6.14.4

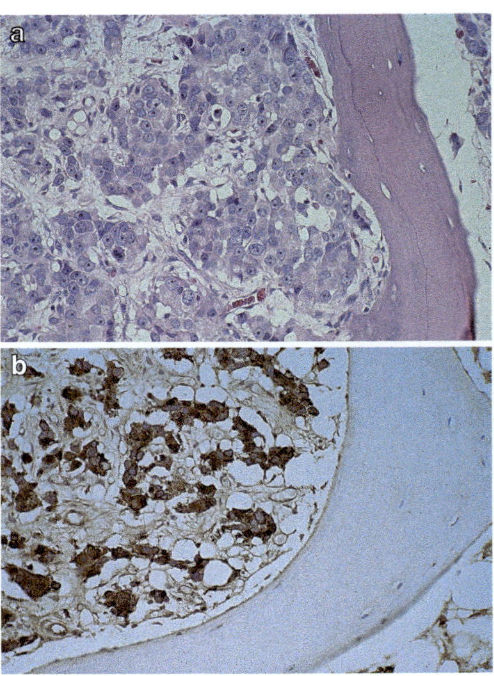

Answers to Case 6.14

1. Bone scans are performed following an intravenous injection of a 99m-Technetium-labelled diphosphonate. This radiopharmaceutical is absorbed onto the normal crystalline matrix of bone with areas of abnormally increased bone activity seen as areas of more intense scintigraphic uptake or 'hot spots' raising the possibility of metastatic disease; although any areas of increased bone turnover, e.g. healing fractures and Paget's disease, will also appear 'hot'. Thus, in the broadest sense, its indication is to confirm and evaluate any area of active bone pathology or metabolism. In urology, the commonest indication is metastatic prostate cancer. The risk of bone metastases rises with increasing PSA and Gleason score, and bone scintigraphy is used to assess the extent of disease and can be used to monitor response to treatment. Bone scan metastases were detected in 2.3%, 5.3% and 16.2% of patients with PSA levels <10, 10.1–19.9 and 20–49.9 ng/ml, respectively. Detection rates were 5.6% and 29.9% for Gleason scores ≤7 and ≥8 respectively.
2. Figure 6.14.1 demonstrates multiple foci of increased tracer uptake in the marrow, indicating increased bone turnover consistent with widespread bone metastases. Plain films of the long bones may be required given the potential risk of pathological fracture. This is not a 'superscan'; which is distinguished by a uniformly high but homogenous uptake by all the bones, with non-visualisation of the kidneys. The implication being that the marrow is so densely infiltrated that all tracer is bound by the marrow and none is available for renal excretion.
3. Figure 6.14.2a, b show sagittal T2 and T1 weighted images through the lower thoracic and lumbar sacral spine. Marrow signal is extremely heterogeneous on the T2W image. Normally, on T1W studies the marrow is of a high signal reflecting the normal high-fat component, but in this case marrow is replaced by abnormal low signal consistent with widespread bone metastases. The body of T12 is expanded and bulges into the spinal canal causing significant compression of the conus, seen best on the T2W image. This is associated with abnormal high signal consistent with oedema within the distal cord.
4. The vertebral bodies are partly replaced by white nodules. The H and E stained microscopic section (Fig. 6.14.4a) shows carcinoma cells invading bone. Figure 6.14.4b shows an immunohistohemical technique demonstrating PSA in the cytoplasm of the malignant cells, confirming prostatic carcinoma metastases in bone.

Further Reading

Abuzallouf S, Dayes I, Lukka H. Baseline staging of newly diagnosed prostate cancer: a summary of the literature. *J Urol*. June 2004;171(6 Pt 1):2122–2127.

Case 6.15

1. What are the images in Fig. 6.15.1a–c and what do they show?
2. What do the arrows in Fig. 6.15.1c demonstrate?
3. Figure 6.15.2 is a post-mortem section across retroperitoneal tissue, what does it show?

Fig. 6.15.1

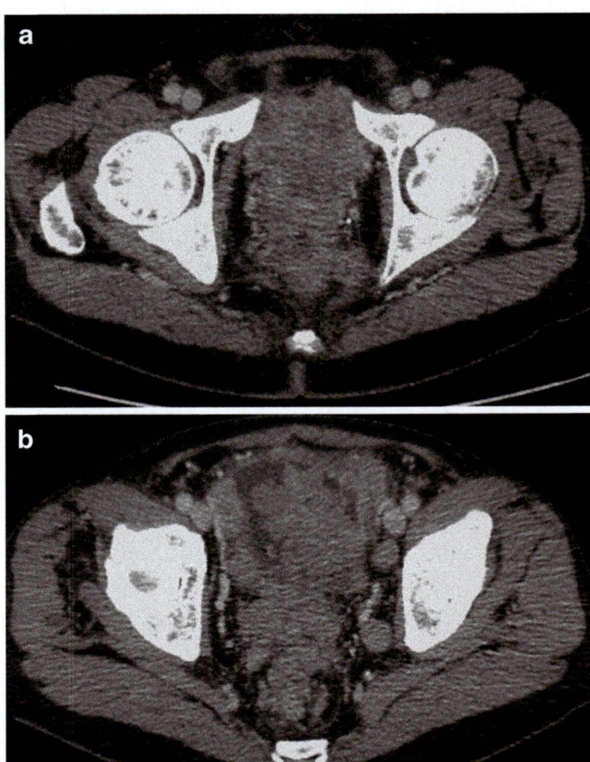

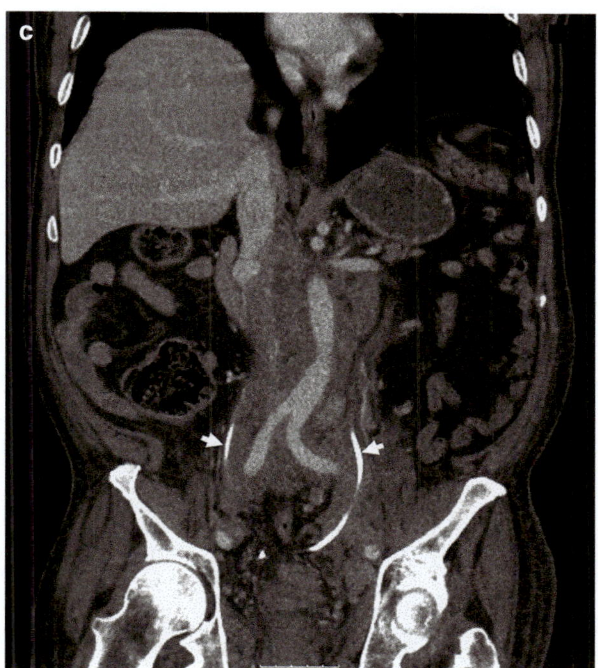

Fig. 6.15.1 (continued)

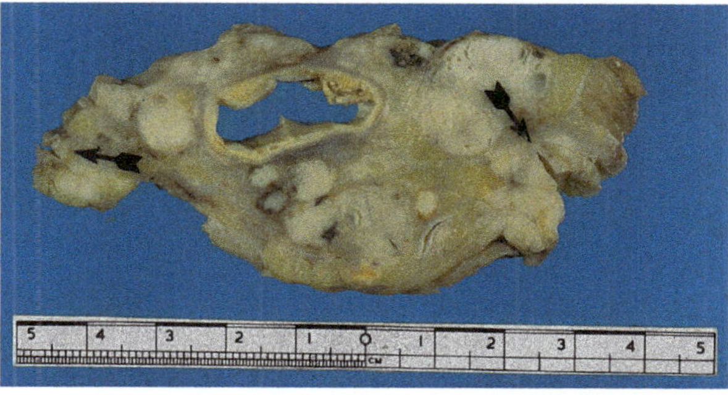

Fig. 6.15.2

Answers to Case 6.15

1. Figure 6.15.1a, b are axial CT scans through the pelvis showing locally advanced disease with an enlarged irregular prostate and invasion of the rectum and mesorectal fat. There is also invasion of the bladder base with a large mass occupying much of the bladder lumen and further perivesical tumour deposits. There are multiple enlarged mesorectal and left iliac lymph nodes along the pelvic side wall.
2. Figure 6.15.1c is a coronal CT image showing extensive retroperitoneal lymphadenopathy encasing the IVC, aorta and common iliac arteries. The high-density tubular structures marked by the arrows are bilateral ureteric stents, introduced to relieve ureteric obstruction by the malignant adenopathy.
3. The post-mortem specimen 6.15.2 shows numerous white deposits in the retroperitoneal fat, confirmed on microscopy to be prostate cancer metastases in both lymph nodes and adipose tissue. The ureters, opened at dissection, are arrowed.

Case 6.16

1. Describe the findings in Fig. 6.16.1a, b and suggest a diagnosis.
2. Describe morphological variants of prostatic adenocarcinoma. Do they have any prognostic significance?

Fig. 6.16.1

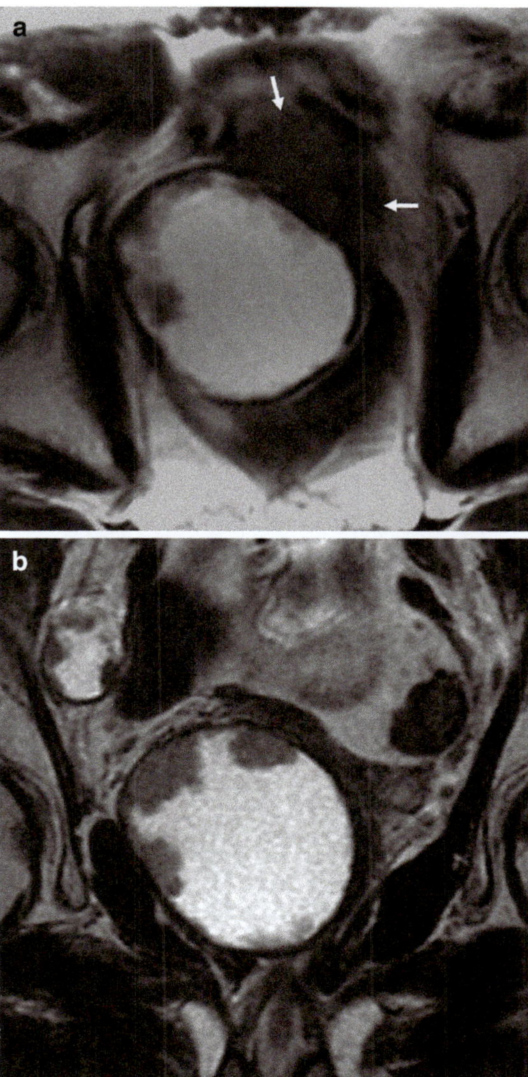

Answers to Case 6.16

1. Figure 6.16.1a, b are axial and coronal MR images showing a large complex prostatic mass. The mass is of high T2 signal centrally (and therefore cystic) with papillary projections of intermediate signal consistent with a complex cyst. The axial image also demonstrates a more solid component anterolaterally (arrows) representing residual prostate gland. A right external iliac node (seen on Fig. 6.16.1b) has been expanded by tissue of similar signal characteristics. The differential diagnosis is similar to that discussed in Case 6.4, but in this patient the presence of a significantly enlarged lymph node would be unexpected for benign and inflammatory cysts, and malignancy is more likely. The microscopic diagnosis was mucinous adenocarcinoma.
2. Morphological variants of adenocarcinoma arising from the acinar secretory cells include ductal, atrophic, foamy cell, pseudo-hyperplastic, carcino-sarcoma, signet ring-like, mucinous, oncocytic, clear cell and lympho epithelioma-like. Assignation of the Gleason grade should be based on pattern rather than any unique variant cytological feature. However, the pseudo-hyperplastic variant is assigned to grade 3 and mucinous/colloid and ductal cancers are regarded as Gleason grade 4.

Further Reading

Chang JM, Lee HJ, Lee SE, et al. Unusual tumours involving the prostate: radiological-pathological findings. *BJR*. 2008;81(971):907–915.

Epstein JI, Allsbrook WC Jr, Amin MB et al. The 2005 International Society of Urologic Pathology (ISUP) consensus conference on Gleason grading of prostatic carcinoma. *AMJ Surg Pathol*. 2005:29;1228–1242.

Case 6.17

Study the figures given below. The last two images represent a study undertaken 6 months after the first two images

1. Describe the changes between images 6.17.1a, b vs. 6.17.1c, d.
2. What is the explanation for these changes and why was this procedure undertaken?

Fig. 6.17.1

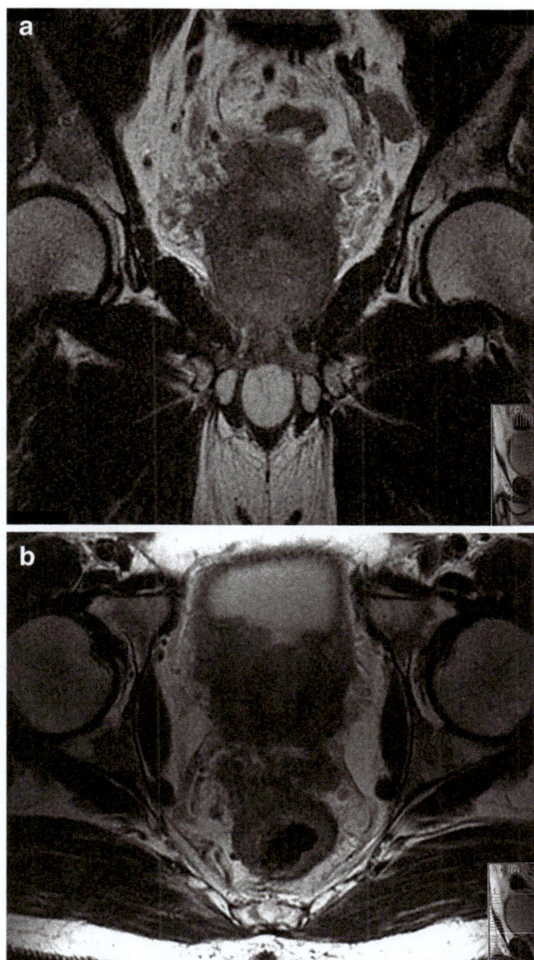

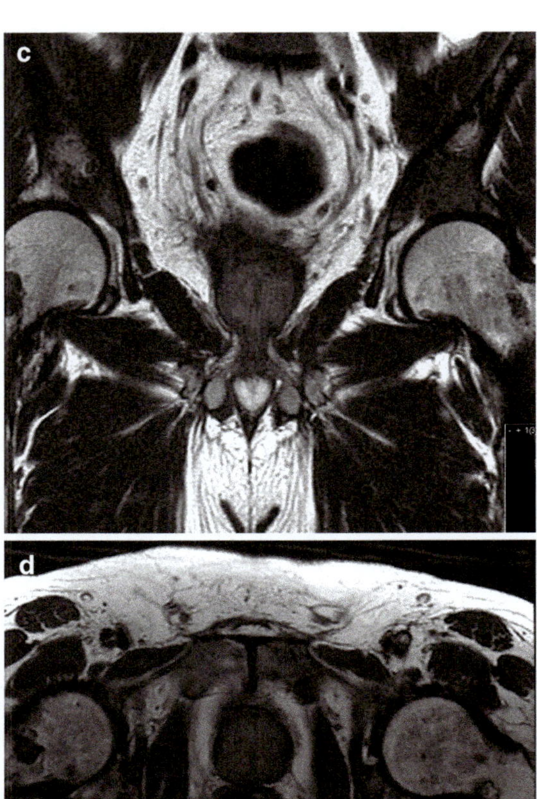

Fig. 6.17.1 (continued)

Answers to Case 6.17

1. Figure 6.17.1a, b show widespread low T2 signal abnormality within the prostate gland, with extension through the capsule, into the seminal vesicles and posteriorly into the rectum as well as local and regional nodal involvement. Also note the low signal focus within the right acetabulum representing a bone metastasis. The appearances are of locally advanced and metastatic prostate carcinoma. In Fig. 6.17.1c, d there has been a reduction in the size and extent of the disease with a decrease in the size of the pelvic nodes. The primary prostatic tumour has become more uniform and lower in signal.
2. These are typical post-radiotherapy changes. Radical radiotherapy (conformal or IMRT) should be offered as one of the treatment options for men with localised prostate cancer, with a life expectancy of more than 10 years. It is also offered with curative intent to men with locally advanced disease in the absence of lymph node metastases with at least a 5-year life expectancy and as palliation in men with locally advanced disease with a shorter life expectancy. Neoadjuvant and adjuvant hormones in addition to radiotherapy improve outcome in high-risk patients. Radiotherapy also has a role in patients with a high risk of recurrence or in the salvage setting after radical prostatectomy.

   Low-dose brachytherapy using implanted Iodine 125 seeds is an option for those with low or intermediate risk disease as long as the gland volume is favourable (usually <50 ml) and there is no history of significant lower urinary tract symptoms. High-dose brachytherapy using Iridium 192 rods is used in men with more unfavourable disease – PSA >10 ng/ml or Gleason score 8–10. Hollow rods are positioned in the prostate using ultrasound guidance and the patient receives two to three separate doses over an 18 h period. Either forms of brachytherapy may be used in conjunction with external beam radiotherapy to give a radiation boost.

Case 6.18

1. This MRI study (Fig. 6.18.1a–c) was performed in a patient who had biochemical relapse following previous radical prostatectomy. What do these images show?
2. What is this study shown in Fig. 6.18.2? How is it performed and what is the role of this imaging modality in the management of prostate cancer?

Fig. 6.18.1

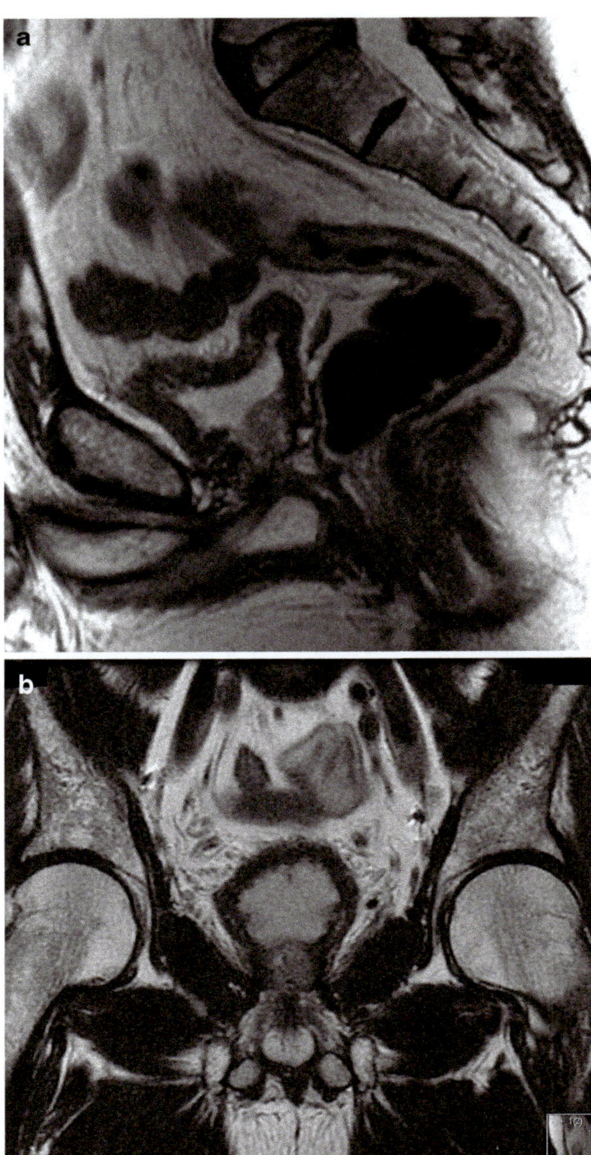

Fig. 6.18.1 (continued)

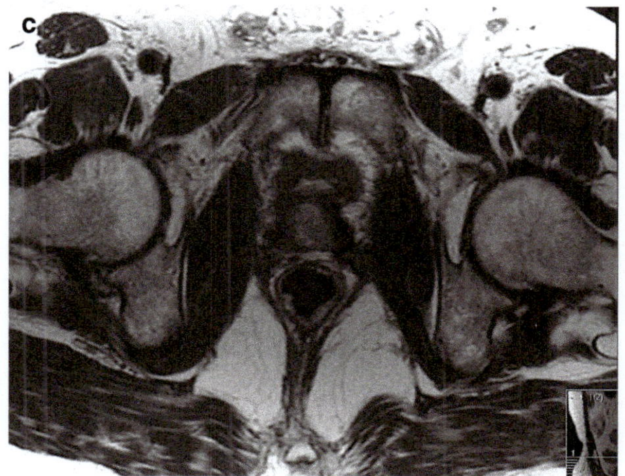

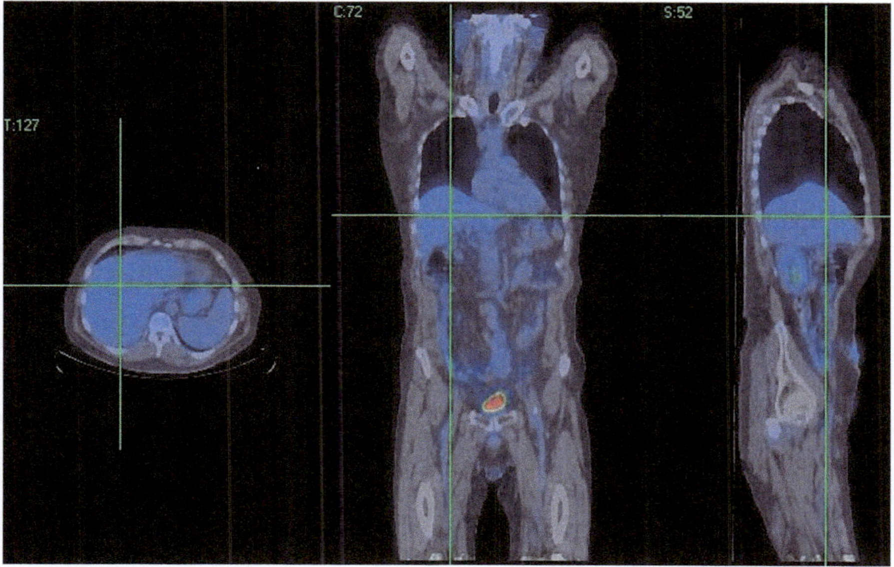

Fig. 6.18.2

Answers to Case 6.18

1. Figure 6.18.1a–c are sagittal, coronal and axial T2W MR images, showing a focus of abnormal intermediate signal tissue in the prostatic bed, in contrast to the usual ring of low signal seen as a result of post-surgical fibrosis. The appearances are of local tumour recurrence. Radiological evaluation for suspected recurrent disease after prostatectomy lacks sensitivity for cancer recurrence when it is still low volume. The PSA is usually significantly elevated (>5 ng/ml) or the doubling time very short (<3 months) before any local or metastatic disease is seen, either on MRI, CT or bone scan.
2. Figure 6.18.2 is a normal fused Positron Emission Tomography (PET) CT image. Routine PET CT imaging with F-18 fluorodeoxyglucose (FDG) relies on malignant tissue being more metabolically active than adjacent benign tissue. Malignant tissue is demonstrated as areas of increased tracer uptake. These foci can then be anatomically localised using the simultaneously acquired CT images. Unfortunately well-differentiated prostate cancer utilises less glucose than other tumour types and there is an overlap between malignant and benign conditions such as BPH. This is further complicated by the urinary excretion of radioisotope into bladder with the potential to obscure pathological uptake (as seen on this image). These factors make PET CT unreliable for routine staging purposes. Some reports have suggested that PET CT can be useful in the assessment of pelvic nodal and recurrent disease using other alternative radioisotopes such as 11-C choline and 11-C acetate.

Further Reading

Choueiri TK, Dreicer R, Paciorek A, Carroll PR, Konety B. A model that predicts the probability of positive imaging in prostate cancer cases with biochemical failure after initial definitive local therapy. *J Urol.* 2008;179(3):906–910.

Takahashi N, Inoue T, Lee J, Yamaguchi T, Shizukuishi K. The roles of PET and PET CT in the diagnosis and management of prostate cancer. *Oncology.* 2007;72:226–233.

Case 6.19

1. Apart from adenocarcinoma, what other malignant neoplasms of the prostate may be encountered?
2. What features are seen in Fig. 6.19.1a, b?

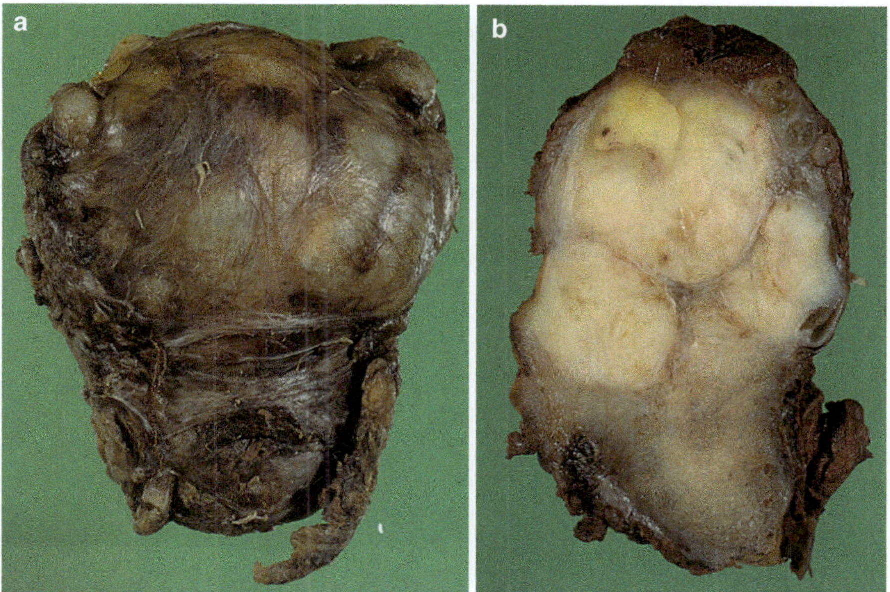

Fig. 6.19.1

Answers to Case 6.19

1. Non-adenocarcinomas of the prostate fall into three main groups:
   - Epithelial, e.g. transitional, basal cell, neuroendocrine
   - Mesenchymal, e.g. leiomyosarcoma, rhabdomyosarcoma, tumours of prostatic stromal origin including phylloides tumours and very rarely the range of sarcomas found in other anatomical sites
   - Haematological, e.g. plasmacytoma, leukaemic deposits and lymphomas.

   The most common primary tumour after adenocarcinoma is transitional cell carcinoma arising from the prostatic ducts, often in association with urethral cancer and to be differentiated from a primary tumour of the bladder invading the prostate. Sarcomas are rare, with rhabdomyosarcoma (embryonal subtype) and leiomyosarcoma being the commonest prostatic sarcomas in children and adults, respectively. Prostatic stromal tumours are an amorphous group in terms of appearances and natural history. Rarity enhances difficulties in interpretation. Leukaemic prostatic infiltrates in patients with chronic lymphatic leukaemia are not uncommon as an incidental microscopic finding. Primary lymphoma is rare.
2. Figure 6.19.1a, b show the outer and parasagittal cut surfaces, respectively, of a radical prostatectomy specimen. The gland is expanded by tumour which has caused obstruction and dilatation of the SVs. Areas of necrosis can be seen within the tumour. The diagnosis on microscopy was leiomyosarcoma. Leiomyosarcoma of the prostate is a rare aggressive tumour usually presenting in the fifth to eighth decades as a large mass with a thin pseudocapsule. Clinically, it may be mistaken for simple BPH. Microscopically, appearances resemble leiomyosarcomas arising in the soft tissues and viscera. Immunohistochemistry may be required to differentiate it from a rectal or gastrointestinal stromal tumour. The other important differential diagnosis is that of post-operative spindle cell nodule (a benign reactive process usually following weeks or months after TURP).

Further Reading

Vandoros GP, Manolidis T, Karamouzis MV, Gkermpesi M, Lambrooulou M, Papaatsoris AG. Leiomyosarcoma of the prostate: case report and review of 54 previously published cases.

Vandoros GP, Manolidis T, Karamouzis MV, Gkermpesi M, Lambropoulou M, Papatsoris AG, Zachos I, Konstantinopoulos PA. Leiomyosarcoma of the prostate: case report and review of 54 previously published cases. Sarcoma 2008; 2008: 458709. Epub 2008 Nov 18.

Case 6.20

1. Describe the main abnormalities demonstrated in Fig. 6.20.1.
2. Describe the histological features seen in Fig. 6.20.2.
3. What is the relevance of this finding at TRUS biopsy?

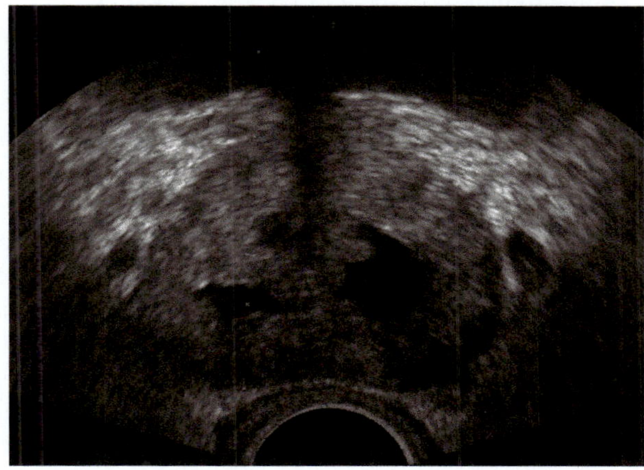

Fig. 6.20.1

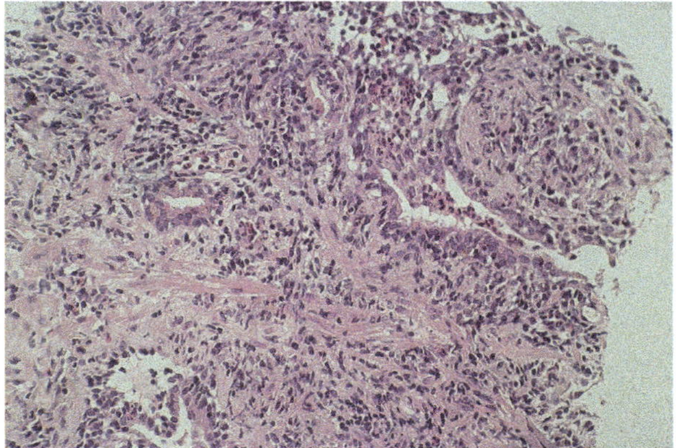

Fig. 6.20.2

Answers to Case 6.20

1. The TRUS image (Fig. 6.20.1) shows irregular cavities, with ill-defined small mixed echoic nodular areas in the peripheral zone and the inner gland. The appearances are those of prostatitis with abscess formation.

   Prostatitis is one of the commonest urologic complaints in men below the age of 50 but the term covers a whole range of symptoms and pathologies, with often little to find on clinical examination, laboratory tests or imaging. If a pathogenic organism is causative the route of infection is usually unknown although indwelling catheters, previous intervention such as TRUS biopsy and urethritis have all been implicated. Severe infection can progress to abscess formation.
2. In Fig. 6.20.2 polymorphonuclear leucocytes and desquamated epithelial cells are seen in distended ducts/acini. Both acute and chronic inflammatory cells are present, predominantly the latter, in an oedematous stroma. The appearances are of acute prostatitis. Gram-negative bacteria are the commonest pathogens but fungi may be the cause, especially in immunosuppressed patients. Rare variants are eosinophilic, allergic, iatrogenic or parasitic prostatitis. Although a close correlation between imaging and microscopy is seen in this case, this association plus that with symptoms and results of clinical investigations does not always occur. Thus histopathologists may refer to acute or chronic inflammatory infiltrates, rather than prostatitis, with the latter being a clinical diagnosis.
3. If prostatitis and especially prostatic abscess is suspected, TRUS biopsy should be deferred as it may exacerbate the infection and lead on to frank septicaemia. A course of antibiotics is appropriate, and a more accurate baseline PSA level obtained post-treatment, although it may take some weeks for the PSA to return to normal. Chronic inflammatory cells are commonly seen in prostate biopsies, a florid inflammatory response may account for an elevated PSA in the absence of prostate cancer.

Further Reading

Benway BM, Moon TD. Bacterial prostatitis. *Urol Clin North Am.* 2008;35:23–32.

Case 6.21

1. This patient presented with fever, suprapubic pain and acute urinary retention. What are these images (Fig. 6.21.1a–c) and what do they show?
2. Describe the main features seen in a study performed 8 weeks later (Fig. 6.21.1d).
3. What are the usual causative organisms of this condition and describe the management?

Fig. 6.21.1

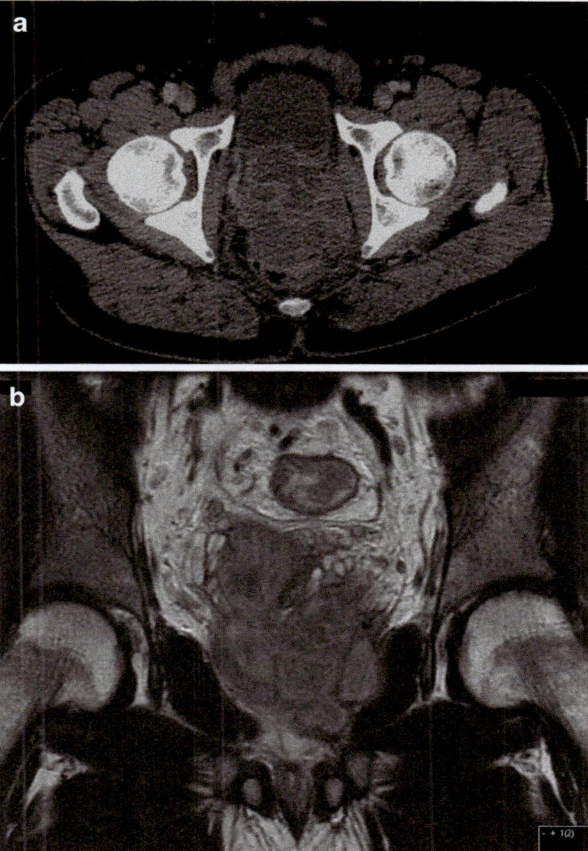

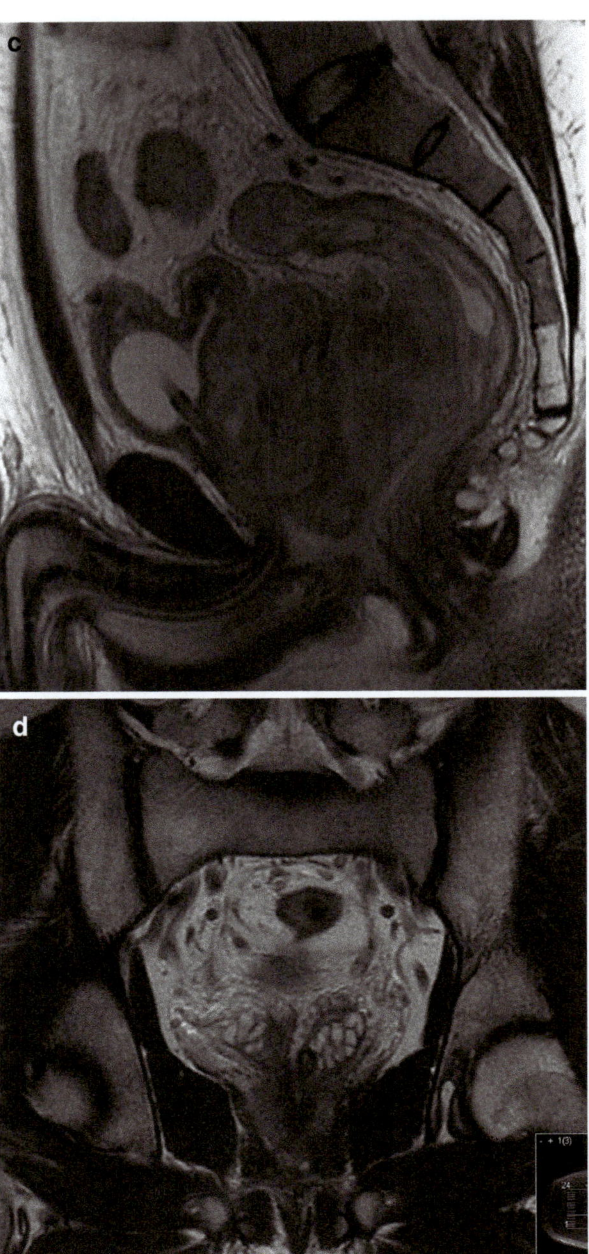

Fig. 6.21.1 (continued)

Answers to Case 6.21

1. Figure 6.21.1a demonstrates a large complex mass on axial CT at the bladder base. Following bladder catheterisation, the MRIs (Fig. 6.21.1b, c) confirm that the normal anatomical zones of the prostate are lost, replaced by a large, complex, partly cystic and loculated mass centred on the prostate, which displaces the rectum posteriorly. The appearances are those of a prostatic abscess.
2. This was proven to be secondary to an *Escherichia coli* infection and following appropriate antibiotics, the patient was re-imaged 8 weeks later. The MRI in Fig. 6.21.1d shows a marked improvement in appearances. Although there is some persistent minor distortion of the seminal vesicles, the prostate is now normal in size and zonal anatomy is definable.
3. The most common causative organisms include *E. coli, Proteus mirabilis, Klebsiella* species, *Enterobacter* species, *Pseudomonas aeruginosa* and *Serratia* though cases due to *S. aureus*, *M. tuberculosis* and *Candida* have been described. The risk of acute bacterial prostatitis and subsequent abscess formation is increased with bacterial colonisation – catheterisation, urethral instrumentation, unprotected anal intercourse and in immunocompromised individuals including diabetics and HIV/AIDS patients. Medical management of prostatic abscess is often unsuccessful. Transrectal or perineal aspiration of the abscess may be undertaken or transurethral resection of the abscess cavity roof may be required.

Case 6.22

This patient had a PSA of 16ng/ml and a hard irregular prostate on DRE. Study these MR and histological images.

1. Describe the abnormalities seen in Figs. 6.22.1a, b and 6.22.2.
2. What is the aetiology of this condition?

Fig. 6.22.1

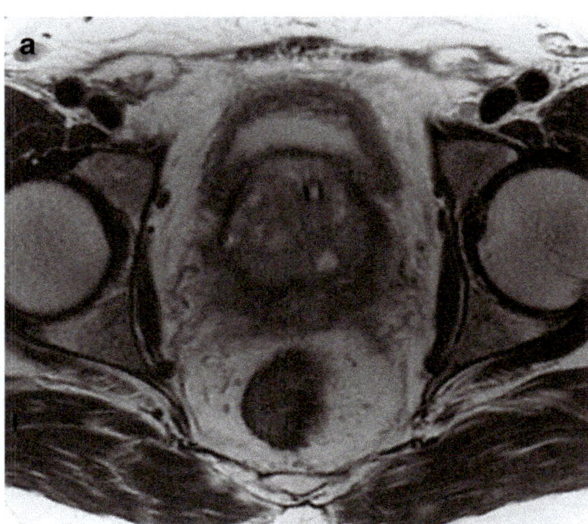

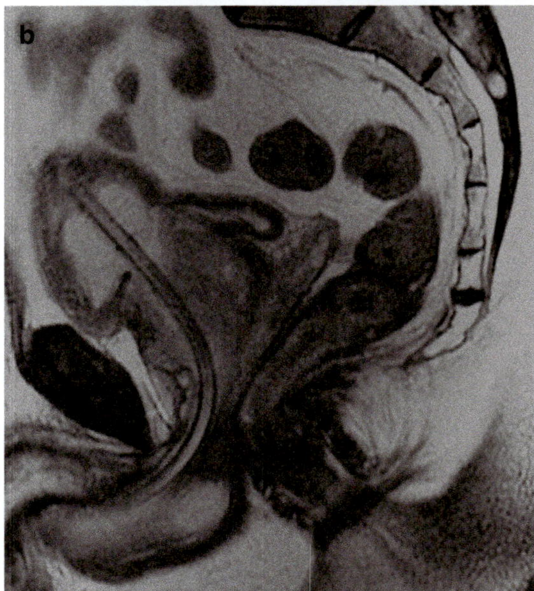

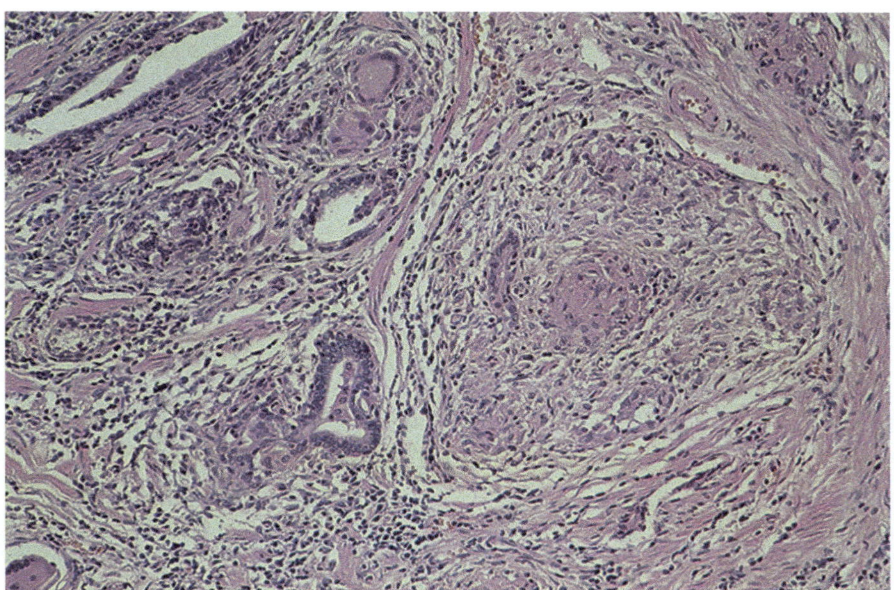

Fig. 6.22.2

Answers to Case 6.22

1. The MRIs (Fig. 6.22.1a, b) show diffuse abnormal low signal throughout the PZ with fine stranding within periprostatic fat. Clinically prostate cancer was suspected and biopsies were undertaken. The H and E section of prostate (Fig. 6.22.2) shows non-caseating granuloma with giant cells adjacent to prostatic ducts and acini. The epithelium of the acini in the lower left and mid right of the field is disrupted. This is granulomatous prostatitis, an uncommon diagnosis, accounting for 0.8–1% of benign inflammatory conditions of the prostate, but it is one which can mimic malignant disease, both clinically and radiologically.
2. The aetiology of granulomatous prostatitis is thought to be a reaction to extravasated acinar or duct contents following obstruction or alternatively an autoimmune response. Eosinophilic forms rarely occur in association with systemic or pulmonary allergic diatheses. Specific infective aetiologies include tuberculosis and various fungi when prostatic involvement is usually a component of disseminated infection. Iatrogenic causes include BCG therapy for transitional carcinoma, peri-urethral Teflon injection and reactions seen at biopsy or TUR sites. Rarely systemic diseases involve the gland, for example both sarcoidosis and Wegener's granulomatosis can cause a granulomatous prostatitis.

Further Reading

Uzoh CC, Uff JS, Okeke AA. Granulomatous prostatitis. *BJU Int*. 2007;99: 510–512.

The Testes and Their Adnexae

7

Arjun Nair and James Pilcher

Case 7.1

1. Examine Fig. 7.1.1a, b and describe the normal anatomy of the testis.
2. What is the blood supply to and from the testes?
3. What are the characteristic appearances of the testis on USS?

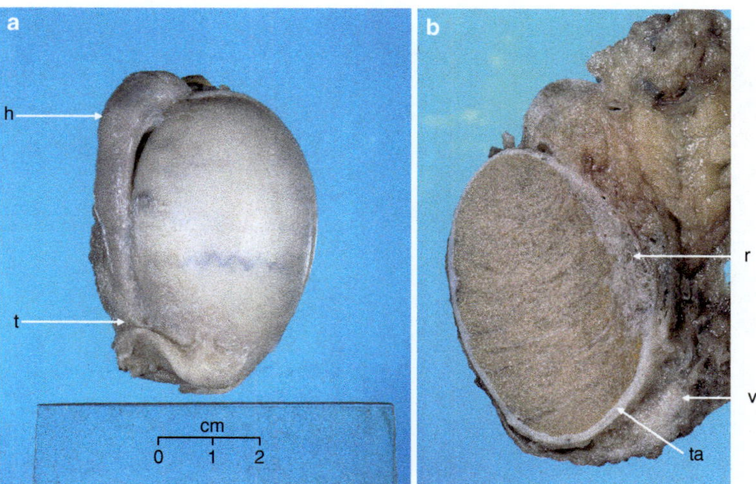

Fig. 7.1.1

S. Bott et al. (eds.), *Images in Urology*,
DOI 10.1007/978-0-85729-769-3_7, © Springer-Verlag London Limited 2012

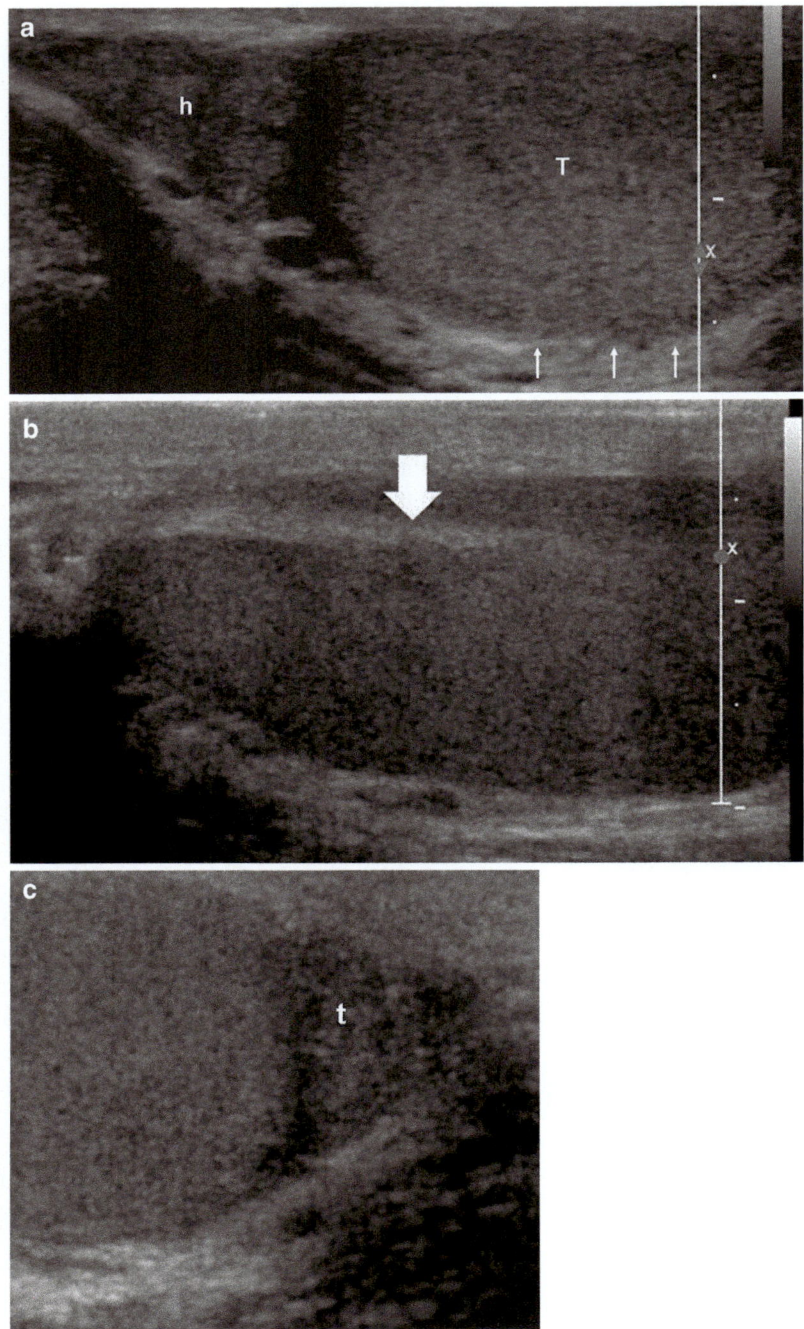

Fig. 7.1.2

Answers to Case 7.1

1. The scrotum is divided by a midline septum into two compartments, each consisting of the testis, epididymis and spermatic cord. The adult testis is an ovoid structure (Fig. 7.1.1a) and is composed of numerous seminiferous tubules. These form 200–300 lobules each separated by fibrous septa. The septa originate from the fibrous capsule, the tunica albuginea, which surrounds the testis and converges at the posterior aspect of the testis to form an incomplete central septum known as the mediastinum testis, where the vessels and ducts perforate the tunica. The seminiferous tubules join in a network of tubules, the rete testis, located towards the upper pole of the testis. These form 12–20 efferent ductules which drain through the mediastinum into the head (caput) of the epididymis. Each ductule opens into the single duct of the epididymis which forms the body and tail terminating in the vas deferens. Figure 7.1.1b shows the cut surface of a normal testis and adjacent adipose tissue of the cord. The tunica albuginea (ta), rete testis (r) and proximal vas deferens (v) are arrowed.

   Figure 7.1.1a shows the outer surface of normal testis and epididymis covered by the smooth visceral layer of the tunica vaginalis. The head (h) and tail (t) of the epididymis are arrowed. The tunica vaginalis is a continuation of the peritoneum that forms with the descent of the testis into the scrotum during development, after which its communication with the peritoneum is usually obliterated. It is composed of an outer parietal and a closely applied inner visceral layer that envelopes the testicle, usually separated by a small amount of fluid. The tunica vaginalis is deficient posteriorly.

   There are five testicular appendages, only three listed below are commonly seen on ultrasound, more easily in the presence of a hydrocele: the appendix epididymis, often a pedunculated structure at the epididymal head; the appendix testis, located near the upper pole of the testis; and the appendix of the epididymal tail, the least commonly identified of the three appendages.
2. The testicular arteries arise directly from the aorta, travel within the spermatic cord and branch out from the mediastinum testis to supply the testis. The deferential artery, a branch of the superior vesical artery, and the cremasteric artery, a branch of the inferior epigastric artery, supply the epididymis, vas deferens and extratesticular scrotal tissue. Venous drainage is via the pampiniform plexus at the upper half of the epididymis, draining into the testicular veins. The right testicular vein drains directly into the inferior vena cava, while the left drains into the left renal vein.
3. Sonography of the testis is performed with a high-frequency (usually between 7 and 12 MHz) linear array transducer. As well as evaluating the testis in transverse and longitudinal planes, ultrasound offers the added advantage of visualising the testis in non-orthogonal planes. On ultrasound, the testis is of slightly increased homogenous reflectivity (Fig. 7.1.2a, labelled T). The tunica albuginea can be identified as an echogenic line (Fig. 7.1.2a, thin arrows), and is usually inseparable from the tunica vaginalis. The layers of the tunica vaginalis itself can only be separately identified in the presence of a hydrocele. The mediastinum testis can be identified as an echogenic line originating from the posterior upper aspect of the testis in the longitudinal plane (Fig. 7.1.2b, block arrow). The head of the epididymis is a pyramidal structure found over the upper pole of the testis (Fig. 7.1.2a, labelled h), while the tail is more curved and located at the inferior pole (Fig. 7.1.2c, labelled t). The epididymis is similar in echogenicity to the testis and is best identified on longitudinal imaging.

Case 7.2

Figures 7.2.1a, b and 7.2.2a, b are images from two different patients who both presented in a similar fashion, with acute painful scrotal swelling and a painful palpable intrascrotal lump, attached to but separate from the testis. The patient in Fig. 7.2.2a, b was febrile. Figure 7.2.3 is a surgical specimen from a patient with a similar problem.

1. Describe the studies performed, and the abnormalities, in each figure.
2. What complication of this condition is additionally illustrated in Figs. 7.2.2a, b and 7.2.3?
3. What are the other imaging findings associated with this condition, and what other complications may be sonographically detected?

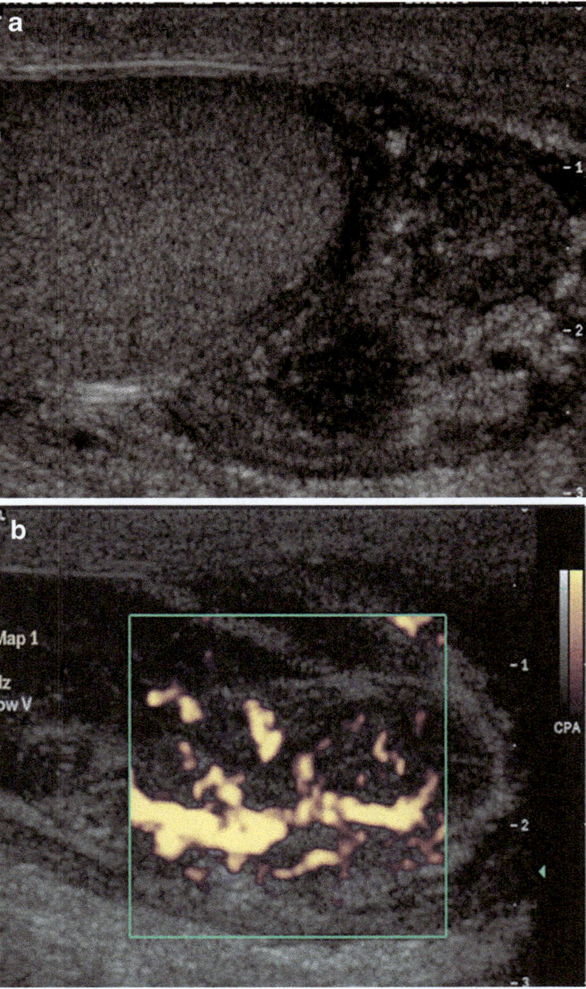

Fig. 7.2.1

Fig. 7.2.2

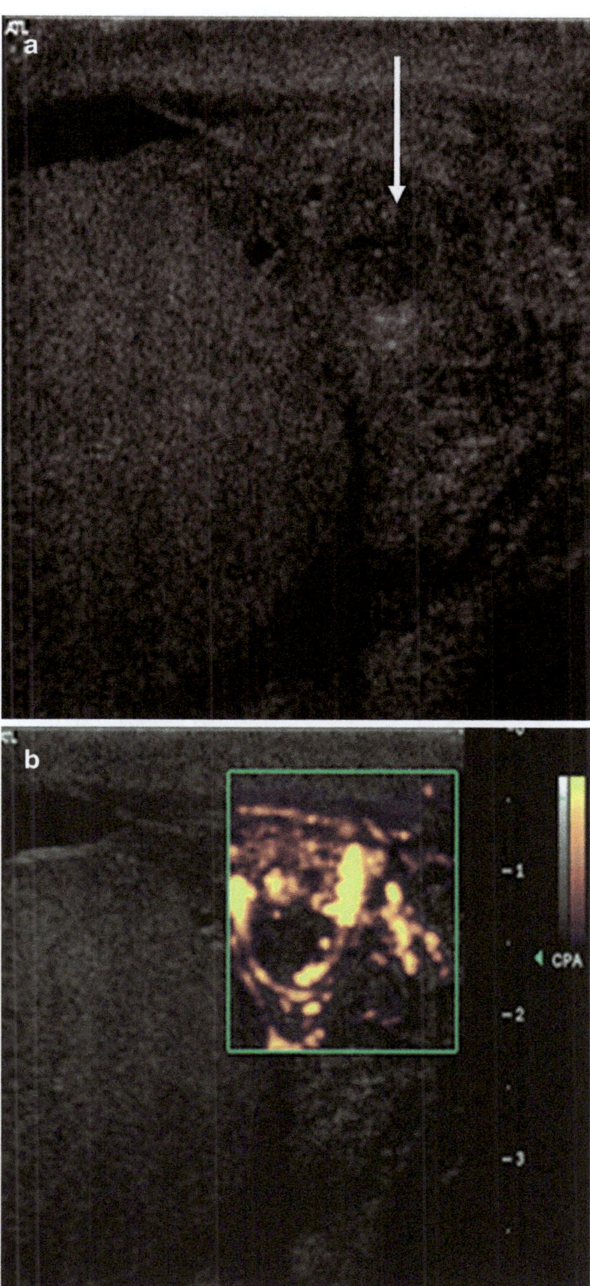

Fig. 7.2.3

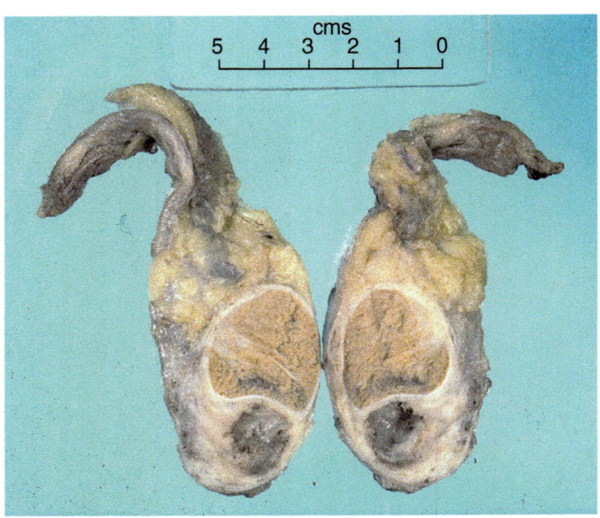

Answers to Case 7.2

1. Figures 7.2.1a and 7.2.2a are longitudinal grey-scale ultrasound images demonstrating an enlarged, heterogeneous epididymal tail, of predominantly low reflectivity. In addition, a more focal rounded area of hyporeflectivity is noted in Fig. 7.2.2a (arrow). The lower pole of each testis is normal. Doppler imaging of the epididymal tails in Figs. 7.2.1b and 7.2.2b demonstrates marked hyperaemia. The grey-scale and power Doppler findings are in keeping with epididymitis.

   Epididymo-orchitis is the most common cause of acute scrotal pain. Epididymitis usually originates in the epididymal head but may involve the entire epididymis in about 50% of cases, and about a third of cases will, to a degree, involve the testis. Sonographic appearances can be non-specific or normal. Colour Doppler evaluation is useful in comparing vascularity with the unaffected side, especially since the infection is usually unilateral.
2. In Fig. 7.2.2b there is a lack of vascularity in the rounded focus, with marked perilesional hyperaemia. These features are in keeping with an evolving epididymal abscess, a rare complication of epididymitis. Figure 7.2.3 is a bi-valved orchidectomy specimen showing an abscess cavity surrounded by fibrosis in the epididymal tail. Scars are present in the testis.
3. Other associated sonographic findings include evidence of orchitis (heterogeneity, hyperaemia and possible enlargement of the ipsilateral testis), hydrocoele and scrotal skin thickening. Haemorrhage into the epididymis due to severe inflammation may manifest sonographically as areas of increased rather than reduced reflectivity. Epididymal or testicular abscesses may rupture, resulting in a pyocele. Testicular ischaemia due to compression of the testicular vessels by

the swollen epididymis is another rare complication that can mimic testicular torsion on ultrasound, although clinical presentation should help distinguish these two conditions.

Further Reading

Amaechi I, Sidhu PS. Ultrasound in the assessment of the "on-call" acute scrotum. *Imaging*. 2008;20(2):131–138.
Cook JL, Dewbury K. The changes seen on high-resolution ultrasound in orchitis. *Clin Radiol*. 2000;55(1):13–18.
Horstman WG, Middleton WD, Melson GL. Scrotal inflammatory disease: colour Doppler US findings. *Radiology*. 1991;179(1):55–59.

Case 7.3

Figure 7.3.1 is an USS from a healthy 3-year-old child noted by his mother to have only a single testis within the scrotum.

1. Describe the abnormality shown in Fig. 7.3.1. What is the most likely associated finding and its anatomical location?
2. What are the complications and comment on the appearances of the H and E section in Fig. 7.3.2, from a 10-year old boy?
3. How accurate is ultrasound and what alternative imaging techniques are available for evaluation of the condition shown in Fig. 7.3.1?

Fig. 7.3.1

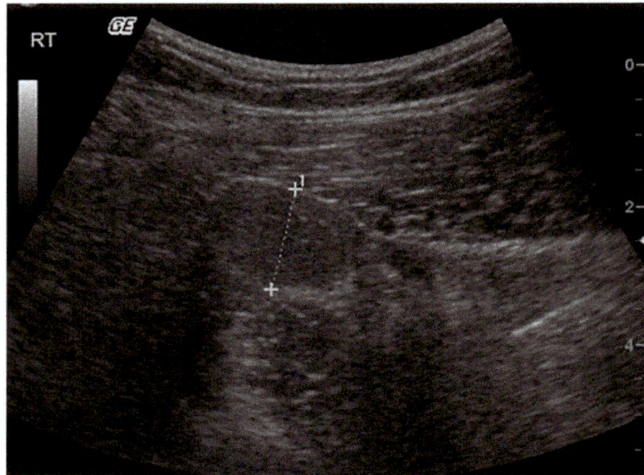

Fig. 7.3.2

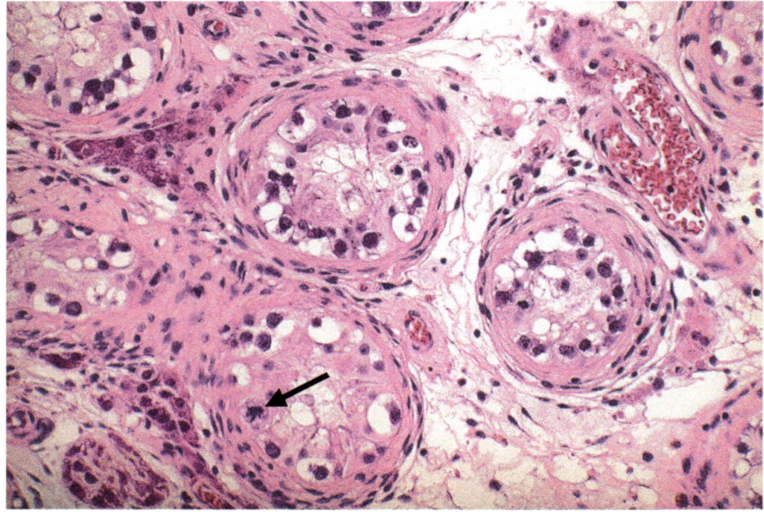

Answers to Case 7.3

1. Figure 7.3.1 is a grey-scale sonographic image of the inguinal region illustrating a well-circumscribed ovoid structure of low echo reflectivity. Given the clinical presentation the appearance is consistent with an undescended right testis (UDT or cryptorchidism). About 80% of undescended testes are found in the inguinal canal. UDT is bilateral in 25% of cases, and more common in premature infants. If the mediastinum testis (a hyperechoic line seen through the centre of the testis on ultrasound, signifying the midline rete) can be visualised, UDT can be confidently diagnosed using ultrasound; this is rarely the case, however, and in practice differentiation from a lymph node can be difficult.
2. There is an increased relative risk (2.75–8) of developing testicular cancer, usually seminoma, within the undescended testis. The timing of orchidopexy influences cancer risk. When orchidopexy is performed before 13 the relative risk is 2.2 compared with 5.4 after the age of 13. Whether or not a 'normal' contralateral testis is at increased risk of malignancy is controversial. Certainly the contralateral intrascrotal testis is often anatomically abnormal and in these cases there is a small increased risk of malignancy. In patients with a Germ cell tumour (GCT) there is certainly an increased risk to the contralateral testis if there is atrophy or a history of maldescent. UDT is also associated with infertility and evidence of germ cell damage is detectable on electron microscopy in testes which remain in an abnormal position after the first year of life. Torsion and trauma, the latter due to compression against the pubis, are more common in UDT.

   The H and E section Fig. 7.3.2 shows seminiferous tubules containing atypical germ cells with ballooned cytoplasm and hyperchromatic nuclei aligned at the periphery. An abnormal mitotic figure is present (arrow) and spermatogenesis is absent. Peritubular fibrosis is present. Appearances are those of intra-tubular germ cell neoplasia, a lesion which precedes invasive tumours.
3. Ultrasound has an accuracy of 90% in detection of the undescended testis. However, MR imaging can be used where ultrasound fails, particularly in cases of intra-abdominal undescended testis. MRI can also differentiate undescended testis from testicular agenesis. In practice, laparoscopic exploration is usually undertaken to identify the site and size of an intra-abdominal undescended testis and then to either excise a vestigial testis or bring down a normally sized testis in one or two stages (Fowler Stephens orchidopexy).

Further Reading

Friedland GW, Chang P. The role of imaging in the management of the impalpable undescended testis. *AJR Am J Roentgenol.* 1988;151(6):1107–1111.

Wood HM, Elder JS. Cryptorchidism and testicular cancer: separating fact from fiction. *J Urol.* 2009;181(2):452–461.

Case 7.4

A 38-year-old man presents with a self-palpated, painless, small firm swelling in his right scrotum. He thinks it has been present for several years. The only abnormality found was within the right epididymal tail. Two focused ultrasound images of the right epididymal tail are presented below in Fig. 7.4.1a, b.

1. Describe the abnormality.
2. What is the differential diagnosis for this lesion?

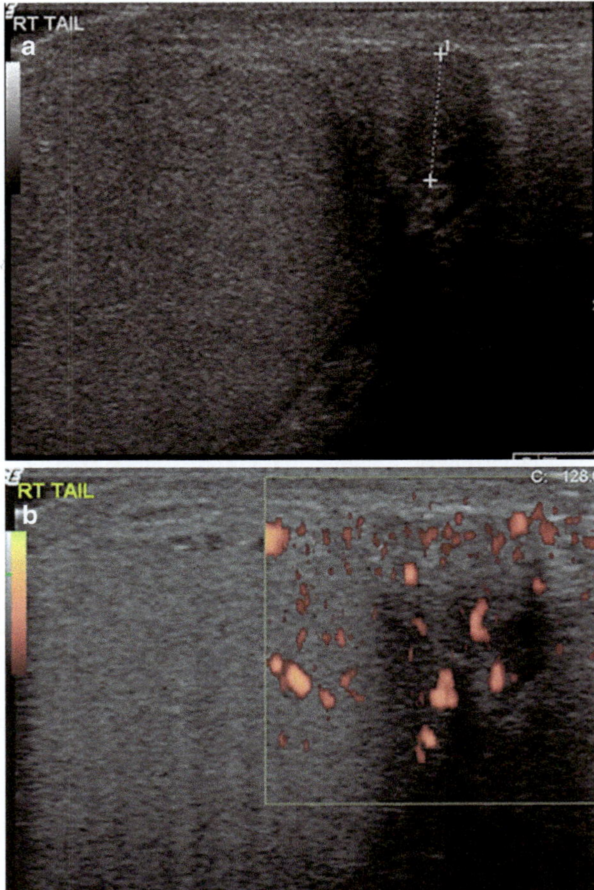

Fig. 7.4.1

Answers to Case 7.4

1. These longitudinal sonographic images reveal a focal, oval, well-circumscribed solid epididymal tail mass (between callipers) of lower echo reflectivity compared to the adjacent testis. There is increased vascularity within the lesion and the tail of the epididymis as a whole.
2. The age, presentation and location of the mass suggest a diagnosis of adenomatoid tumour of the epididymis. Adenomatoid tumours are the commonest tumour associated with the epididymis but arise from mesothelial cells. They range in size from 1 to 5 cm. Sonographically they are commonly well-circumscribed, but vary in echogenicity being hypo-, iso- or hyperechoic with respect to the adjacent testis. Other benign epididymal lesions include papillary cystadenomas, which are found in 17% of men with von Hippel-Lindau disease but are rare in the general population. More common are sperm granulomas of the epididymis. Malignant tumours at this site are rare and include adenocarcinoma, melanotic neuro-ectodermal tumour (usually in infants and having limited metastatic ability), and a variety of primary mesenchymal and hematopoietic neoplasms. Metastases from other organs are uncommon but can occur especially from the left kidney (via the left testicular vein).

Further Reading

Akbar SA, Sayyed TA, Jafri SZ, Hasteh F, Neill JS. Multimodality imaging of paratesticular neoplasms and their rare mimics. *Radiographics*. 2003;23(6): 1461–1476.

Perez-Ordonez B, Srigley JR. Mesothelial lesions of the paratesticular region. *Semin Diagn Pathol*. 2000;17(4):294–306.

Case 7.5

A 14-year old boy was referred for testicular ultrasound because of precocious puberty and suspected adrenal insufficiency. Selected transverse (Fig. 7.5.1a, b) and longitudinal (Fig. 7.5.1c, d) ultrasound images of his left testis are presented below.

1. Describe the abnormality.
2. What is the likely diagnosis and what condition is this associated with?

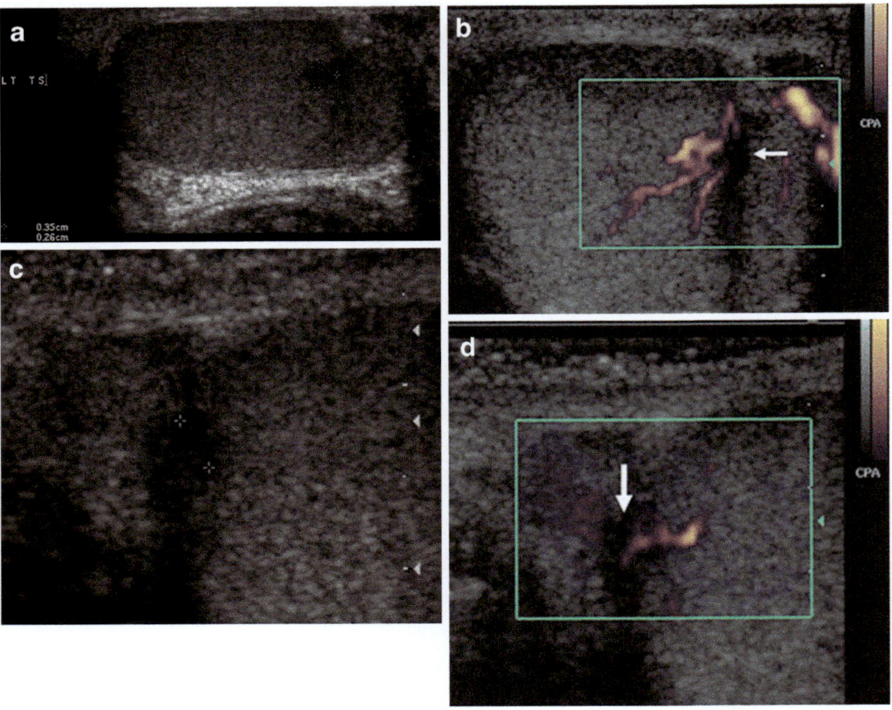

Fig. 7.5.1

Fig. 7.5.2

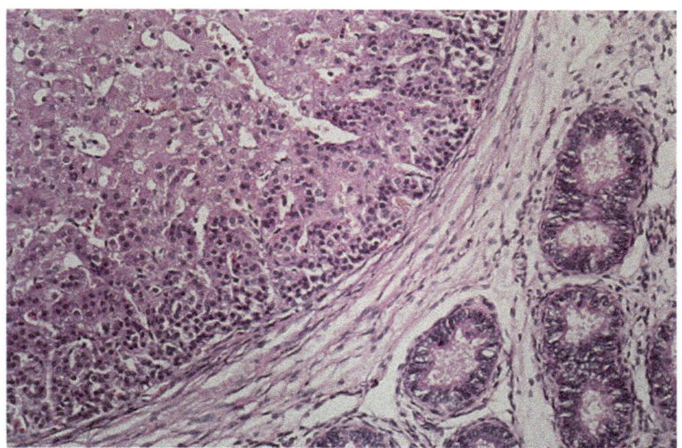

Answers to Case 7.5

1. There is a focal 3.5×2.6 mm hypoechoic oval lesion located close to the mediastinum testis (Fig. 7.5.1a, b) and a second in the upper pole adjacent to the head of the epididymis (Fig. 7.5.1c, d). Doppler ultrasound demonstrates normal vascularity at the mediastinum testis where the testicular vessels enter and leave the testis, but no vascularity is seen within the lesion itself (white arrow in Fig. 7.5.1b) while with the second lesion a branching vessel passes through its margin (Fig. 7.5.1d).
2. The most likely diagnosis is steroid cell nodules associated with congenital adrenal hyperplasia (CAH).These nodules are intratesticular, multiple, brown and microscopiclly resemble Leydig cells. They are adrenocorticotrophic hormone (ACTH) dependent and disappear on hydrocortisone therapy. There is some debate as to their cell of origin, the majority favour the Leydig cells or multipotent testicular stromal cells capable of producing different steroids according to the hormonal milieu. The terminology used reflects this debate – tumours associated with CAH, steroid cell nodules and adrenal cell rest tumour. Such nodules are found in up to 94% of boys with CAH and have also been reported in patients with Addison's disease and Cushing's syndrome.

   Sonographically, testicular nodules associated with CAH are usually hypoechoic and bilateral. They are located close to the mediastinum testis and are usually of normal vascularity, though vascularity is difficult to detect in small lesions, Vessels running through the lesion are not usually deviated in their course, and this may be an important feature in distinguishing these lesions from other small testicular tumours such as Leydig cell tumours, or small metastatic deposits. These nodules can impair spermatogenesis and testicular endocrine function, and may therefore require routine sonographic surveillance but surgical excision is not required.

Adrenal rests (or more correctly aberrant or ectopic adrenals) in contrast to the findings in CAH, occur in 1–2% of the normal adult population, as bright yellow nodules in the spermatic cord, adjacent to the epididymis and rarely in the tunica. They have a fine fibrous capsule and the characteristic layers of the adrenal cortex (Fig. 7.5.2) The presence of adrenal vestiges adjacent to the testis reflects the close proximity of these two organs in early development. (A similar rationale also accounts for gonado–splenic fusion in the left scrotum) Based on the anatomical site and microscopic appearance of adrenal rests, their relationship to the intratesticular nodules of CAH is debatable.

Further Reading

Avila NA, Premkumar A, Shawker TH, Jones JV, Laue L, Cutler GB, Jr. Testicular adrenal rest tissue in congenital adrenal hyperplasia: findings at Gray-scale and color Doppler US. *Radiology*. 1996;198(1):99–104.

Stikkelbroeck NMML, Otten BJ, Pasic A, Jager GJ, Sweep CGJ, Noordam K & Hermus ARMM. High prevalence of testicular adrenal rest tumours, impaired spermatogenesis, and Leydig cell failure in adolescent and adult males with congenital adrenal hyperplasia. *J. Clin. Endocrinol. Metab.* 2001;86:5721–5728.

Case 7.6

Figures 7.6.1 and 7.6.2 are longitudinal grey-scale sonographic images of the left testis taken from two healthy patients. Figure 7.6.3 is the orchidectomy specimen from a third patient who had the same condition.

1. Describe the main abnormalities shown?
2. What is the diagnosis and its clinical significance?

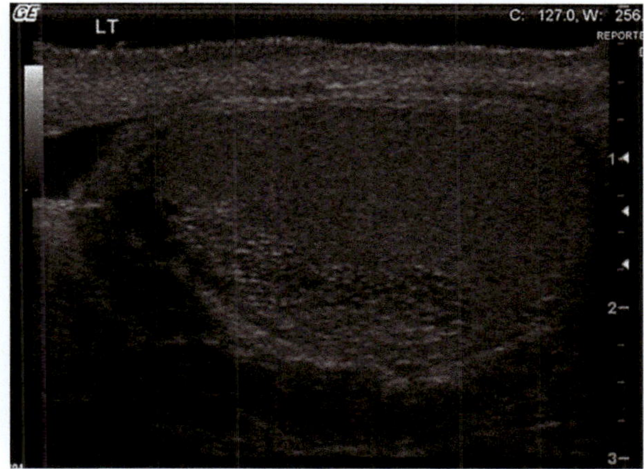

Fig. 7.6.1

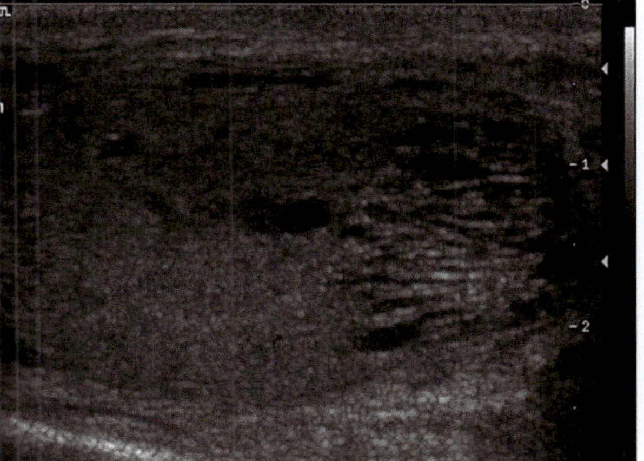

Fig. 7.6.2

Fig. 7.6.3

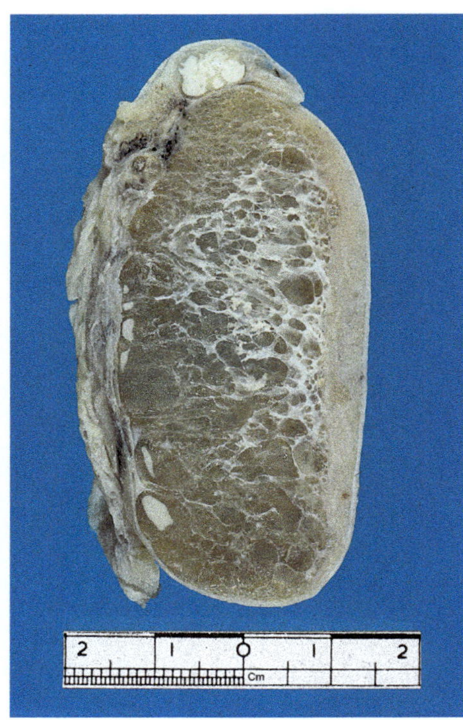

Answers to Case 7.6

1. Figure 7.6.1 demonstrates multiple anechoic tubules along the posterior aspect of the left testis, and aligned along the mediastinum of the testis. Figure 7.6.2 depicts similar but more severely dilated tubular structures in association with anechoic circular lesions. Figure 7.6.3 is the cut surface of a testis including numerous cystic spaces, seen microscopically to be dilated rete testis. The residual testis is compressed to a rim (on the right).
2. This is tubular ectasia of the rete testis, also known as cystic transformation of the rete testis. This is a benign condition that occurs as a consequence of partial or total obliteration of the efferent ducts, usually as a consequence of inflammation or trauma. It often occurs in men over the age of 50, and can frequently be bilateral and asymmetrical. It is often associated with epididymal cysts, and remains unchanged over time. Recently a more specific association has been described in patients on dialysis for chronic renal failure, in whom the rete ectasia is thought to result from the presence of oxalate crystals. The appearance of elongated tubules replacing and paralleling the mediastinum testis is diagnostically characteristic, such that confusion with a cystic malignant testicular tumour can usually be avoided.

The above condition in adults differs from cystic dysplasia in infants and children which may cause testicular enlargement and be associated with congenital renal anomalies.

Further Reading

Brown DL, Benson CB, Doherty FJ, Doubilet PM, DiSalvo DN, Van Alstyne GA, et al. Cystic testicular mass caused by dilated rete testis: sonographic findings in 31 cases. *AJR Am J Roentgenol*. 1992;158(6):1257–1259.

Tartar VM, Trambert MA, Balsara ZN, Mattrey RF. Tubular ectasia of the testicle: sonographic and MR imaging appearance. *AJR Am J Roentgenol*. 1993;160(3): 539–42.

Case 7.7

These two ultrasound images of the right testis were obtained from a 24-year-old patient with sickle-cell disease who was referred to urology out-patients with a sudden onset of acute right testicular pain, following a recent upper respiratory tract illness.

1. Describe the abnormalities. What is the differential diagnosis for this appearance and the likely diagnosis in this case?
2. What are the important management considerations?
3. Comment on the orchidectomy specimens in Fig. 7.7.2a, b.

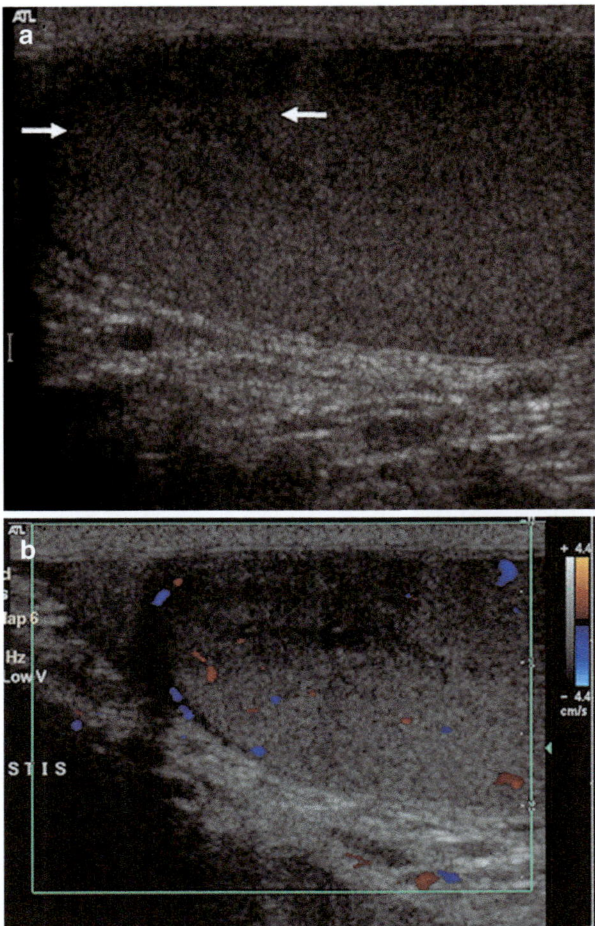

Fig. 7.7.1

Fig. 7.7.2

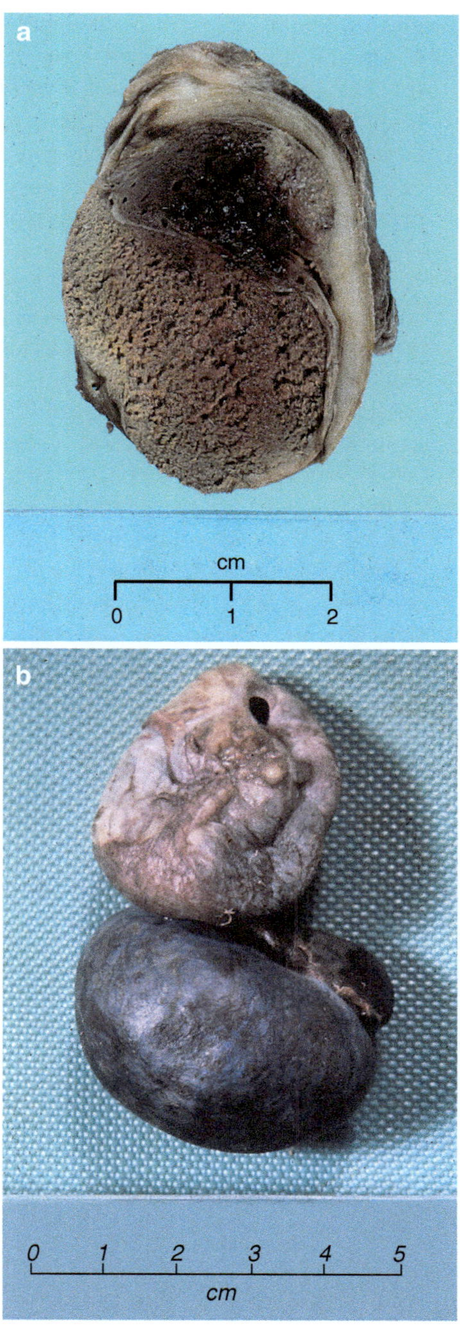

Answers to Case 7.7

1. There is a focal oval rounded region of low echoreflectivity with ill-defined margins within the periphery of the upper right testis on the longitudinal grey-scale image (Fig. 7.7.1a; between arrows). This is avascular on colour Doppler (Fig. 7.7.1b). The adjacent epididymal head (best seen in Fig. 7.7.1b) is normal in appearance and vascularity. These features could reflect an acute focal testicular infarction, but any cause of an avascular hypoechoic mass in the testis, such as a testicular tumour or abscess could give this appearance. In this case however, the history of sickle cell disease and a predisposing infection triggering a vasoocclusive crisis, makes focal infarction the likely diagnosis.
2. Acute focal infarction can occur as a consequence of epididymo-orchitis, surgical trauma (e.g., following inguinal hernia repair), hypercoagulable states such as polycythaemia rubra vera and sickle cell disease, and also the vasculitides. However, testicular torsion can also rarely give rise to focal infarction. A thorough history should be sought, and if there is any suspicion of torsion, surgical exploration is required. In cases where there is no obvious predisposing factor for infarction, it would not be unreasonable to perform sonographic surveillance of the lesion, or to proceed to biopsy, to exclude the possibility of a testicular tumour, as there are no distinguishing features on ultrasound alone.
3. Figure 7.7.2a shows the cut surface of an orchidectomy specimen with an area of haemorrhage in the epididymis. Microscopy revealed recent infarction resulting from arteritis. The testis showed older foci of ischaemic change.

   Figure 7.7.2b shows florid recent infarction following torsion.

Further Reading

Bilagi P, Sriprasad S, Clarke JL, Sellars ME, Muir GH, Sidhu PS. Clinical and ultrasound features of segmental testicular infarction: six-year experience from a single centre. *Eur Radiol.* 2007;17(11):2810–2818.

Dogra VS, Gottlieb RH, Rubens DJ, Liao L. Benign intratesticular cystic lesions: US features. *Radiographics.* 2001;21 Spec No:S273–S281.

Flanagan JJ, Fowler RC. Testicular infarction mimicking tumour on scrotal ultrasound—a potential pitfall. *Clin Radiol.* 1995;50(1):49–50.

Case 7.8

The ultrasound image (Fig. 7.8.1) below was taken from a 16-year-old patient with painless gradual enlargement of the scrotum. The macroscopic picture (Fig. 7.8.2a) is from a different patient with the same condition. Figure 7.8.2b represents a complication.

1. Describe the abnormality shown in Figs. 7.8.1 and 7.8.2, and name the layers labelled a and b.
2. In what conditions may this occur?

Fig. 7.8.1

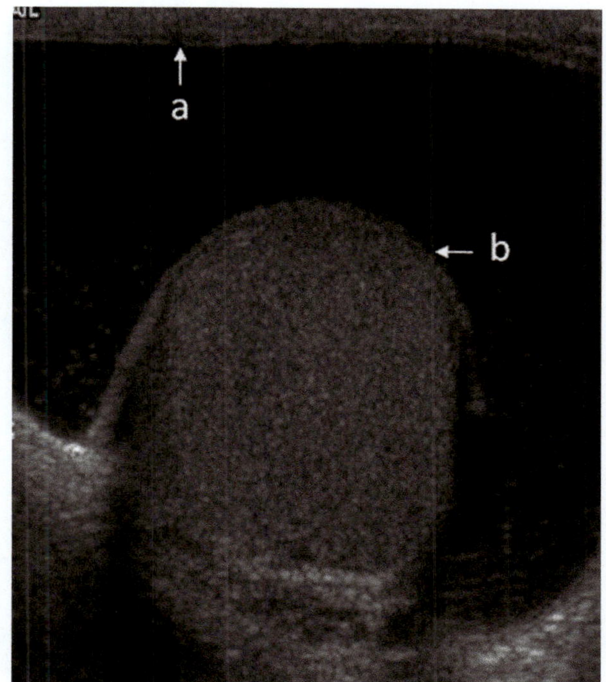

Fig. 7.8.2

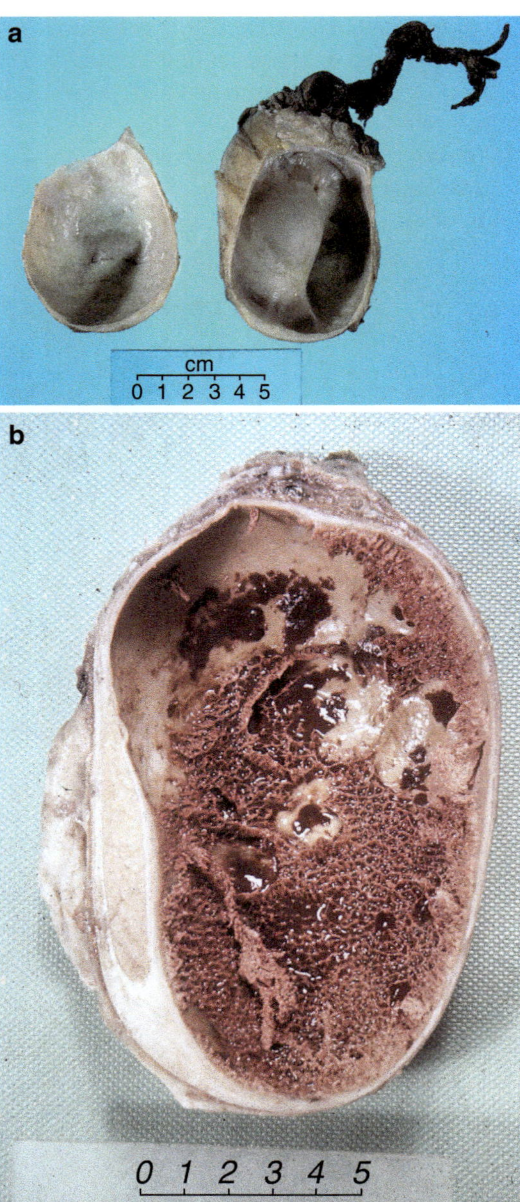

Answers to Case 7.8

1. Figures 7.8.1 and 7.8.2a demonstrate a hydrocele. Figure 7.8.1 is single transverse grey-scale sonogram demonstrating a large, anechoic fluid collection, with some low level internal echoes, surrounding the testis. This fluid is located between the parietal and visceral layers of the tunica vaginalis, which have been labelled a and b respectively. Figure 7.8.2a demonstrates a hydrocele, where the anterior parietal layer of the tunica vaginalis has been removed to reveal the visceral layer overlying the testis. A small amount of fluid, usually only a few millimetres in thickness, is normally present within this space, but such a large collection is consistent with a hydrocele. A hydrocele is the most common cause of scrotal swelling, and may be bilateral. The low level echoes seen in Fig. 7.8.1 are due to protein or cholesterol content, or less commonly to the presence of blood (Fig. 7.8.2b) or inflammatory debris, in a haematocele or pyocele, respectively. More marked septations or loculation may be seen in chronic hydroceles.
2. A hydrocele may occur for a variety of reasons. In children, congenital hydroceles are usually the result of a patent processus vaginalis that communicates with the peritoneal cavity, thereby allowing free flow of fluid. The patent processus vaginalis usually closes within the first 2 years of life, but after this it is unlikely to resolve, and a high ligation of the processus is usually required.

   In adults, hydroceles are usually idiopathic, but they may occur as a consequence of other pathology such as trauma, infection, testicular torsion or malignancy. Initial treatment is aimed at the underlying condition, but idiopathic or refractory hydroceles may be treated surgically. Aspiration and sclerotherapy have also been described but the recurrence rates are high. A large hydrocoele may occasionally compromise the blood flow to the testis, or lead to testicular atrophy if chronic, and these features may also be observed sonographically.

Further Reading

Bhatt S, Rubens DJ, Dogra VS. Sonography of benign intrascrotal lesions. *Ultrasound Q*. 2006;22(2):121–136.

Lau ST, Lee YH, Caty MG. Current management of hernias and hydrocoeles. *Semin Pediatr Surg*. 2007;16(1):50–57.

Case 7.9

A 14-year-old boy presented with a mass in his scrotum. Examine the figures below (Fig. 7.9.1). What is the diagnosis?

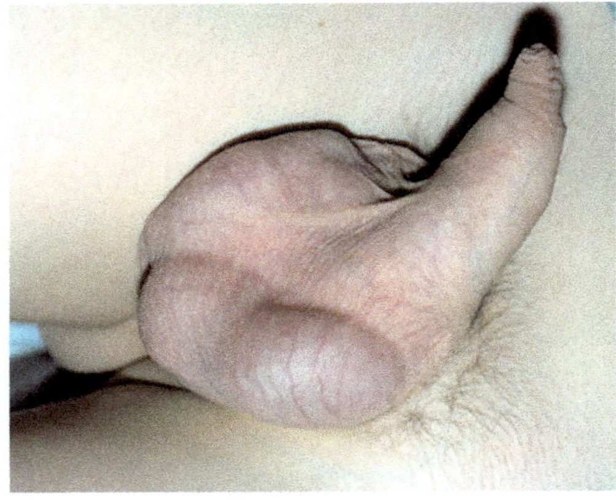

Fig. 7.9.1

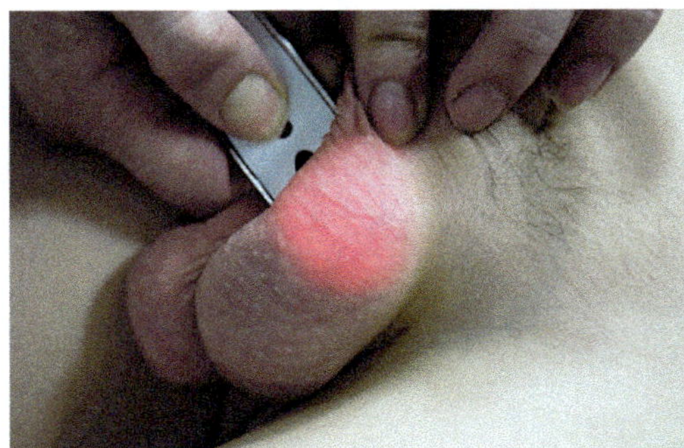

Fig. 7.9.2

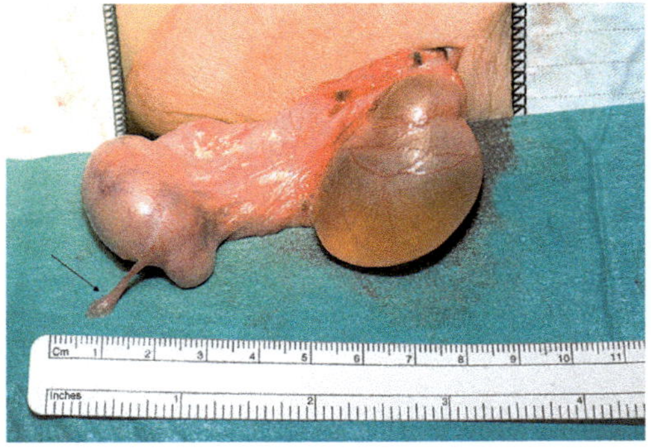

Fig. 7.9.3

Answers to Case 7.9

1. There is a 3 cm fluctuant mass superior to and separate from the left epididymis, it transilluminates (Fig. 7.9.2).This is a hydrocoele of the spermatic cord and the treatment is surgical excision. Figure 7.9.3 also demonstrates a testicular appendage (arrow), which is present on 90% of testes.

Case 7.10

A 28-year-old man was referred for a scrotal ultrasound with a history of chronic left sided scrotal discomfort. Ultrasound examination demonstrated a normal right testis. Two ultrasound images of the left testis are presented in the figures below.

1. Describe the sonographic findings and the likely diagnosis.
2. What are some of the usual sonographic characteristics of this lesion? How was the image in Fig. 7.10.1b obtained?

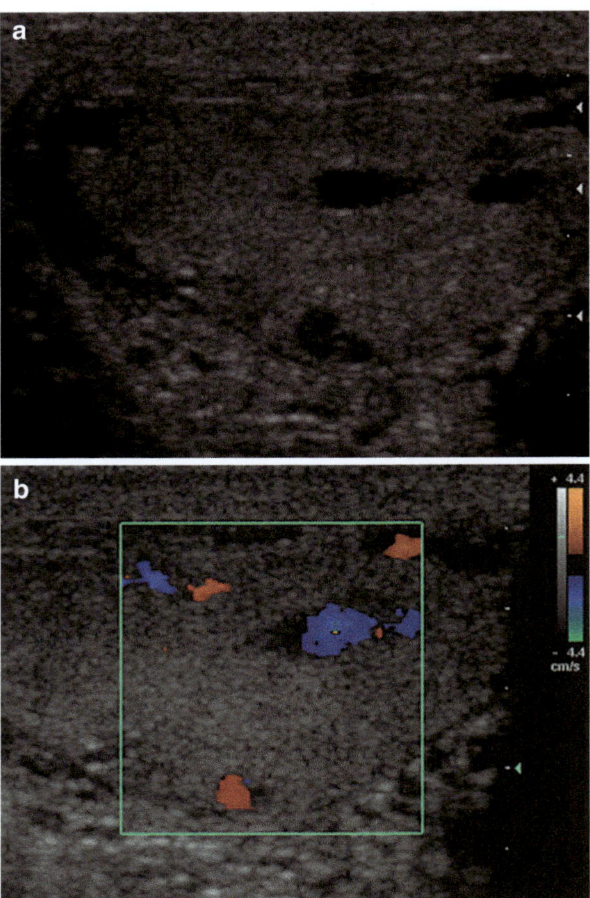

Fig. 7.10.1

Answers to Case 7.10

1. The grey-scale sonographic image (Fig. 7.10.1a) shows multiple tubular or/oval, anechoic dilated structures within the left testis, some of which are located close to the tunica albuginea. Colour Doppler imaging (Fig. 7.10.1b) reveals vascular flow within these vessels, which was venous in nature, being non-pulsatile. The most likely diagnosis is an intratesticular varicocele. The differential diagnosis for vascular lesions of this nature would include an intratesticular pseudoaneurysm, but this can normally be quite easily distinguished by its high velocity, turbulent flow. No extratesticular varicocoele was noted in this case.
2. Intratesticular varicocele has been described relatively recently. They are similar in sonographic characteristics to extratesticular varicocoele, being composed of multiple intratesticular anechoic tubular or oval structures with venous flow on colour Doppler imaging, especially during Valsalva manoeuvre. Up to 40% of patients may have flow demonstrated only with Valsalva manoeuvre. Imaging the patient standing and/or with a Valsalva manoeuvre is therefore crucial, and the colour Doppler image in Fig. 7.10.1b has been obtained this way. They appear to occur closer to the mediastinum testis, and, like extratesticular varicocele, have a left-sided preponderance. Recent reports suggest that intratesticular varicoceles occur more frequently in the presence of extratesticular varicoceles, and that there is an association with ipsilateral testicular atrophy, but the clinical relevance of this condition is still speculative.

Further Reading

Das KM, Prasad K, Szmigielski W, Noorani N. Intratesticular varicocoele: evaluation using conventional and Doppler sonography. *AJR Am J Roentgenol.* 1999;173(4):1079–1083.

Tetreau R, Julian P, Lyonnet D, Rouviere O. Intratesticular varicocoele: an easy diagnosis but unclear physiopathologic characteristics. *J Ultrasound Med.* 2007;26(12):1767–1773.

Case 7.11

A 63-year-old man presented with a one-month history of low-grade fever and night sweats together with a left-sided scrotal swelling that was occasionally painful. Images from an ultrasound examination of his left testis (Fig. 7.11.1a, b), a single axial image from a CT of his pelvis (Fig. 7.11.2) and an orchidectomy specimen from a different patient with the same condition (Fig. 7.11.3a and b) are presented below.

1. Describe the main sonographic findings in Fig. 7.11.1a, b.
2. What are the abnormalities highlighted by the straight arrow in Fig. 7.11.2 and seen in Fig. 7.11.3a and what is the likely diagnosis?
3. How should this patient be further investigated?
4. What haematological malignancies may be seen in the testis?

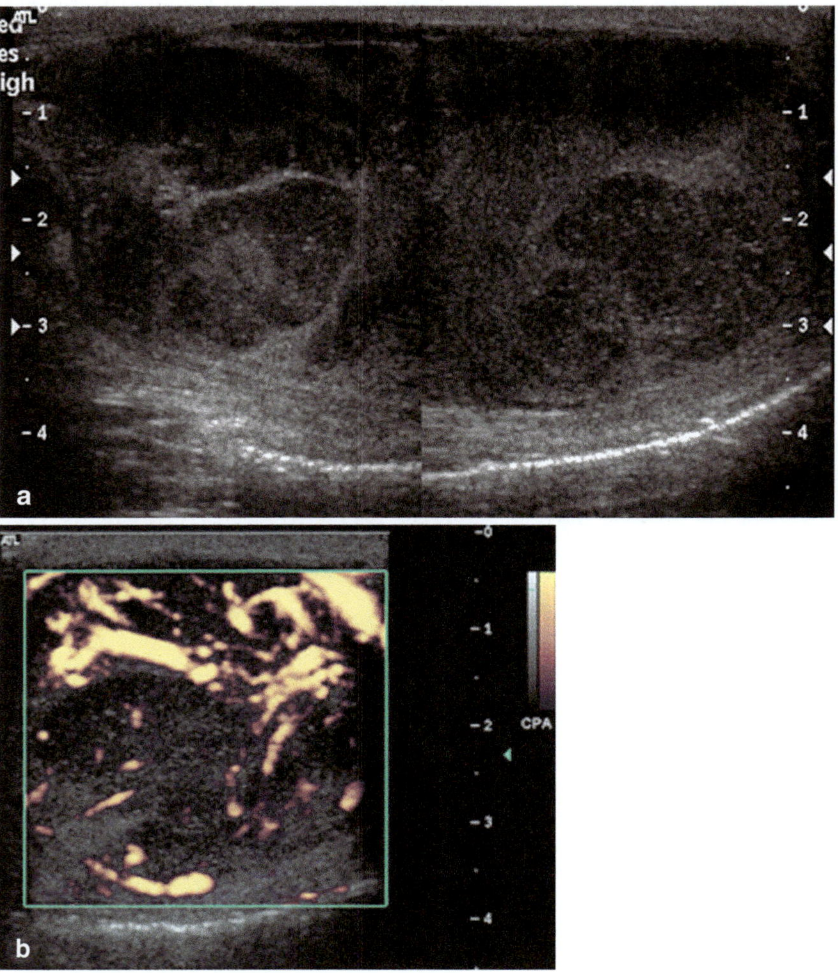

Fig. 7.11.1

Fig. 7.11.2

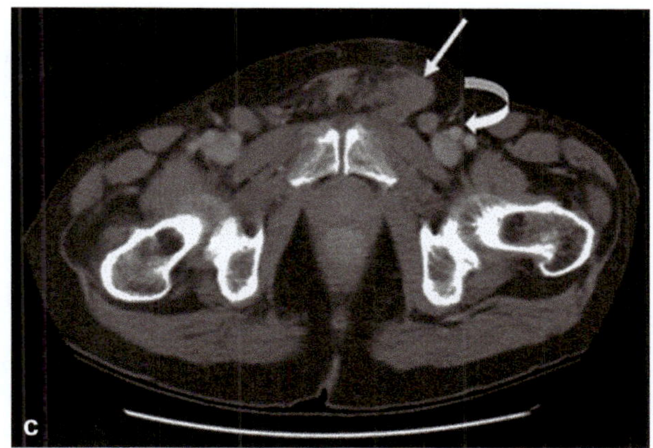

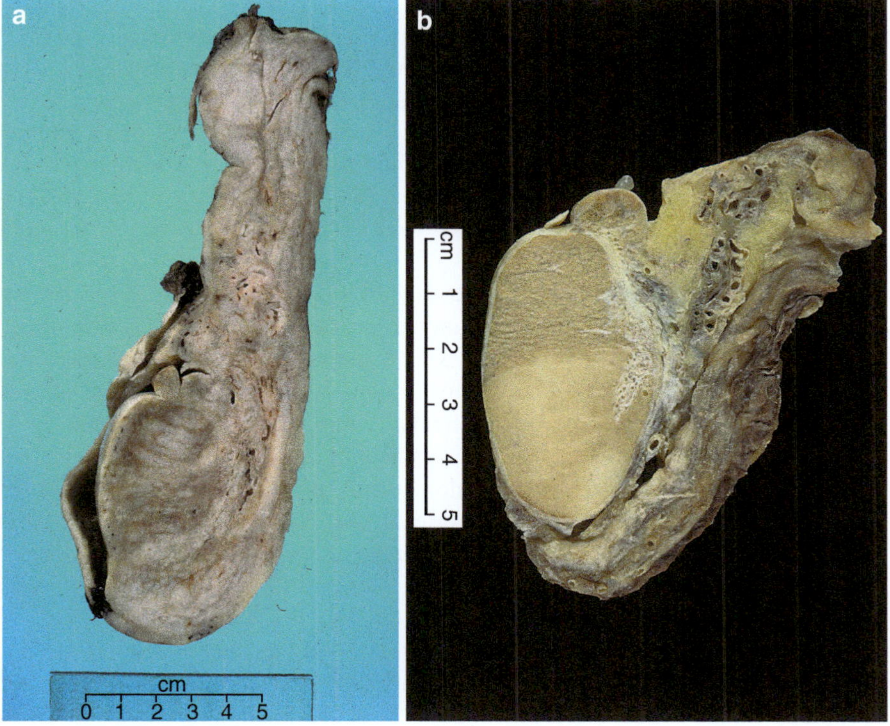

Fig. 7.11.3

Answers to Case 7.11

1. Figure 7.11.1a is a composite image of an enlarged left testis, in which there are multiple discrete hypoechoic masses which have almost completely replaced the testis. These masses do not have easily definable margins, with foci of increased echo reflectivity. They are hypervascular on Doppler imaging (Fig. 7.11.1b). There are no cystic or calcific foci present.
2. Figure 7.11.2 is a single axial CT image of the patient's pelvis at the level of the pubic symphysis. The straight arrow highlights gross enlargement of the left spermatic cord, medial to the left femoral vessels within the femoral sheath (curved arrow). The patient's age, clinical presentation and imaging features point to testicular lymphoma as the likely diagnosis. Figure 7.11.3a shows the cut surface of an orchidectomy specimen showing extensive infiltration of the testis epididymis and cord by ill-defined grey/white tissue classified microscopically as diffuse large B-cell lymphoma.

   Primary testicular lymphoma is the most common testicular neoplasm in men over the age of 50 (spermatocytic seminoma being next most common), and is most frequently of the type diagnosed in both these patients. Lymphoma is the most common bilateral testicular tumour, with bilateral, usually metachronous, tumours detected in up to 35% of patients. Spread to the epididymis, spermatic cord (as in Figs. 7.11.2a and 7.11.3a), and retroperitoneal lymph nodes are often seen.

   Grey-scale sonographic appearances vary from ill-defined enlargement of the entire testis, with decreased echoreflectivity, only appreciated when compared with the normal contralateral testis, to multiple discrete hypoechoic masses. They usually demonstrate avid intralesional vascularity. However, these imaging features are not specific enough to be considered diagnostic of testicular lymphoma.
3. Subsequent investigations are similar to those performed for any suspected testicular tumour (see NSGCT and seminoma sections), with histological confirmation obtained at orchidectomy. However, staging investigations similar to those performed for any lymphoma are also crucial. Bone marrow aspiration will therefore be imperative. Primary testicular lymphoma has a high propensity for spread to uncommon extranodal sites such as central nervous system, skin and Waldeyer's ring. Thus, CT of the abdomen and pelvis should be extended to the neck and thorax to accurately detect nodal and Waldeyer's ring disease, while MRI of the brain and CSF examination may also be necessary. Unfortunately there is still a high rate of relapse, and overall prognosis remains poor with a median survival of 12–24 months.
4. Testicular involvement by leukaemic infiltrates is not uncommon but rarely clinically apparent. Plasmacytoma is usually an extramedullary manifestation of multiple myeloma and is seen presenting as a testicular mass in the lower half of the testis in Fig. 7.11.3b.

Further Reading

Mazzu D, Jeffrey RB, Jr., Ralls PW. Lymphoma and leukaemia involving the testicles: findings on gray-scale and color Doppler sonography. *AJR Am J Roentgenol.* 1995;164(3):645–647.

Moller MB, d'Amore F, Christensen BE. Testicular lymphoma: a population-based study of incidence, clinicopathological correlations and prognosis. The Danish Lymphoma Study Group, LYFO. *Eur J Cancer.* 1994;30A(12):1760–1764.

Vitolo U, Ferreri AJ, Zucca E. Primary testicular lymphoma. *Crit Rev Oncol Hematol.* 2008;65(2):183–189.

Case 7.12

These two images are from a high-frequency ultrasound study of a 27- year old man presenting with a painless palpable lump of the right testis (Fig. 7.12.1a, b) and both macroscopic and microscopic illustrations from orchidectomy specimens from a patient with a similar problem (Fig. 7.12.2a, b).

1. Describe the abnormalities seen, and state the most likely diagnosis.
2. What further investigations should be performed, and how do they help direct management?

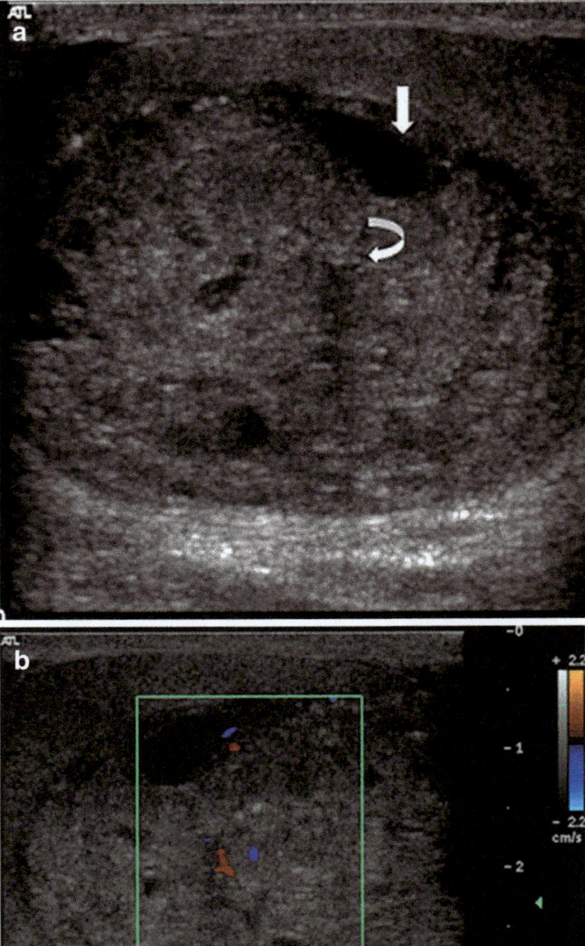

Fig. 7.12.1

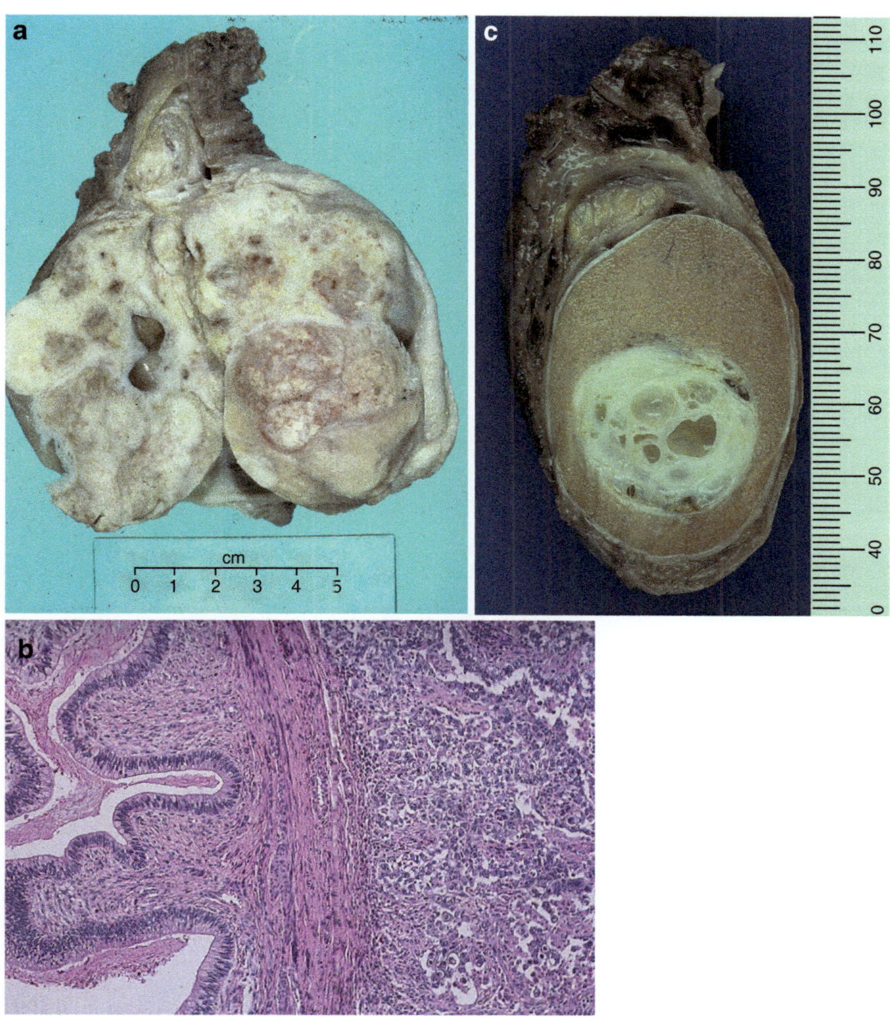

Fig. 7.12.2

Answers to Case 7.12

1. In Fig. 7.12.1a, there is large heterogeneous testicular mass with well-defined irregular margins, areas of cystic change (arrow) and punctate calcification with some acoustic shadowing (curved arrow). Figure 7.12.1b demonstrates its poor vascularity. The mass is consistent with a testicular tumour, and given the cystic and calcific foci, a non-seminomatous germ cell tumour (NSGCT) is favoured, although tumour types are not reliably distinguished on imaging. Pure embryonal cell carcinomas often appear to have multiple cystic areas on USS, and invade the tunica albuginea, giving the testis a lobulated outline. Pure differentiated teratomas tend to be more well-defined, but may have similar cystic areas, and demonstrate calcification (with or without posterior acoustic shadowing).

   The tumour in Fig. 7.12.1 proved to be a mixed germ cell tumour with predominantly embryonal cell carcinoma elements, as seen in Fig. 7.12.2a, b. The former shows a bivalved orchidectomy extensively replaced by a heterogeneous nodular, solid and cystic mass. Microscopically (Fig. 7.12.2b) this was composed of teratomatous elements (left) and embryonal carcinoma (right). For comparison with Fig. 7.12.2a, in Fig. 7.12.2c the testis contains a well circumscribed fibro cystic mass which microscopically was composed of mature somatic elements typical of Teratoma.
2. Further investigations are aimed at securing a histopathological diagnosis and clinical staging, using serum tumour markers, plain chest radiography and cross-sectional imaging to decide treatment strategy. Mixed NSGCTs are the second most common type of germ cell tumour encountered after seminomas. The most common histological subtype seen within mixed NSGCTs is embryonal cell carcinoma (up to 87%), followed by differentiated teratoma, yolk sac tumour, and choriocarcinoma. Serum tumour markers, especially α-fetoprotein (AFP) and β-human chorionic gonadotrophin (β-HCG) are likely to be raised in up to 90% of NSGCT. In contrast only 20% of seminomas are associated with an elevated β -HCG at presentation. Alpha fetoprotein is not produced by pure classical seminomas. Tumour markers provide a prognostic index, and help in assessment of treatment response, though there is still disagreement over whether the rate of initial decrease of tumour markers correlates with prognosis.

   CT of thorax and abdomen is used for nodal staging. A retroperitoneal node >8 mm in short axis is considered a positive node on conventional CT criteria. Enlarged nodes will generally be seen ipsilateral to the tumour, but crossover nodal enlargement can be identified, with crossover metastases from right to left observed much more frequently than left to right. However, CT may have a false-negative rate of up to 30% due to small volume disease. MRI is comparable to CT in staging accuracy for nodes, but cannot stage the lungs. Distant metastases are seen in the lung, liver, brain and bone, in order of decreasing frequency. Patients with high β-HCG levels (>10,000 IU/L) or multiple (>20) pulmonary metastases are considered at high-risk of cerebral metastases and would benefit from MR imaging of the brain.

The overall cure rate of stage I germ cell tumour remains excellent, at about 99%, though the rate of relapse after orchidectomy alone is approximately 25–30% for stage I NSGCT and 15–20% for stage 1 seminoma. Relapse occurs mostly within the first 2 years following orchidectomy for NSGCT, though there is a small but clinically significant risk of relapse more than 5 years after orchidectomy for stage I seminoma which supports the need for long term follow-up. Patients with NSGCT at higher risk of relapse include those with lymphovascular invasion, the presence of embryonal cell carcinoma, and the absence of yolk sac tumour. Tumour size >4 cm and tumour involvement of the rete testis increases the likelihood of relapse in men with seminoma.

Primary treatment of stage 1 NSGCT involves orchidectomy and in high risk patients adjuvant chemotherapy usually with bleomycin, etoposide and cisplatin. For patients with stage 1 seminoma orchidectomy alone is used or if there are adverse pathological findings adjuvant carboplatin or dog-leg radiotherapy.

Further Reading

Albers P. Management of stage I testis cancer. *Eur Urol.* 2007;51(1):34–43.

Horwich A, Shipley J, Huddart R. Testicular germ-cell cancer. *Lancet.* 2006;367 (9512):754–765.

Sohaib SA, Koh DM, Husband JE. The role of imaging in the diagnosis, staging, and management of testicular cancer. *AJR Am J Roentgenol.* 2008; 191(2): 387–395.

Woodward PJ, Sohaey R, O'Donoghue MJ, Green DE. From the archives of the AFIP: tumors and tumorlike lesions of the testis: radiologic-pathologic correlation. *Radiographics.* 2002;22(1):189–216.

Case 7.13

A 75-year-old man presented with a palpable lump in the right inguinal region, as well as a right-sided scrotal swelling. He gave no prior history of trauma, and had otherwise been well.

Figure 7.13.1a, b are focused ultrasound images of the lump within the right inguinal canal, while Fig. 7.13.1c is a single axial pelvic image from his CT scan performed on the same day. Examples of resection specimens for similar conditions are shown in Fig. 7.13.2a–c

1. Describe the abnormalities seen below.
2. What is the differential diagnosis in this patient?

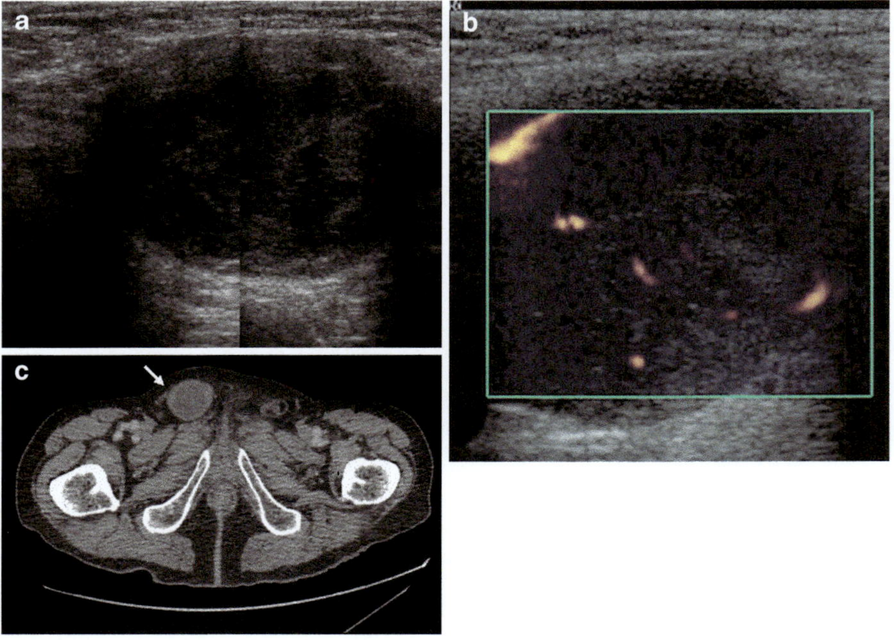

Fig. 7.13.1

Fig. 7.13.2

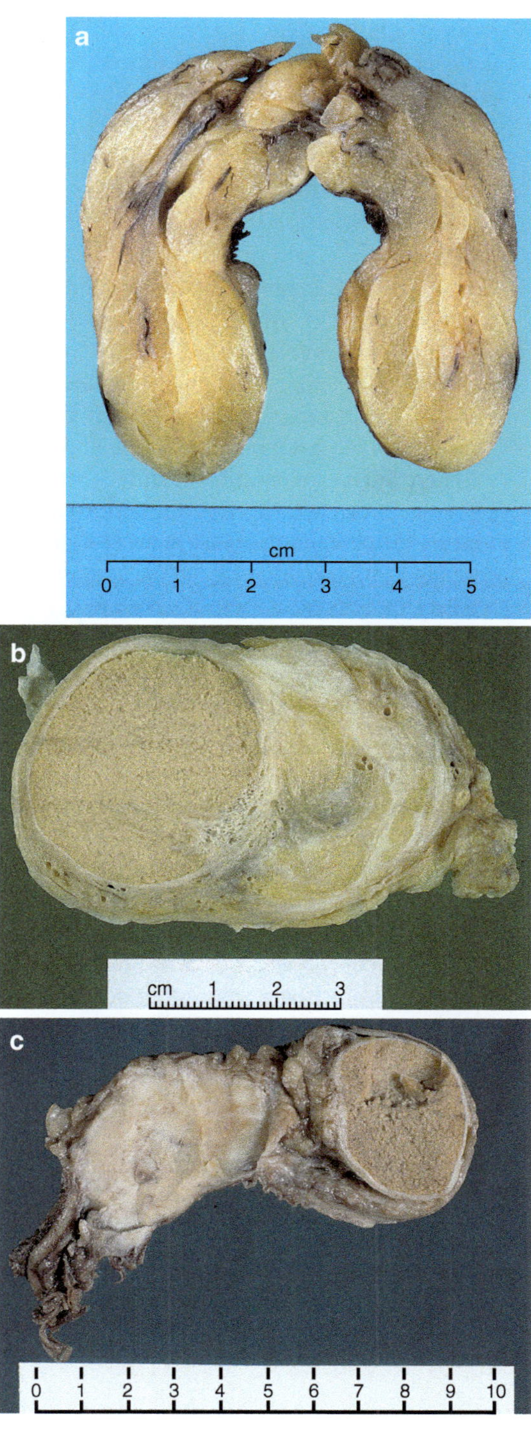

Answers to Case 7.13

1. Figure 7.13.1a, b demonstrate a slightly vascular focal well-circumscribed ovoid mass within the right inguinal canal. The mass could be traced into the right hemiscrotum, where swelling of the right epididymis was also noted. Both testes and left epididymis were normal. The single CT image in Fig. 7.13.1c demonstrates the same lesion, which can now be clearly seen to lie in the right spermatic cord (arrow). It is of slightly low density with respect to muscle and soft tissue, but much higher density than the adjacent fat.
2. The appearances are in keeping with a tumour of the spermatic cord. As the spermatic cord is embryologically derived from mesoderm, the malignant tumours most frequently seen at this site are sarcomas. In this older age group, the most common type of sarcomatous tumour is a liposarcoma. However, fatty elements of a liposarcoma are usually easy to identify as tissue of fat density on CT or MRI. As no such elements are present here, other sarcomas such as leiomyosarcoma, malignant fibrous histiocytomas and undifferentiated sarcoma should be considered in the differential diagnosis.

   There are no sonographic features that help to distinguish the various types of sarcoma. It can also be very difficult to distinguish a malignant tumour from a benign lipoma on ultrasound alone. Lipoma is the most common extratesticular neoplasm and usually arises in the spermatic cord. MR imaging is very useful to identify fat content within these lesions. Figure 7.13.2a is a bisected lipoma of the cord, with a fine fibrous capsule and microscopically composed of benign mature adipose tissue. Figure 7.13.2b is a transverse section of an orchidectomy specimen in which the paratestis is expanded by fibro fatty tissue seen microscopically to be liposarcoma. Figure 7.13.2c is the cut surface of an orchidectomy specimen in which the cord is replaced and expanded by a white fibrous mass, macroscopically found to be a malignant fibrous histiocytoma.

Further Reading

Cramer BM, Schlegel EA, Thueroff JW. MR imaging in the differential diagnosis of scrotal and testicular disease. *Radiographics*. 1991; 1(1):9–21.

Woodward PJ, Schwab CM, Sesterhenn IA. From the archives of the AFIP: extratesticular scrotal masses: radiologic-pathologic correlation. *Radiographics*. 2003; 23(1):215–240.

Case 7.14

These two ultrasound images have been obtained from examination of a 42-year-old patient, presenting with a painless palpable lump of the left testis. The right testis was normal on palpation and sonography. Figure 7.14.2a, b show surgical resections for a similar condition.

1. Describe the abnormalities seen in Fig. 7.14.1a, b state your most likely diagnosis and give a differential diagnosis.
2. Describe your subsequent management of this patient.

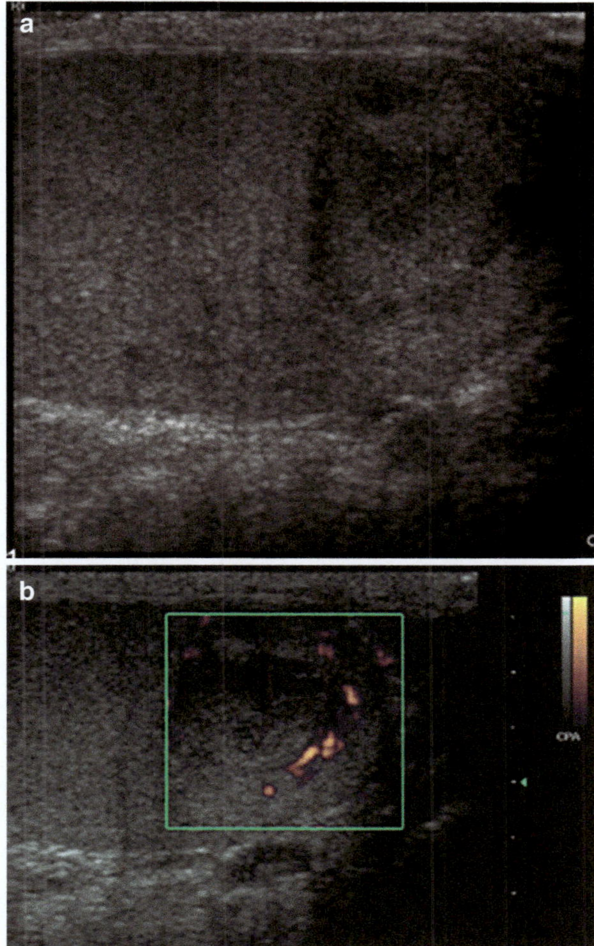

Fig. 7.14.1

Fig. 7.14.2

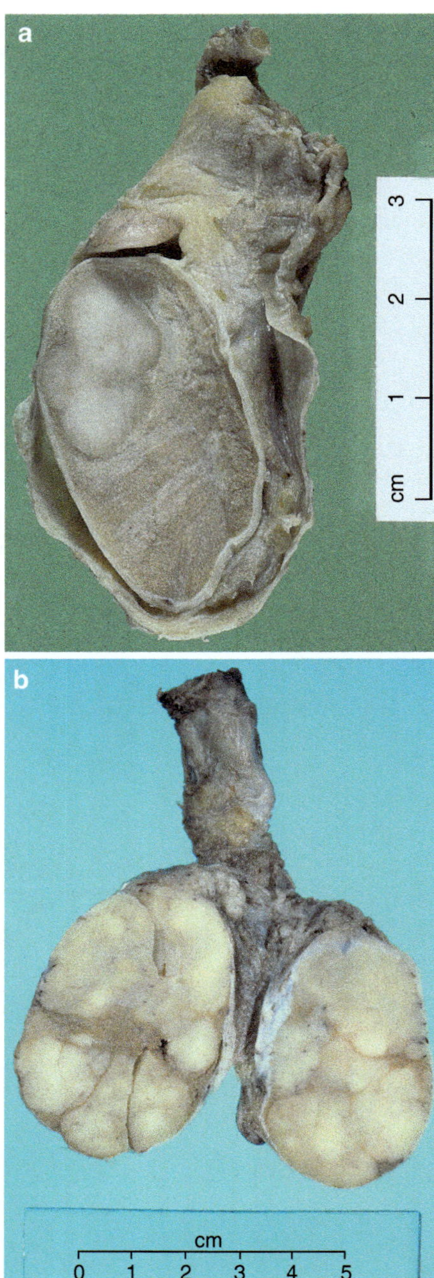

Answers to Case 7.14

1. The longitudinal grey-scale image of the testis (Fig. 7.14.1a) demonstrates a solitary, slightly heterogeneous but predominantly low reflective mass with a well-defined hypoechoic rim. Calcification and cystic areas are absent. Vascularity is predominantly peripheral on the Doppler image (Fig. 7.14.1b). In the absence of any history of trauma, inflammation or pain, the most likely diagnosis is a primary testicular tumour. The well-defined nature of the mass, and the absence of cystic change make seminoma the most likely diagnosis, although neither ultrasound nor MR imaging appearances are accurate in distinguishing testicular tumour types. Seminomas may also be multinodular or lobulated, simulating multifocal masses and may rarely be bilateral (2% of patients), when they are usually metachronous. However, the imaging appearances alone could also be compatible with a chronic testicular abscess. This case thus illustrates the inability of ultrasound to differentiate malignancy from focal inflammation within the testis. Clinical correlation is thus important. Doppler ultrasound can be useful in distinguishing these focal masses from a post-traumatic haematoma, which would be avascular. This can help identify incidental tumours in patients with scrotal trauma.

   The orchidectomy specimens (Fig. 7.14.2a, b) are from two different patients both of which were seen to be invaded by classical seminoma on microscopy.
2. As imaging and clinical features are non-specific, the subsequent management is aimed at securing an accurate pathological diagnosis and clinical staging to guide treatment and for prognostication.

   Testicular tumours are broadly classified as Testicular neoplasms are broadly classified as germ cell tumours (TGCT) or gonadal stromal tumours. The two main groups of TGCT are seminomas and non-seminomatous germ cell tumours (NSGCTs). Seminomas are the most common testicular tumour in adults (approximately 50%). Measurement of serum alpha-fetoprotein (α-FP), beta- human chorionic gonadotrophin (β-HCG) and lactate dehydrogenase (LDH) levels provide valuable staging information. α-FP is not produced by pure seminomas, while β-HCG is secreted by both tumour groups, (see Case 7.12) with high levels (>10,000 IU/L) seen in aggressive NSGCT types, including choriocarcinomatous elements. Up to 25% of patients with seminoma have metastatic disease at presentation, and thus CT staging of the thorax and abdomen should be performed to identify metastatic and nodal spread, to retroperitoneal nodes in particular. Whole body 18-Flurodeoxyglucose positron-emission tomography (18FDG PET) adds no further value to the detection of metastases. Similarly to staging of NSGCT, MR imaging of the abdomen is comparable to CT, and has the advantage of avoiding exposure to ionising radiation, but cannot stage the lungs.

Further Reading

Albers P. Management of stage I testis cancer. *Eur Urol.* 2007;51(1):34–43.

Dalal PU, Sohaib SA, Huddart R. Imaging of testicular germ cell tumours. *Cancer Imaging.* 2006;6:124–134.

Woodward PJ, Sohaey R, O'Donoghue MJ, Green DE. From the archives of the AFIP: tumors and tumorlike lesions of the testis: radiologic-pathologic correlation. *Radiographics.* 2002;22(1):189–216.

Case 7.15

A 38-year-old man presents with a painless scrotal swelling 3 months after undergoing a vasectomy. On examination, there is a firm, discrete painless lump. Two images from the subsequent ultrasound examination of this lump are presented below.

Describe the findings and the most likely diagnosis.

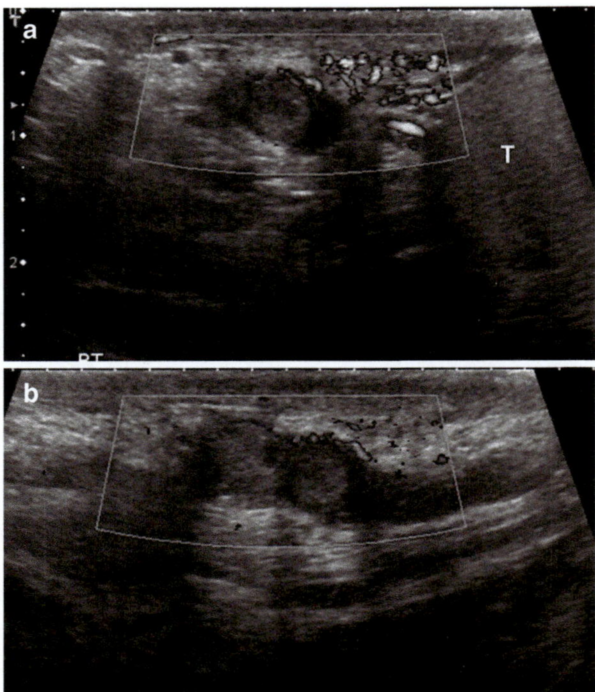

Fig. 7.15.1

Answers to Case 7.15

The longitudinal (Fig. 7.15.1a) and transverse (Fig. 7.15.1b) images demonstrate a discrete, solid and avascular hypoechoic mass, adjacent to the upper pole of the testis (testis labelled T in Fig. 7.15.1a). This is the typical appearance of a sperm granuloma.

Sperm granulomata are a reaction to spermatozoa that have escaped from the epididymis or vas into surrounding soft tissues. They may be intra- or extra-epididymal in location and occur in up to 40% of post-vasectomy patients, but are only rarely painful. Sonographic follow-up is usually unnecessary if the diagnosis has been confidently made. However, a follow-up ultrasound in 3–4 months to demonstrate no growth or change in the lesion is not an uncommon approach for reassurance or in equivocal cases.

Further Reading

Dogra VS, Gottlieb RH, Oka M, Rubens DJ. Sonography of the scrotum. *Radiology*. 2003;227(1):18–36.

Ramanathan K, Yaghoobian J, Pinck RL. Sperm granuloma. *J Clin Ultrasound*. 1986;14(2):155–156.

Reddy NM, Gerscovich EO, Jain KA, Le-Petross HT, Brock JM. Vasectomy-related changes on sonographic examination of the scrotum. *J Clin Ultrasound*. 2004;32(8):394–398.

Case 7.16

The images in Fig. 7.16.1a–c are grey-scale ultrasound images taken from three different patients, and depict the same incidental finding.

1. Describe the findings.
2. What conditions are associated with this?
3. What is the clinical significance of this abnormality?

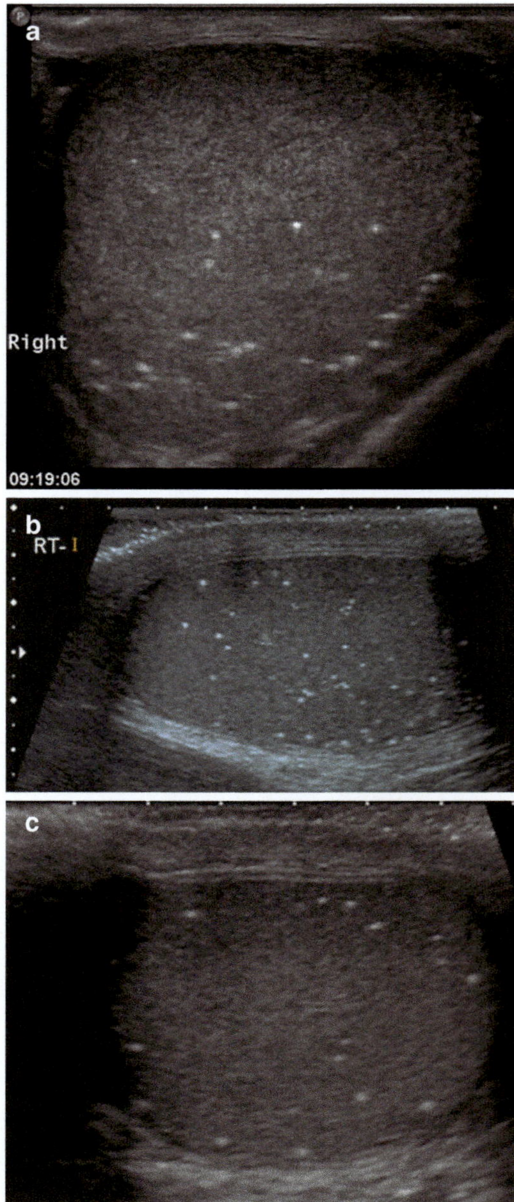

Fig. 7.16.1

Answers to Case 7.16

1. Figure 7.16.1a–c demonstrate multiple punctate echogenic foci. The appearances are consistent with testicular microlithiasis (TM). The prevalence of microlithiasis varies between 0.5 and 9%, with a higher prevalence noted in African American males. Sonographic definitions of testicular microlithiasis vary, but it is broadly accepted that five or more hyperechoic foci measuring <3 mm, with absent posterior acoustic shadowing, in either or both testes on at least one image is in keeping with this condition.
2. Most patients do not have an underlying associated condition, although it has been described in association with a multitude of conditions, including Klinefelter syndrome, undescended testis and Acquired Immune Deficiency Syndrome (AIDS).
3. The clinical significance of testicular microlithiasis arises from the observation that in patients with germ cell tumours areas of calcification (<200 μm) may be found in the seminiferous tubules. The issue of whether TM is associated with a predisposition to GCT has been addressed in a number of studies. Many of these studies were performed in groups already at high risk of testicular malignancy, and are further limited by their retrospective nature and short follow-up period. The number of reports documenting testicular cancer following previous ultrasound evidence of microlithiasis remains low. Thus, no causal relationship between testicular microlithiasis and malignancy has been proven. Although follow-up strategies are still debated, it is now acceptable to recommend careful self-examination, with repeat referral to the urologist reserved for any palpable abnormality, as the financial costs of an ultrasound-based screening programme are not justified.

Further Reading

Costabile RA. How worrisome is testicular microlithiasis? *Curr Opin Urol.* 2007;17(6):419–423.

Janzen DL, Mathieson JR, Marsh JI, Cooperberg PL, del RP, Golding RH, et al. Testicular microlithiasis: sonographic and clinical features. *AJR Am J Roentgenol.* 1992;158(5):1057–1060.

Peterson AC, Bauman JM, Light DE, McMann LP, Costabile RA. The prevalence of testicular microlithiasis in an asymptomatic population of men 18 to 35 years old. *J Urol.* 2001;166(6):2061–2064.

Case 7.17

These images of the right testis were taken from an emergency scrotal ultrasound performed on a 28-year-old motorcyclist who presented with a painful swollen scrotum, after collision with a car, resulting in impact with the motorcycle handlebars.

1. Describe the abnormalities and the likely diagnosis.
2. How should this patient be managed?

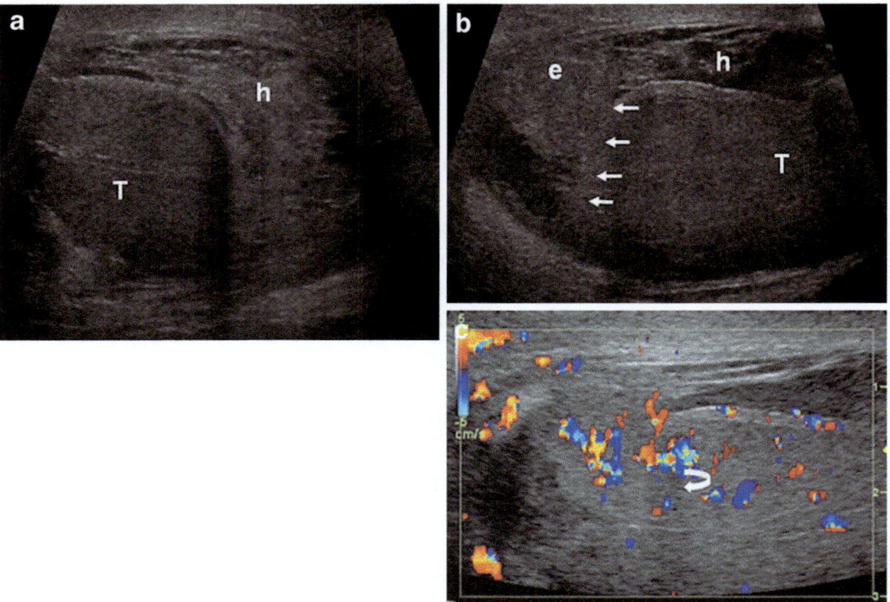

Fig. 7.17.1

Answers to Case 7.17

1. The transverse (Fig. 7.17.1a) and longitudinal (Fig. 7.17.1b) grey-scale ultrasound images demonstrate a large heterogeneous, extratesticular collection (h) within the scrotal sac in keeping with a haematocele. The right testis (T) has poorly defined margins at its upper pole (Fig. 7.17.1b, straight arrows), with extrusion of the testicular contents (e). Colour Doppler imaging (Fig. 7.17.1c; curved arrow) demonstrates preserved vascularity. The appearances are those of testicular rupture.
2. This patient requires immediate surgical exploration. Other indications for exploration include non-perfusion of the testis, or a high clinical suspicion in the presence of an equivocal ultrasound study. It can sometimes be difficult to distinguish testicular extrusion from haematocele, or the tunica albuginea may not be easily visualised, and subtle breaches may be missed. Studies have suggested that using a single criterion of heterogeneous testicular echotexture with loss of definition of the tunica albuginea, even in the absence of testicular extrusion or haematocele provide a specificity and sensitivity of over 90% for testicular rupture. Nevertheless, surgical exploration should be performed at the earliest suspicion of testicular rupture to maximise testicular salvage rates, as the salvage rate can fall from 90% in the first 72 h to 45% after this point.

Further Reading

Amaechi I, Sidhu PS. Ultrasound in the assessment of the "on-call" acute scrotum. *Imaging*. 2008;20(2):131–138.

Buckley JC, McAninch JW. Use of ultrasonography for the diagnosis of testicular injuries in blunt scrotal trauma. *J Urol*. 2006;175(1):175–178.

Guichard G, El AJ, Del CC, Cellarier D, Loock PY, Chabannes E, et al. Accuracy of ultrasonography in diagnosis of testicular rupture after blunt scrotal trauma. *Urology*. 2008;71(1):52–56.

Case 7.18

The two ultrasound images (below) are of the left testis in an 80-year old patient presenting with an initially painful, palpable lump, which had progressed to an exudative boggy swelling. In his youth, the patient had spent a number of years serving as an officer with the British Army in Southeast Asia. He was afebrile and had sterile pyuria on urinalysis. An orchidectomy specimen from a patient with the same condition is seen in Fig. 7.18.2.

1. Describe the ultrasound and pathology images and what is the most likely diagnosis?
2. Which categories of patients may be at risk of this condition?
3. What complications may arise from this condition, and how should this condition be managed?

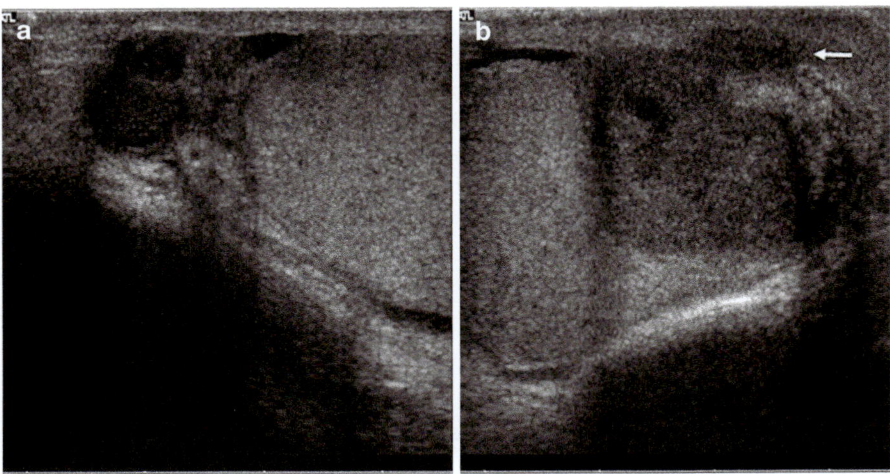

Fig. 7.18.1

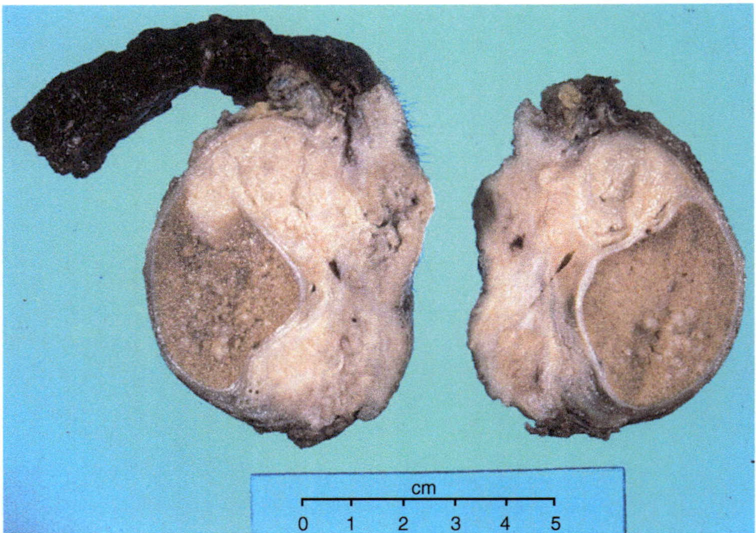

Fig. 7.18.2

Answers to Case 7.18

1. Figure 7.18.1a is a longitudinal grey-scale USS image of the left epididymal head and upper pole of the left testis. This demonstrates multiple heterogeneous, hypoechoic nodular masses of varying sizes in the epididymal head. Figure 7.18.1b confirms these findings in the transverse plane, but additionally a fistulating track can be seen extending out from the mass (arrow). The findings are in keeping with an epididymal abscess, and in the context of this patient's history, the most likely diagnosis is tuberculous epididymo-orchitis. Figure 7.18.2 shows a bi-valved orchidectomy specimen in which the epididymis is effaced by fibro-caseous tissue. A sinus necessitated excision of scrotal skin. Microscopically in the testis there were multiple granulomas, in which the presence of Ziehl - Neelsen positive bacilli confirmed a diagnosis of tuberculosis.

   Tuberculous epididymo-orchitis usually results from haematogenous spread of tuberculosis (TB). While genitourinary TB is rare, it represents the most common form of extrapulmonary TB, with tuberculous epididymo-orchitis accounting for up to 22% cases of genitourinary TB. The latent period between pulmonary TB and the development of genitourinary TB can be as long as 30 years. There is a propensity for tuberculous epididymitis to originate at the epididymal tail. Isolated tuberculous orchitis without epididymal involvement is rare, though the converse may be seen. On sonography, there may be a diffusely enlarged heterogeneous or homogenous hypoechoic epididymis or nodular masses as in this case, due to a combination of caseating necrosis, granuloma formation, calcification and fibrosis. Other associated findings include scrotal skin thickening, hydrocoele, and intrascrotal but extratesticular calcification.
2. Patients at risk include: the immunocompromised, such as patients with Human Immunodeficiency Virus (HIV) infection, immunosuppressed organ transplant recipients and the elderly. Travellers to, and immigrants from, endemic areas are also at risk, as well as those who have received Bacille Calmette-Guérin (BCG) therapy for transitional cell carcinoma of the bladder.
3. Tuberculous epididymo-orchitis is more likely to lead to epididymal and testicular abscesses. Abscesses may in turn rupture into the scrotal sac, forming a pyocoele, or form sinus tracts through the scrotal skin.

Further Reading

Lee IK, Yang WC, Liu JW. Scrotal tuberculosis in adult patients: a 10-year clinical experience. *Am J Trop Med Hyg*. 2007;77(4):714–718.

Madeb R, Marshall J, Nativ O, Erturk E. Epididymal tuberculosis: case report and review of the literature. *Urology*. 2005;65(4):798.

Muttarak M, Peh WC, Lojanapiwat B, Chaiwun B. Tuberculous epididymitis and epididymo-orchitis: sonographic appearances. *AJR Am J Roentgenol*. 2001;176(6):1459–1466.

Case 7.19

A 45 year-old man presented with a small, painless, palpable and non-mobile lump in his left testis, and the relevant ultrasound image is shown below (Fig. 7.19.1).

1. Describe the abnormality and state the diagnosis.
2. What difficulties may arise in the ultrasound diagnosis of these lesions?

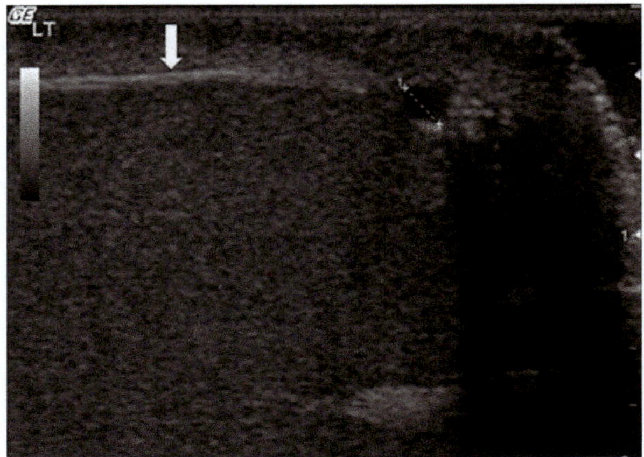

Fig. 7.19.1

Answers to Case 7.19

1. There is a single well-defined, 2 mm anechoic lesion (right side of image, being measured) with no discernible wall and with posterior acoustic enhancement. It is located on the periphery of the testicle, within the tunica albuginea itself. The tunica appears as a thin line of increased reflectivity (arrow). This lesion is characteristic of a tunica albuginea cyst.
2. Tunica albuginea cysts are benign cysts thought to be of mesothelial origin. They present at a mean age of 40 years, often as palpable lumps on self-examination, and can thus be a source of anxiety to the patient. The diagnosis can be made with confidence on sonography when they are small (2–5 mm), and located at the upper anterior or lateral aspects of the testis. However, differentiation from an intratesticular cyst can be difficult when tunica albuginea cysts are large. Conversely, they may be very small (<2 mm) and can be easily overlooked, unless ultrasound examination is focused directly over the palpated abnormality. They may also be multilocular or calcified.

Further Reading

Martinez-Berganza MT, Sarria L, Cozcolluela R, Cabada T, Escolar F, Ripa L. Cysts of the tunica albuginea: sonographic appearance. *AJR Am J Roentgenol.* 1998;170(1):183–185.

Poster RB, Spirt BA, Tamsen A, Surya BV. Complex tunica albuginea cyst simulating an intratesticular lesion. *Urol Radiol.* 1991;13(2):129–132.

The Penis

8

Dan Magrill and Nick Watkin

Case 8.1

1. What type of studies are these and what do they show?
2. What other investigations may be used to investigate this condition?
3. What are the causes and treatment of this condition?

S. Bott et al. (eds.), *Images in Urology*,
DOI 10.1007/978-0-85729-769-3_8,

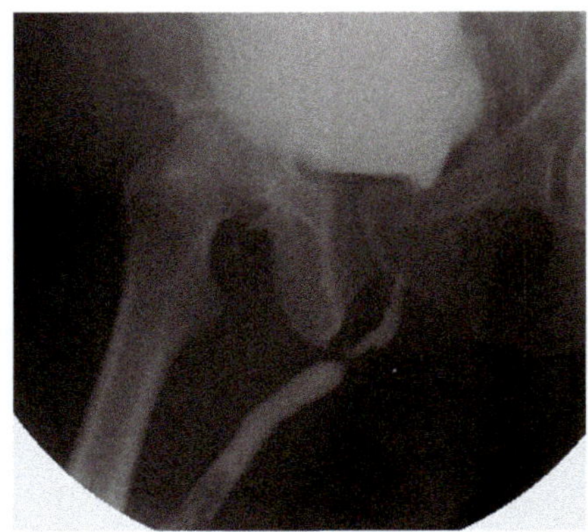

Fig. 8.1.1

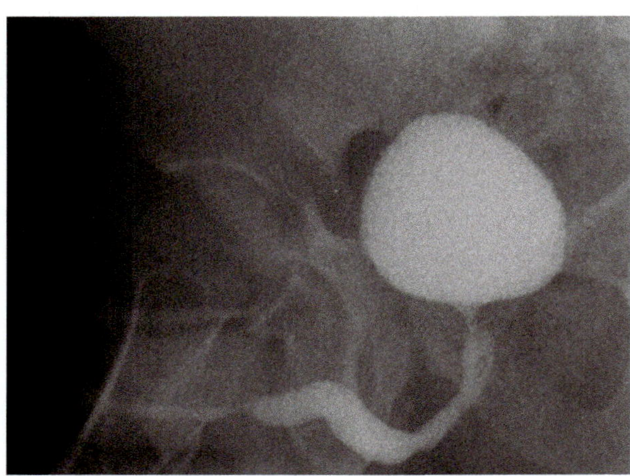

Fig. 8.1.2

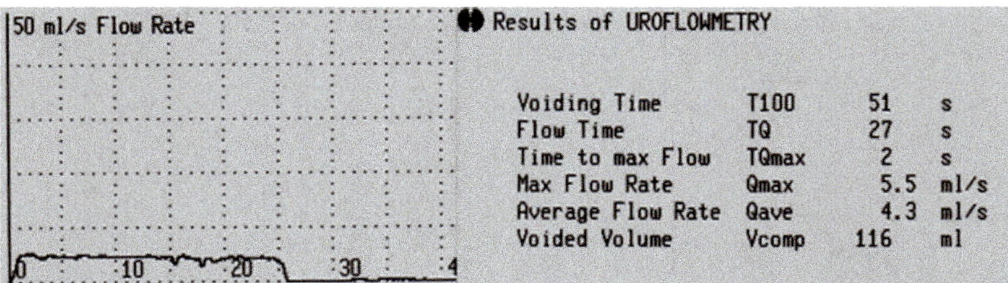

Fig. 8.1.3

Answers to Case 8.1

1. Figure 8.1.1 is an ascending urethrogram (note the tip of balloon catheter in the glans penis) demonstrating a bulbar urethral stricture. Figure 8.1.2 is a descending cystourethrogram (note that being a micturition study, the bladder neck and external sphincter are now wide open), showing a dilated bulbar urethra proximal to a stenosis at the peno-scrotal junction. The bulbar urethra also looks affected by stricture disease, and the bladder has a 'moth eaten' appearance, seen in chronic obstruction. Figure 8.1.3 is a uroflow tracing, demonstrating a reduced maximum flow rate (5.5 ml/s) and the characteristic 'plateau-shaped curve' of a fixed outflow obstruction such as a urethral stricture. This is in contrast to the reduced maximum flow rate and 'flattened bell-shaped curve' typically seen secondary to urethral compression due to benign prostatic hyperplasia.
2. Urethrography can provide information about how many strictures are present, their length and location. It cannot provide information about the health of the non-strictured mucosa either side of the narrowing. If required this is obtained by urethroscopy.
3. The commonest causes of anterior urethral strictures are traumatic and iatrogenic, but infection, lichen sclerosus, malignant and congenital strictures can also occur. Endoscopic treatment is with urethral dilatation or optical urethrotomy. Both techniques have similar outcomes and recurrence rates of 50–80% are seen, usually within 12 months. Recurrence is less common in shorter strictures (<2 cm recur less than >2 cm), in strictures of the bulbar urethra and if only one stricture is present. If an initial dilation or urethrotomy fails, a subsequent attempt has very little chance of success. Catheterisation after this procedure is usually for 3–5 days, there is no benefit in prolonging this, though the use of intermittent catheterisation does prevent recurrence at least until the patient stops.

   Urethroplasty is the gold standard treatment of male urethral strictures and shows the lowest relapse rate, if the diseased segment is excised and an end-to-end anastomosis performed. This is only possible in short (<2 cm), bulbar urethral strictures, as the effect of a shortened urethra in longer strictures and strictures of the penile urethra would result in curvature during erection. In these instances, the excised segment is bridged by a substitution urethroplasty, either by a free graft (e.g. buccal mucosa) or less commonly by a vascularised flap. Recurrence rates should be less than 10%. Aside from this the complication rate is very low, with most complications, e.g. urinary incontinence and erectile dysfunction, reflecting the original injury rather than the surgery.

Further Reading

Andrich DE, Mundy AR. Urethral strictures and their surgical management. *BJUI.* 2000;86:571–580.

Steenkamp JW, Heynes CF, Kock MLS. Internal urethrotomy versus dilation as the treatment for male urethral strictures: a prospective, randomized comparison. *J Urol.* 1997;157:98–101.

Case 8.2

These are urethrogram studies from two different patients

1. What abnormalities do they show and what is the most likely aetiology?
2. Which patients are most at risk of this type of urethral disease?

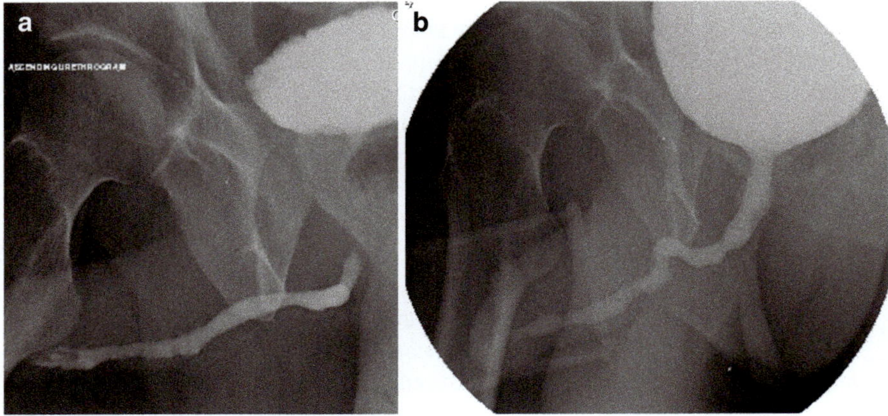

Fig.8.2.1

Fig. 8.2.2

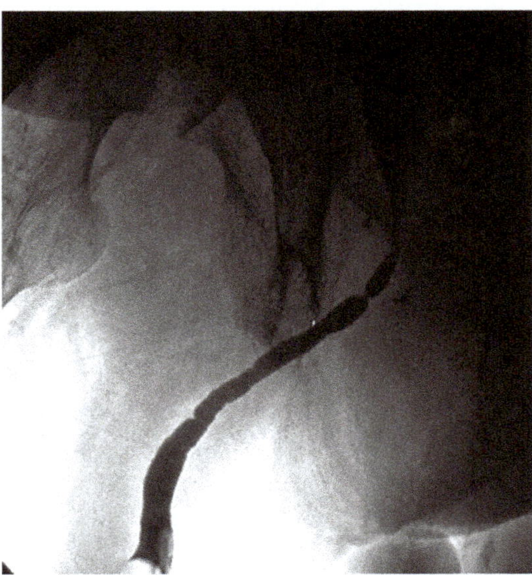

Answers to Case 8.2

1. On urethrography, the normal healthy urethral epithelium is seen as a smooth outline, well delineated by the injected contrast. In both these cases (Figs. 8.2.1a, b and 8.2.2) almost the entire anterior urethra demonstrates an irregularity of the urethral epithelium outline, with scattered areas of focal narrowing. These appearances are of pan urethral stricture disease. Inflammatory and/or infective processes may result in this appearance, the most common pathogen being gonococcus.
2. Risk factors for gonococcal urethritis include:
   - Multiple sexual partners
   - Low socio-economic status
   - Previous sexually transmitted infection.

Case 8.3

Study these images from various radiological studies undertaken in four men after major trauma.

1. What injuries can you see in Fig. 8.3.1a, b. What types of fracture are associated with urethral injury?
2. What is the initial management and investigation of suspected urethral trauma?
3. What is shown in Figs. 8.3.2 and 8.3.3?

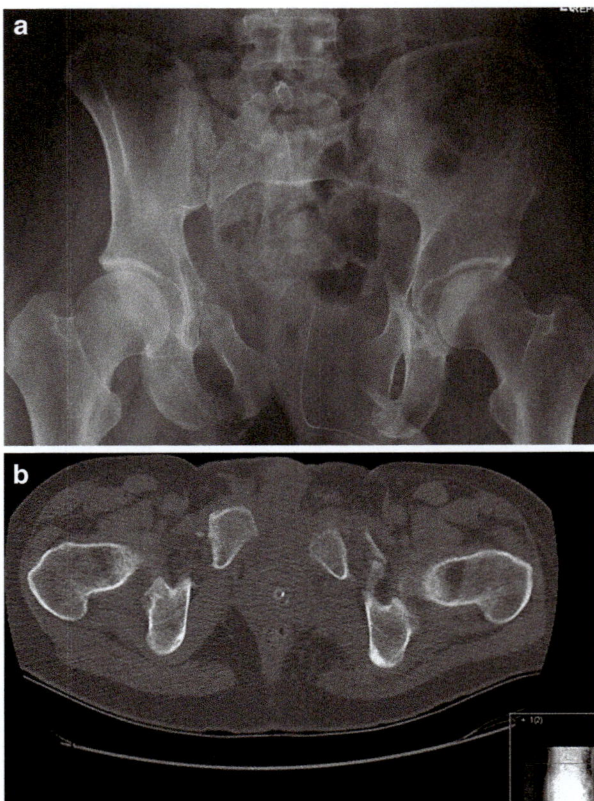

Fig. 8.3.1

Fig. 8.3.2

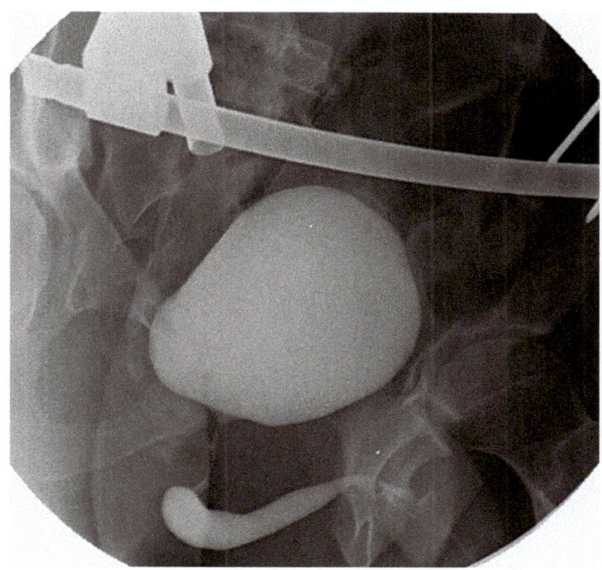

Fig. 8.3.3

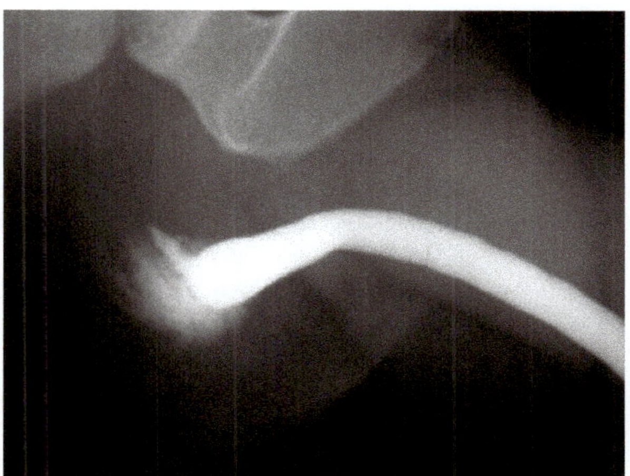

Answers to Case 8.3

1. The first image (Fig. 8.3.1a) shows a diastasis through the pubic symphysis and also fractures through both pubic rami and widened sacro-iliac joints (i.e. an open book fracture). A urethral catheter has been inserted. Figure 8.3.1b is an axial CT scan showing a left-sided pubic ramus fracture. Posterior urethral (including the membranous and prostatic urethra) injuries occur usually in association with unstable pelvic fractures, bilateral ischiopubic rami fractures ('straddle fracture') and symphysis pubis diastasis. Lower urinary tract injury has been reported in 16% of patients with unilateral rami fractures and in 41% of patients with bilateral rami fractures. In contrast, anterior urethral (bulbar and penile urethra) injuries are not usually associated with a pelvic fracture but are more often associated with blunt injury to the perineum. The direct force compresses the relatively immobile bulbar urethra against the inferior surface of the symphysis pubis.
2. After initial assessment and resuscitation, the external urethral meatus is inspected. Absence of blood at the meatus or genital haematoma means a lower urinary tract injury is very unlikely and to confirm this catheterisation may be undertaken. In approximately 75% of urethral injuries blood is present at the meatus. In these cases an ascending urethrogram should be undertaken prior to urethral catheterisation or a suprapubic catheter should be inserted. It is extremely unlikely that gentle passage of a urethral catheter will do any additional damage, although this may, theoretically at least, convert a partial to a complete tear.

   Retrograde urethrography is the recommended investigation for suspected urethral injuries. A scout film is initially taken to detect boney injuries and foreign bodies. A size 14 Fr Foley catheter is placed so the balloon is at the level of the fossa navicularis, 1-2ml of saline is inserted into the balloon. 20–30 ml of contrast is injected into the catheter, and ideally films taken with the patient in the 30° oblique position. If the posterior bladder is not well visualised, a suprapubic catheter and antegrade study may be required. Plain films and CT may be used to define boney and other associated injuries, but cannot be used to assess urethral injuries. Endoscopy has no place in the initial assessment of urethral injuries in men. In women where urethrography is not usually helpful, due to the short urethra, urethroscopy does play a role in the initial assessment of suspected urethral injuries.
3. Figure 8.3.2 shows a normal antegrade urethrogram in a patient with an external fixator in position and Fig. 8.3.3 demonstrates complete traumatic transection of the bulbar urethra. In the first patient urethral catheterisation would be safe but the latter needs a supra-pubic catheter.

Further Reading

Djakovic N, Plas E, Martínez-Piñeiro L, Lynch TH, Mor Y, Santucci RA, Serafetinidis E, Turkeri LN, Hohenfellner M. EAU guidelines Urological Trauma. *Eur Urol.* 2010;57(5):791-803.

McAninch JW, Resnick MI, eds. Genitourinary trauma. *Urol Clin N Am.* 2006;33.

Zorn G. Fractures of the pelvis with urethral injuries, their treatment and results. *Bruns Beitr Klin Chir.* 1960;201:147-155.

Case 8.4

1. Patient 1 (Fig. 8.4.1) developed severe pain in his penis whist having sexual intercourse; he immediately lost his erection and noticed blood at his urethral meatus. Patient 2 (Fig. 8.4.2a, b) had a similar history but there was no blood at the meatus. What do the images below demonstrate and what is the diagnosis?
2. What is the role of imaging in these patients?
3. What is the optimal management and what complication may occur?

Fig. 8.4.1

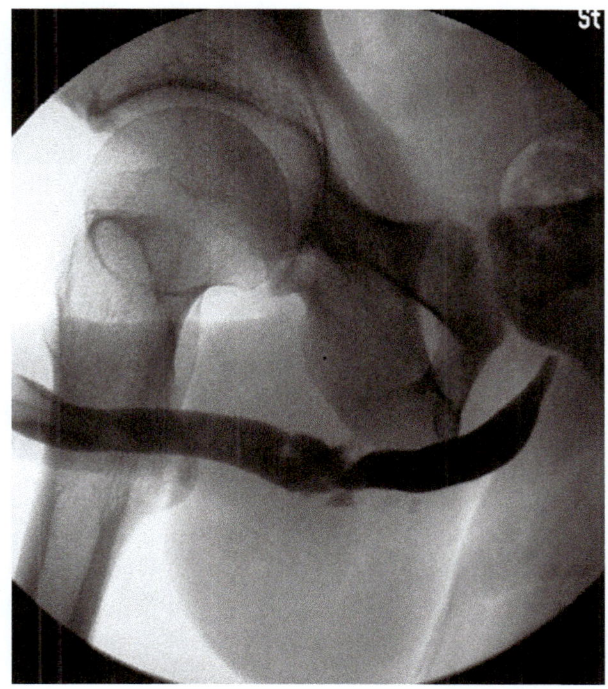

Fig. 8.4.2

a
H989687
L10-5 38mm SmPart/Testi
14 Sep 06
2:49:25 pm
F# 23
+ 6.4
- 6.4
cm/s
SV Angle 0°
Dep 2.6 cm
Size 2.0 mm
Freq 6.0 MHz
WF Low
Dop 80% Map 2
PRF 2500 Hz
12
8
4
cm/s
-4
-8
-12

b

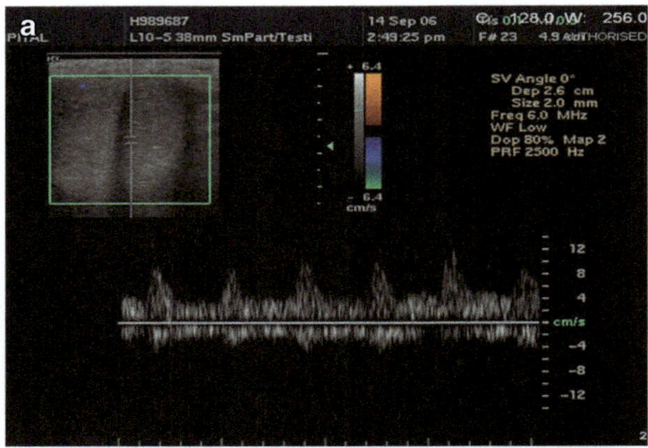

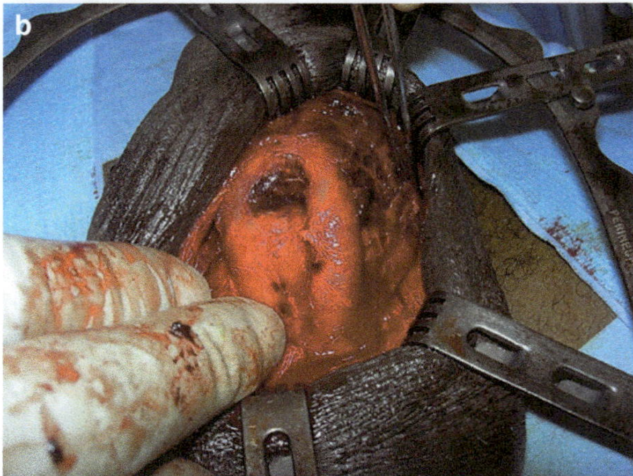

Answers to Case 8.4

1. The history in both patients is consistent with a diagnosis of a fractured penis. In patient 1 the history suggests a concomitant urethral injury and the urethrogram (Fig. 8.4.1) confirms this by showing a urethral distraction injury. In patient 2 the history, Doppler ultrasound (Fig. 8.4.2a) and intraoperative findings (Fig. 8.4.2b) show an intact urethra, a transverse tear is seen on the ventral surface of the corporal bodies.

   Fractured penis occurs due to blunt trauma to the erect penis, usually following sexual intercourse. The corpora cavernosum is surrounded by the tunica albuginea. During tumescence as the corpora fill with blood and become more rigid the tunica albuginea thins to 0.25-0.5mm. Sudden blunt trauma to the erect penis may result in an audible 'crack' as the thinned tunica tears. Typically sudden detumescence occurs due to leakage of blood into the surrounding tissues, resulting in the so-called 'egg-plant (aubergine) deformity'. Up to 30% of patients have blood at the urethral meatus; these patients need investigation with either a preoperative urethrogram or intraoperative urethroscopy. If both corpora are involved urethral injury is more likely.
2. Ultrasonography and MR image may help identify tunical rupture, though with a good history and typical examination findings their negative predictive value may not negate the need for surgery. Retrograde urethrography is useful to exclude a urethral injury, finally corporal cavernosography may confirm a tear, though is seldom used.
3. Immediate surgical exploration is the treatment of choice; good outcomes were reported in 92% of men treated surgically versus 59% treated conservatively. Operative intervention involves either a circumferential incision 1 cm proximal to the glans down to Buck's fascia and then degloving the penis or an incision directly over the defect. The haematoma is evacuated and after careful inspection to assess the degree of injury the corporal bodies and if necessary the urethra are repaired. Complications arising from penile fracture include erectile dysfunction (which may be due to a cavernosal-spongiosal fistula), penile curvature, painful nodular fibrotic plaques and urethral-cutaneous or corporo-urethral fistulae.

Further Reading

Muentener M, Suter S, Hauri D, Sulser T. Long-term experience with surgical and conservative treatment of penile fracture. *J Urol.* 2004;172(2):576–579.

Wessels H, Long L. Penile and genital injuries. *Urol Clin N Am.* 2006;33: 117–126.

Case 8.5

1. A 43-year-old man presents with spraying of his urinary stream. What is the likely diagnosis and how may this be treated (Fig. 8.5.1a, b)?
2. A 65-year man presents with white patches on his glans penis (Fig. 8.5.2a) and says his foreskin splits during sexual intercourse. What is the diagnosis, what are the typical pathological appearances seen in Fig. 8.5.3 and what are the treatment options?
3. Study Fig. 8.5.2b, c. Describe the procedure undertaken.

Fig. 8.5.1

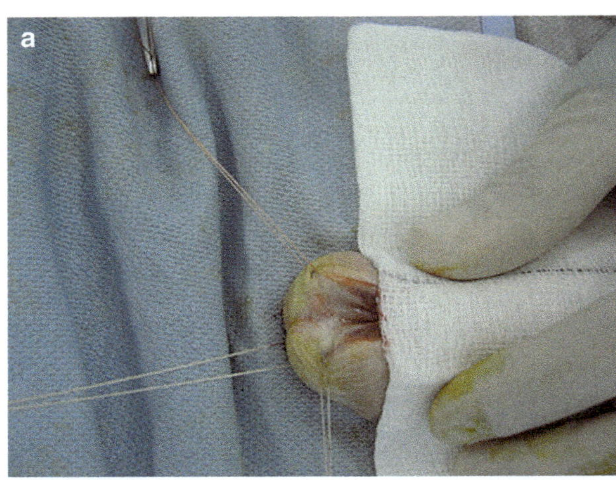

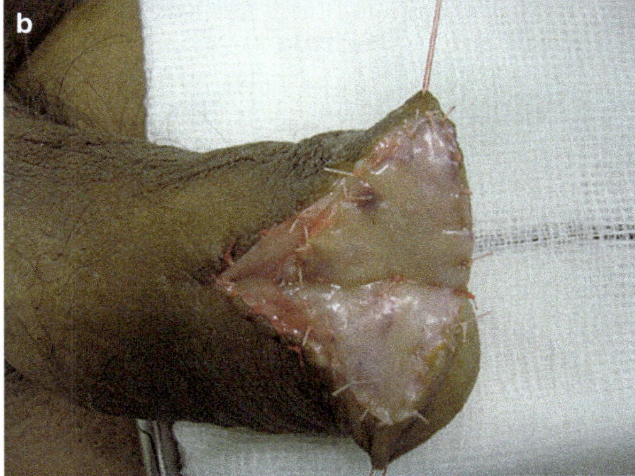

Fig. 8.5.2

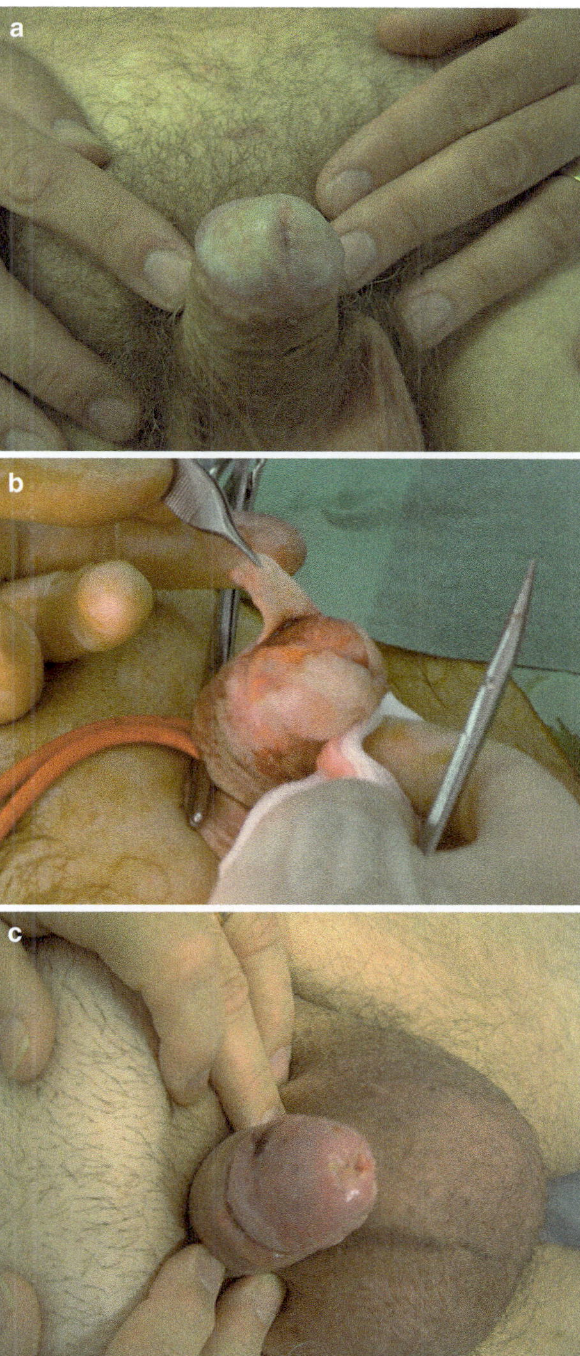

Fig. 8.5.3

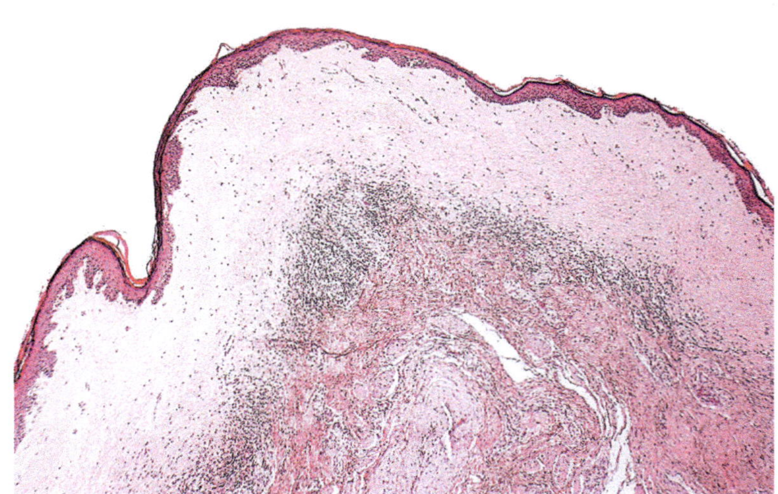

Answers to Case 8.5

1. This patient describes meatal stenosis. Meatal stenosis is more common in children than in adults and is almost exclusively as a result of circumcision. It is seen in 7% of children who have been circumcised, though the exact aetiology is not known. It is likely to be due to trauma and ammoniacal dermatitis from the nappy or underpants on the exposed meatus – meatal stenosis after circumcision is more common if the child is not potty trained. Alternatively damage to the frenular artery during circumcision may lead to ischaemia and subsequent stenosis.

   In adults meatal stenosis may follow trauma, previous catheterisation, lichen sclerosus or failed hypospadias repair. Meatal stenosis is treated by simple dilatation, a ventral slit, the recently described plastic dorsal and ventral meatotomy or in cases with proximal extension to the navicular fossa meatoplasty. Figure 8.5.1a, b show a case of meatal stenosis undergoing meatoplasty. In Fig. 8.5.1a the meatus has been divided ventrally, Fig. 8.5.1b shows a buccal mocosa onlay graft. This can then be closed over a catheter as part of the primary surgery or after the graft has taken at a later date.
2. Lichen sclerosus or balanitis xerotica obliterans (BXO) is a chronic, progressive, sclerosing inflammatory dermatosis of unknown aetiology. As seen in Figs. 8.5.2a and 8.5.3 the prepuce and glans have a whitened or hypopigmented appearance and fibrosis may lead to phimosis and fissuring of the prepuce. In more advanced cases the prepuce becomes adherent to the glans and the urethral meatus and more proximal urethra may become scarred and strictured.

   The histological appearance of typical lichen sclerosus includes a thinned epidermis with hyperkeratosis and basal cell vacuolisation; stromal oedema and hyalinisation of collagen in the upper dermis; a band-like lympho-histiocytic infiltrate just deep to the dermal changes. These features vary with the age of the lesion, the inflammatory infiltrate being more superficial in early disease.

Lichen sclerosus may be treated with topical steroid with a slowing or in some cases regression of the disease process, but surgical intervention is the mainstay of treatment. Circumcision offers excellent cure rates, especially if a phimosis is present; however, an adherent prepuce may make this more difficult.

3. Skin graft techniques such as glans resurfacing (as being undertaken in Fig. 8.5.2b with a good cosmetic result – Fig. 8.5.2c) or split skin grafting of the shaft skin are of benefit in replacing the diseased tissue, if required.

There is increasing evidence that lichen sclerosus is associated with the development of squamous carcinoma, particularly in those variants in which the human papilloma virus (HPV) does not have a role.

Further Reading

Das S, Tunuguntla HS. Balanitis Xerotica Obliterans – a review .*World J Urol.* 2000;18(6):382–387.

Malone P. A new technique for meatal stenosis in patients with lichen sclerosus. *J Urol.* 2004;172:949–952.

McKee PH, Calonje E, Granter SR, eds. *Pathlogy of the skin with clinical correlations*. 3rd edn. Vol 1. Elsevier Mosby; 2005.

Van Howe RS. Incidence of meatal stenosis following neonatal circumcision in a primary care setting. *Clin Pediatr (Phila).* 2006;45(1):49–54.

Velasquez EF, Cubilla AL. Lichen Sclerosus in 68 patients with squamous cell carcinoma of the penis: frequent atypias and correlation with special carcinoma variants suggests a pre cancerous role. *Am J Surg Pathol.* 2003;27(11): 1448–1453.

Case 8.6

1. What is shown in Figure 8.6.1a, b ?
2. What are the predisposing aetiological factors for this condition?
3. What are the principle features and associated anomalies?

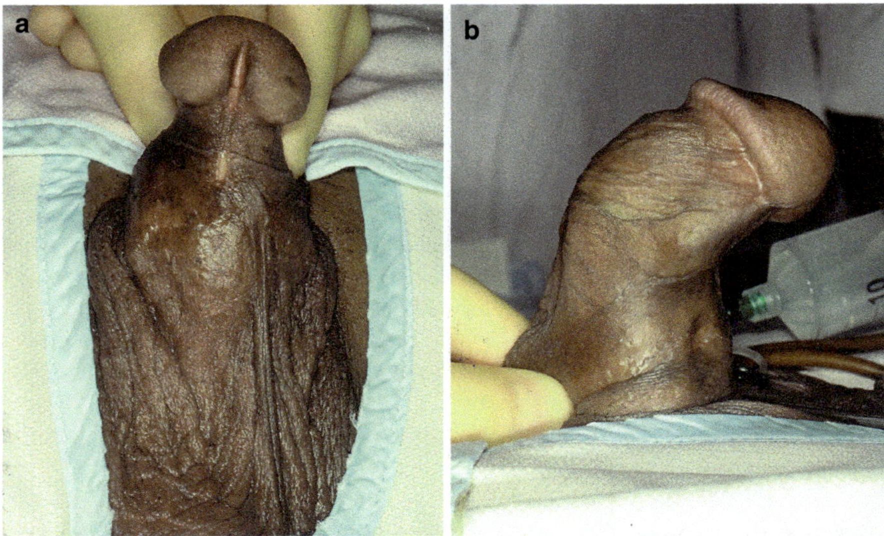

Fig. 8.6.1

Answers to Case 8.6

1. Figure 8.6.1a, b are photographs of a patient with hypospadias. Hypospadias is defined as hypoplasia of the ventral penile structures. There are a number of classifications, but hypospadias is broadly split into anterior (glanular, sub-coronal and distal-penile), middle (penile shaft) and posterior (proximal penile, penoscrotal, scrotal and perineal).
2. Low birth weight and babies of young and older mothers are at greater risk. An increase in the incidence over the last two decades suggests an environmental role – possibly due to pesticides and hormones.
3. The triad of symptoms which occur to varying degrees include a proximal ventrally located urethral meatus (Fig. 8.6.1a), hooded prepuce and chordee, the latter causing ventral curvature as shown in the artificial erection test (Fig. 8.6.1b). Other associated anomalies include cryptorchidism (10%), patent processus vaginalis/inguinal hernia (10%). Undescended testes and severe hypospadias may be associated with congenital adrenal hyperplasia and it is important to exclude this as well as other intersex abnormalities. Associated upper tract anomalies are rare.

Further Reading

Duckett JW. The current hype in hypospadiology. *Br J Urol.* 1995;76 (Suppl 3):1–7.

Case 8.7

1. Study Fig. 8.7.1 and describe the chronic abnormality shown.
2. How can the causes of this condition be classified?
3. What treatment options are available, and when is surgery indicated?

Fig. 8.7.1

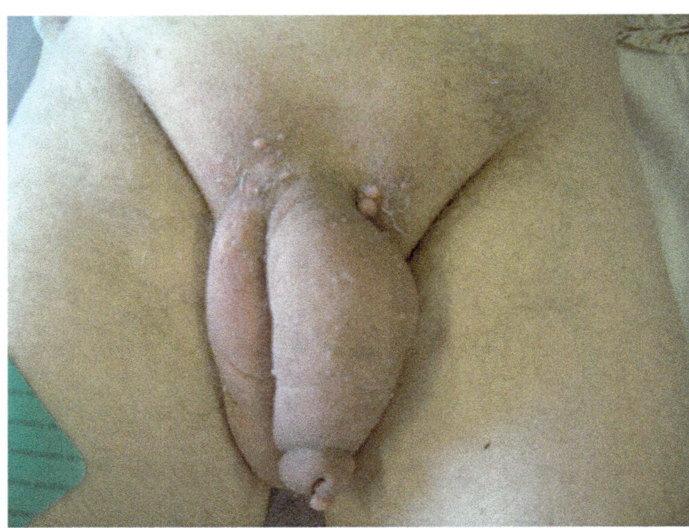

Answers to Case 8.7

1. In Fig. 8.7.1 the penis is generally swollen, and this is an example of penile (or genital) lymphoedema.
2. Lymphoedema is the abnormal collection of fluid in the interstitium. Primary lymphoedema results from an abnormality present at birth and is due to absent or poorly functioning or maldeveloped lymphatics. Secondary lymphoedema is more common and is due to acquired obstruction or infiltration of lymphatics and can follow:
   - Trauma
   - Cellulitis
   - Surgery
   - Radiotherapy
   - Crohn's disease
   - Infections (such as filariasis in the developing world).
3. There are four cornerstones of lymphoedema management, namely meticulous skin care, compression garments, exercise and lymph drainage with massage. Surgery is indicated after failure of conservative management and involves removal of the affected tissue and occasionally skin grafting.

Further Reading

Garaffa G, Christopher N, Ralph DJ. The management of genital lymphoedema. *BJU Int.* 2008;102(4):480–484.

McDougal WS. Lymphoedema of the external genitalia. *J Urol.* 2003;170(3): 711–716.

Case 8.8

1. Two separate uncircumcised men in their 60s presented with a lesions on their glans (Figs 8.8.1a, b). What is the likely diagnosis in each case and how is this confirmed?
2. How is this condition treated?
3. What premalignant conditions of the penis are there?

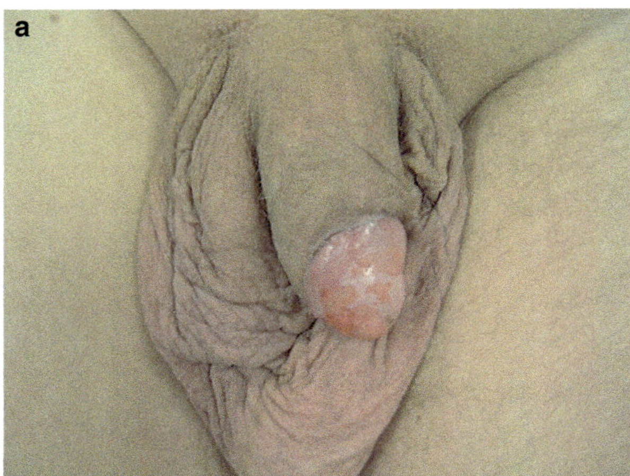

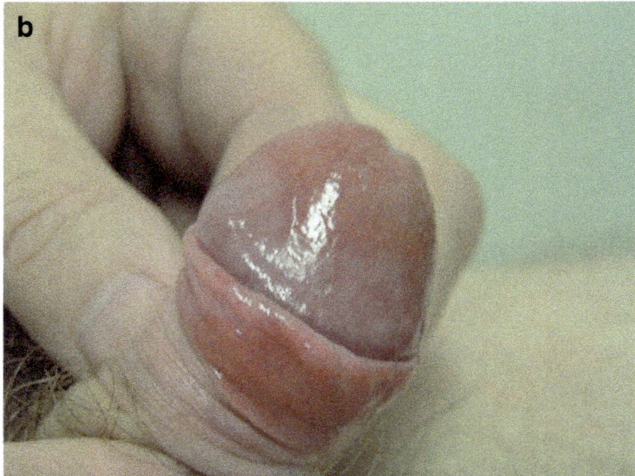

Fig. 8.8.1

Fig. 8.8.2

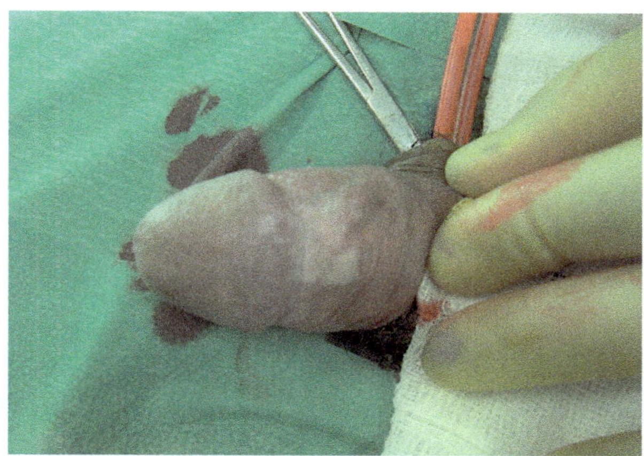

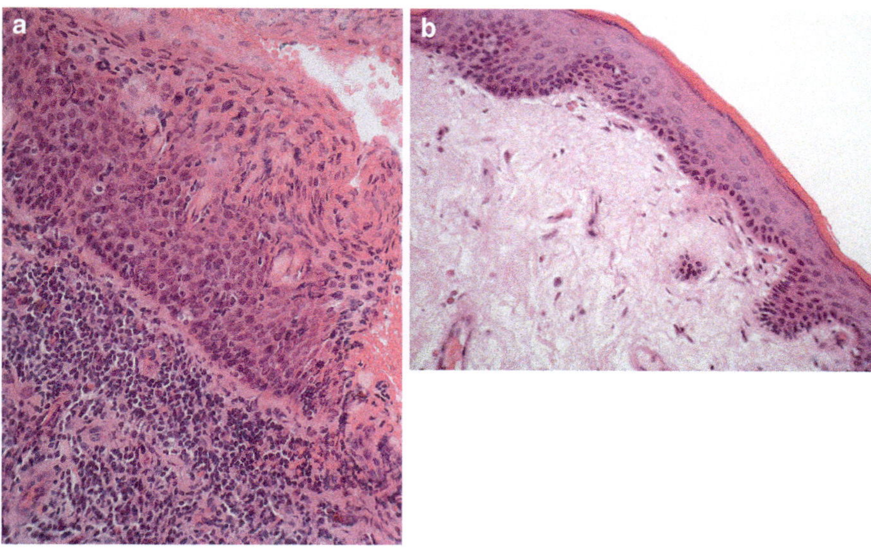

Fig. 8.8.3

Answers to Case 8.8

1. Figure 8.8.1a shows intra-epithelial neoplasia (IN) (carcinoma in situ/severe dysplasia) of the glans. This diagnosis is strongly suggested by white staining with application of acetic acid (Fig. 8.8.2) and is confirmed by biopsy (Fig. 8.8.3a). The microscopic features of IN seen on H and E section (Fig. 8.8.3a) include loss of normal maturation, loss of cellular polarity, cellular pleomorphism and hyperchromatic nuclei. The mitotic figures frequently seen are not easily identified in this particular field. A dense sub-epithelial chronic inflammatory infiltrate is present. These abnormal features are emphasised by comparison with the normal squamous epithelium (Fig. 8.8.3b). It is important to obtain sufficient depth on biopsy to exclude invasion.

   The second man (Fig. 8.8.1b) has Zoon's (plasma cell) balanitis, a condition which my mimic penile IN. Zoon's balanitis is usually an asymptomatic condition in uncircumcised men probably due to chronic irritation, it is not premalignant. Lesions are characterised by erythematous, shiny 'ink blot' areas over the glans often with associated kissing lesions on the prepuce. Biopsy is recommended to confirm the diagnosis and then topical treatment with steroids, antibacterials and antifungals may be tried, though the definitive treatment is circumcision.
2. Conservative and surgical treatments for IN are used. The former include topical therapy with 5-fluorouracil (5-FU) or immunomodulation with 5% imiquimod cream. These are associated with high rates of recurrence. Alternatively, laser ablation with CO_2 laser or Nd:YAG may be undertaken with less risk of recurrence. Surgical treatment includes local excision with or without circumcision or glans resurfacing with a split skin graft.
3. The major established precursor lesion for penile cancer is IN, the histopathological synonyms being carcinoma in situ and severe dysplasia. Other terms for the identical histopathological appearances reflect clinical distinctions. Bowen's disease usually occurs as a solitary lesion on the shaft skin in patients aged>50 years, when present on the glans it is called Erythroplasia of Queyrat. In both these sites IN progresses to invasive carcinoma in up to 30% of patients.

   Cutaneous horn, so-called because of excessive keratin production, may also have a propensity to progress to invasive cancer when IN is present in the underlying epithelium.

   The role of lichen sclerosus in penile cancer is discussed in Case 8.5.

   Bowenoid Papulosis occurs in men aged<30 years and is induced by human papilloma virus (particularly subtype 16). It appears as multicentric maculopapular lesions usually on the penile shaft which usually remit spontaneously in<2 years and very rarely progress to invasive cancer (<3%).

There is increasing evidence of an association between penile IN and the presence of cervical intraepithelial neoplasia (CIN) in sexual partners. The rate of penile IN in those whose female partner has CIN is 33% compared with 1.4% in men whose female partner has condyloma.

Further Reading

Crispen PL, Mydlo JH. Penile intraepithelial neoplasia and other premailignant lesions of the penis. *Urol Clin N Am*. 2010;37:335–342.

Pizzocaro G, Algaba F, Solsona E, Tana S, Van Der Poel H, Watkin NA, Horenblas S. EAU Guidelines on Penile Cancer. *Eur Urol*. 2010;57(6):1002–1012.

Case 8.9

1. What is shown in Fig. 8.9.1a–c? What are the risk factors for this condition?
2. What are the subtypes of this disease? Which subtype is shown in Fig. 8.9.2a–c?
3. What is the common pattern of spread and what are poor predictors?
4. What does the MRI (Fig. 8.9.3) show and describe the staging of this condition.

Fig. 8.9.1

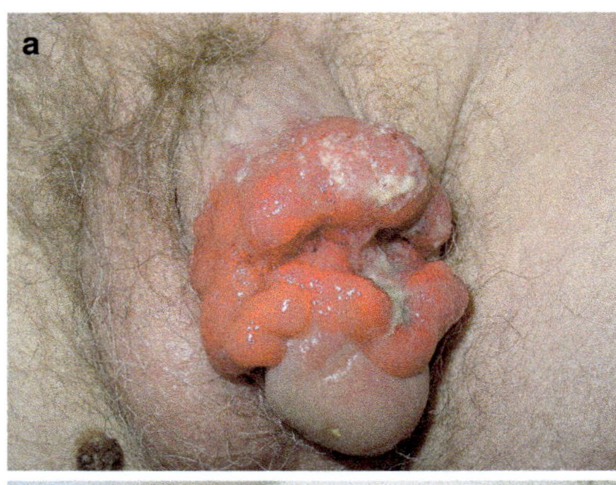

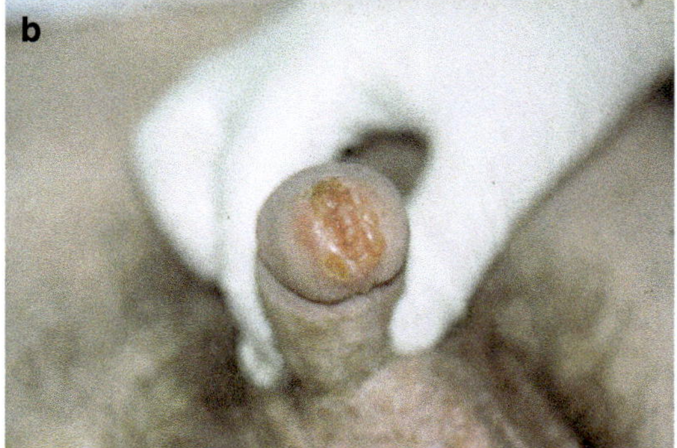

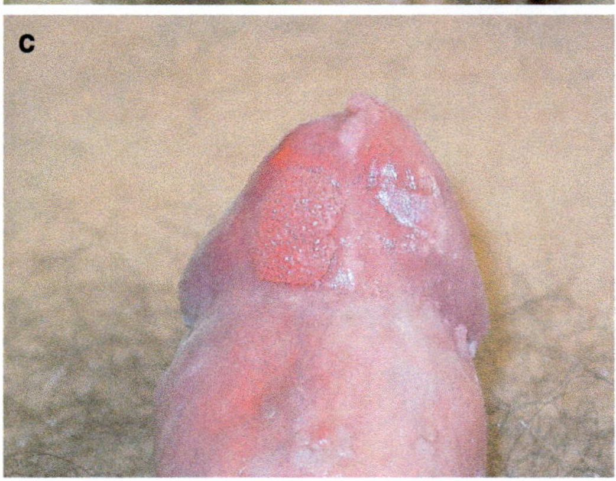

Fig. 8.9.2

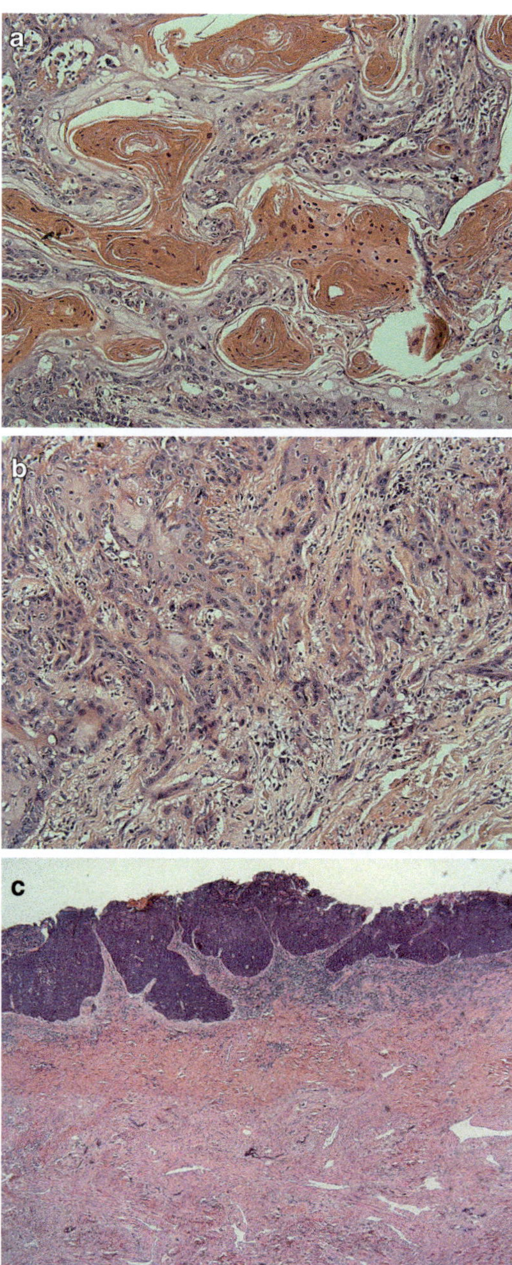

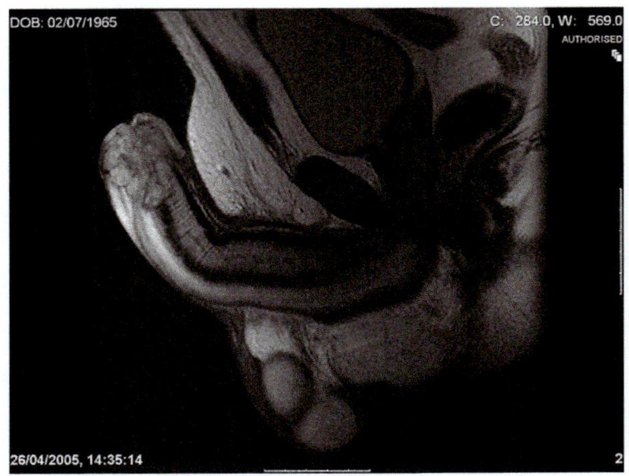

Fig. 8.9.3

Answers to Case 8.9

1. Figure 8.9.1 illustrates invasive penile cancers. Figure 8.9.1a is a fungating squamous cell cancer (SCC), Fig. 8.9.1b is an SCC arising from the urethral meatus and Fig. 8.9.1c is a papillary SCC. In excess of 95% of tumours of the penis are SCC, the majority arising on the glans, prepuce or coronal sulcus, the glans being the commonest site. Less than 2% of SCC present as isolated tumours on the shaft. The remaining rare tumours in the penile skin include malignant melanoma, basal cell carcinoma and metastases primarily from carcinoma of bladder or prostate. Mesenchymal tumours occasionally arise within the corpora.

   The risk factors for SCC penis include phimosis, poor hygiene, smoking, HPV-16 and -18 and chronic inflammatory conditions including balanoposthitis and lichen sclerosus. Multiple sexual partners, early age of first sexual intercourse and a history of condylomata (genital warts) also increase the risk of developing penile cancer.
2. The major subtypes of penile cancer defined by the WHO, and their frequency in brackets include SCC not otherwise specified (NOS) (48–65%); Papillary (5–15%); Warty (7–10%); Basaloid (4–10%); Verrucose (3–8%). Mixed forms of the above occur and rare variants have been described (Sarcomatoid, Adenosquamous, Pseudohyperplastic, Cuniculatum and Acantholytic).

   The subtypes illustrated are well-differentiated SCC (NOS) showing prominent keratinisation (Fig. 8.9.2a), poorly differentiated SCC with atypical cytology, failure of maturation and no obvious keratin (Fig. 8.9.2b) and Basaloid carcinoma composed of uniform small cells giving a basophilic appearance to the invasive solid cell nests (Fig. 8.9.2c).

   The clinical relevance of this classification relates to aetiology and prognosis. The cancers associated with HPV (commonly types 16 and 18) are predominantly Warty and Basaloid forms and occur in a younger age group (45–55 years) than the other subtypes. Basaloid, Sarcomatoid and Acantholytic tumours are the most aggressive in terms of local invasion and are associated with a high incidence of regional metastases and mortality. Squamous cell cancer NOS is associated with a local metastatic rate and mortality of 28–39% and 20–35%, respectively. The mortality is only slightly lower than that of patients with Basaloid cancer. Warty and papillary cancers metastasise locally in 18% and 12% and have an associated mortality of 0–9% and 0–6%, respectively. Verrucose, Cuniculatum and pseudo-hyperplastic cancers have an excellent prognosis, local metastases are not recorded.

3. Penile SCC spreads preferentially by lymphatics (which cross the mid-line) to superficial and subsequently deep inguinal nodes followed by pelvic nodes. Metastases to distant sites (lungs, liver, bone and brain) are rare and usually occur late in the disease course.

   The most significant predictors for lymph node metastases are lymphovascular invasion, perineural invasion and high tumour grade. Other commonly cited factors influencing prognosis include primary tumour size and site; tumour subtype; depth of invasion; growth pattern; positive margins of resection and urethral invasion.

4. Staging of the primary lesion is essentially by clinical examination. In men with suspected corporal invasion an artificial erection with prostaglandin E1 (alprostadil) in combination with penile MRI may exclude corporal invasion allowing penile preserving surgery, with glansectomy. The MRI in Fig. 8.9.3 is a sagittal T2-weighted study and demonstrates corporal invasion by a primary penile cancer, necessitating partial penectomy. Nodal staging is best performed with physical examination. Where the inguinal nodes are impalpable an USS may detect abnormal nodes and allow ultrasound guided fine needle aspiration. In patients with impalpable nodes and negative inguinal USS dynamic sentinel lymph node biopsy is increasingly becoming the preferred approach to lymph node staging, though it is only available in a few centres. Iliac lymph node involvement does not occur in the absence of inguinal lymph node metastases, so MRI/CT staging of the abdomen and pelvis is only indicated if inguinal node metastases are suspected. FDG PET/CT scanning can be utilised in the detection of regional and distant metastases.

Further Reading

Chaux A, Velasquez EF, Algaba F, Ayala G, Cubilla AL. Developments in the pathology of penile squamous carcinomas. *Urology*. 2010;76(2 Suppl 1):S7–S14.

Cubilla AL. The role of pathologic prognostic factors in squamous cell carcinoma of the penis. *World J Urol*. 2009;27(20):169–177.

Heyns CF, Mendoza-Valdes A, Pompeo AC. Diagnosis and staging of penile cancer. *Urology*. 2010;76(2 Suppl 1):S15–S23.

Case 8.10

1. What is the investigation shown in Fig. 8.10.1a, b, and what are the intraoperative images (Fig. 8.10.2)?
2. What are the advantages and accuracy of this technique?
3. How are palpable lymph nodes managed?

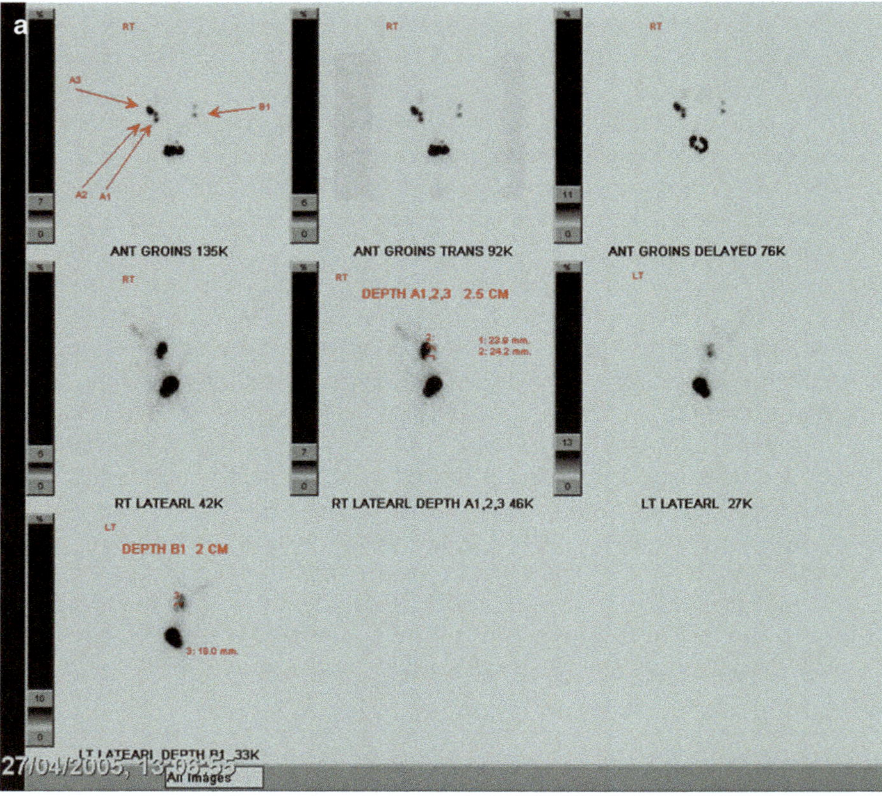

Fig. 8.10.1

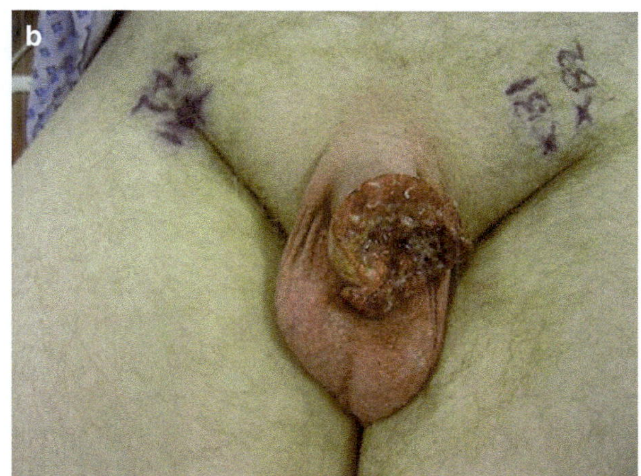

Fig. 8.10.1 (continued)

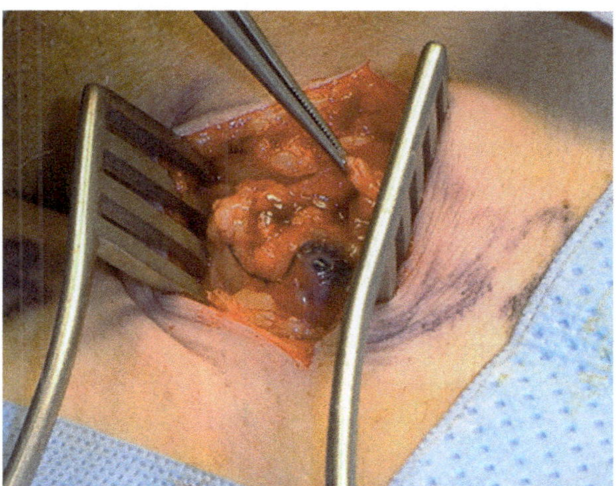

Fig. 8.10.2

Answers to Case 8.10

1. These three images correspond to three different patients. The investigation shown in Fig. 8.10.1a is the result of a dynamic sentinel lymph node biopsy study (DSNB). Tc99m nanocolloid is injected into the penis the day before surgery. On the day of surgery a gamma(γ) probe is used to identify the sentinel nodes and the patient is marked accordingly (Fig. 8.10.1b). Patent blue is also injected into the penis prior to surgery (Fig. 8.10.2) and a γ probe may be used intraoperatively along with direct visualisation to identify the sentinel node or group of nodes and these are then excised.
2. The advantage of DSNB is the avoidance of inguinal lymphadenectomy and subsequent high morbidity. Wound infection, flap necrosis, prolonged lymph leak, lymphocoele, scrotal and leg lymphoedema occur in 30–70% of patients after lymphadanectomy. The modified lymphadenectomy results in less morbidity, but increases the chance of a false-negative result. Sentinel node biopsy is associated with virtually no morbidity, it has a short learning curve and prospective studies demonstrate 100% specificity and 95% sensitivity.
3. Palpable nodes are managed depending on the features of the primary lesion. USS guided FNA may be undertaken to confirm nodal involvement, but a negative result does not exclude metastases. Lymphadenectomy or modified lymphadepathy is performed in high-risk patients and where metastases are extensive skin reconstruction with a flap may be required. In low-risk patients early review of enlarged lymph nodes after resection of the primary tumour may avoid unnecessary lymphadenectomy in men with reactive lymphadenopathy. Persistent lymphadenopathy is almost certainly due to metastatic disease necessitating surgery. Antibiotics were given to assess whether the lymphadenopathy was reactive, but this proved to be the case in less than 20% of palpable nodes in recent series and with enhanced sampling techniques and predictive nomograms this is seldom required. Adjuvant cisplatin-based chemotherapy is of benefit in men with N2+ disease.

Further Reading

Akduman B, Fleshner NE, Ehrlich L, Klotz L. Early experience in intermediate-risk penile cancer with sentinel node identification using the gamma probe. *Urology*. 2001;58(1):65–68.

Hadway P, Smith Y, Corbishley C, Heenan S, Watkin NA. Evaluation of dynamic lymphoscintigraphy and sentinel lymph-node biopsy for detecting occult metastases in patients with penile squamous cell carcinoma. *BJU Int*. 2007;100(3):561–565.

Tanis PJ, Lont AP, Meinhardt W, Olmos RA, Nieweg OE, Horenblas S. Dynamic sentinel node biopsy for penile cancer: reliability of a staging technique. *J Urol*. 2002;168(1):76–80.

Case 8.11

1. What is shown in the artificial erection test below (Fig. 8.11.1), what is the diagnosis and what are the features of this condition?
2. How is this condition assessed?
3. How might imaging options (Fig. 8.11.2) differ in acquired as opposed to congenital penile curvature?

Fig. 8.11.1

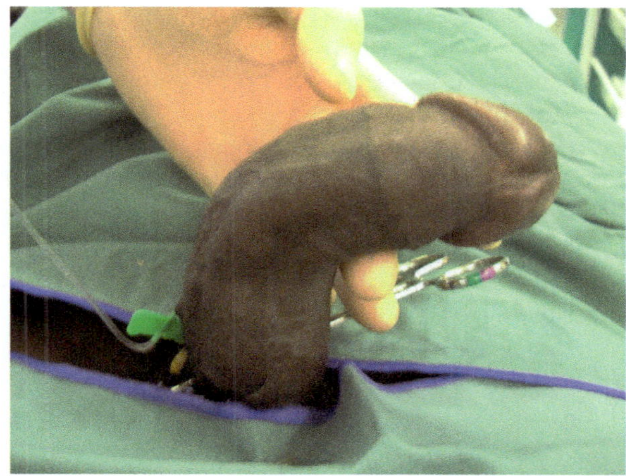

Fig. 8.11.2

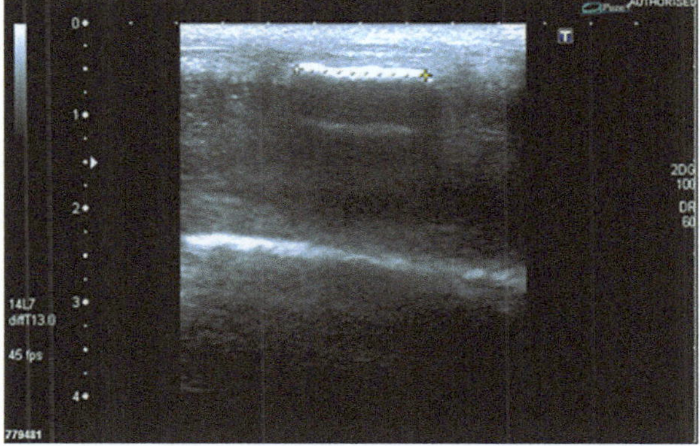

Answers to Case 8.11

1. Figure 8.11.1 shows a near 90° lateral curvature of the midshaft of the penis. The diagnosis is Peyronie's disease. The features include penile pain, curvature and flaccidity distal to the curve. A fibrous plaque may be palpable on the tunica albuginea.
2. A good history of the curvature should include duration of problem, associated pain, degree of curvature (and whether stable) and erectile function. Palpation for a plaque in the flaccid state and photography or injection of the penis with a vasoactive agent may be required to formally document curvature.
3. Cavernosography, plain radiography and CT have all been used to assess acquired penile curvature. Ultrasonography, with or without intra-cavernosal injection of a vasoactive substance, is the most useful and readily available imaging investigation. It can help define the anatomy of the plaque, especially if calcified, and evaluate the corporal bodies for scar tissue. It is also useful for haemodynamic evaluation of the erectile circuit and gives functional information to help in management decisions. Figure 8.11.2 is a longitudinal grey-scale ultrasound image showing a long calcified tunical plaque along the dorsal surface of the cavernosa. MRI of the penis can also be used for anatomical information, but has not been as thoroughly studied.

Further Reading

Smith JF, Walsh TJ, Lue TF. Peyronie's disease: a critical appraisal of current diagnosis and treatment. *Int J Impot Res.* 2008;20(5):445–459.

Taylor FL, Levine LA. Peyronie's Disease. *Urol Clin N Am.* 2007;34:517–534.

Case 8.12

1. What study is shown below? How is the study carried out? Which drug is administered before the study, by which route and what is the mode of action?
2. What are the diagnostic parameters used during this study?
3. What other radiological investigations can be used for further diagnostic evaluation?

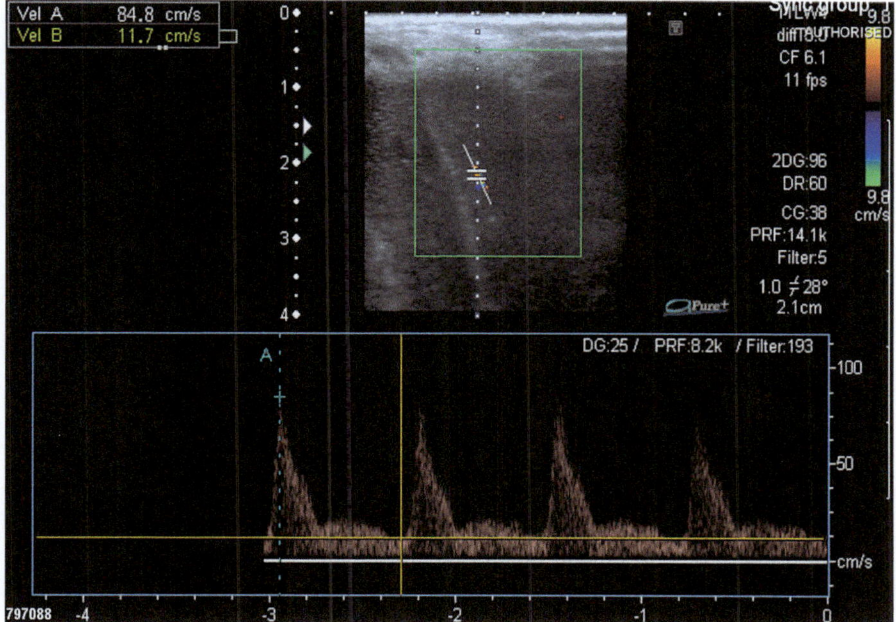

Fig. 8.12.1

Answers to Case 8.12

1. Figure 8.12.1 is a colour Doppler ultrasound image of a Penile Doppler study. This is a dynamic study of the penile haemodynamics and carried out by repeated Doppler ultrasound measurements of the systolic and diastolic velocities of the cavernosal artery flow after artificial pharmacostimulation. The commonest agent used for pharmacostimulation in modern practice is intra-cavernosal Prostaglandin E1. This is administered as an intra-cavernosal injection and has a vasodilatory and relaxing effect on the smooth muscle of the corpora cavernosum. This triggers a rapid increase in the cavernosal artery inflow. Reduced inflow after stimulation is the hallmark of arteriogenic erectile dysfunction. Whilst venous leak or the failure of the veno-occlussive mechanism is characterised by sustained high diastolic outflows.
2. Normal cavernosal velocities are a systolic inflow >30 or >35 cm/s (different thresholds are recommended by different authors) and a diastolic velocity <5 cm/s after pharmacostimulation. Arteriogenic erectile dysfunction is diagnosed if systolic velocity does not rise >30 cm/s and venous leak if the diastolic velocity remains >5 cm/s throughout the study. Figure 8.12.1 shows an example of an elevated diastolic velocity (11.7 cm/s as shown in the upper left hand corner of the image) which is seen with venous leak.
3. Cavernosometry with cavernosography can be used to confirm venous leak. Arteriography will help define whether the arterial obstruction is at the level of the larger arteries, e.g. the anterior division of the internal iliac artery or the internal pudendal artery that may be amenable to endovascular or surgical correction; or whether the arterial defect is at the level of the cavernosal artery.

Further Reading

Eid JF. What is new for inflatable penile prostheses? *Curr Opin Urol.* 2009;19(6):582–588.

Halls J, Bydawell G, Patel U. Erectile dysfunction: the role of penile Doppler ultrasound in diagnosis. *Abdom Imaging*. 2009;34(6):712–725.

Case 8.13

1. What condition is illustrated by this images (Fig. 8.13.1), and what advice regarding patient contact should be offered?
2. What treatment options are available for this condition and is vaccination available?

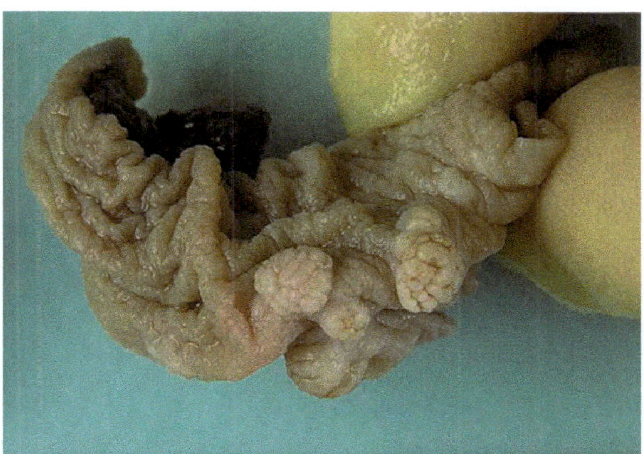

Fig. 8.13.1

Answers to Case 8.13

1. Figure 8.13.1 is a piece of foreskin showing exophytic polypoid nodules. On microscopy, the growth pattern, hyperkeratosis and koilocytosis supported the diagnosis of benign viral warts. These are caused by HPV infection, of which there are numerous varieties. Although many strains have been implicated, 90% of genital warts are caused by types 6 and 11. Human papilloma viruses can be sexually transmitted and are involved in the pathogenesis of cervical cancer and pre-cancerous states. The use of barrier protection (such as condoms) before sexual intercourse should be advised as well as contact tracing and treatment.
2. A vaccine protecting against HPV 6 and 11 (implicated in Genital Warts) and 16 and 18 (implicated in cervical cancer) is currently being administered in some countries.
3. Treatments include patient applied creams such as podophyllotoxin or the immune-modulating imiquimod can be used. Cryosurgery, surgical excision, laser ablation and interferon have also been adopted.

Case 8.14

1. A 73-year-old man presents 2 weeks after abdominal surgery with a blackened ulcer at the base of his penis and surrounding cellulitis and crepitus (Fig. 8.14.1). What is the likely condition?
2. What does his plain abdominal X-ray (Fig. 8.14.2) show?
3. What is the appropriate management (Fig 8.14.3a, b)?

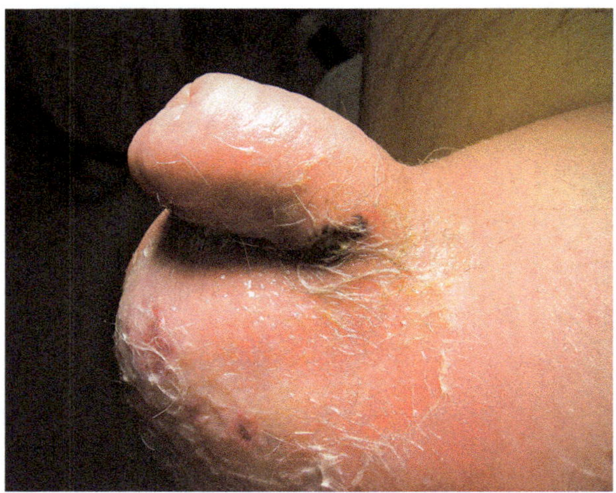

Fig. 8.14.1

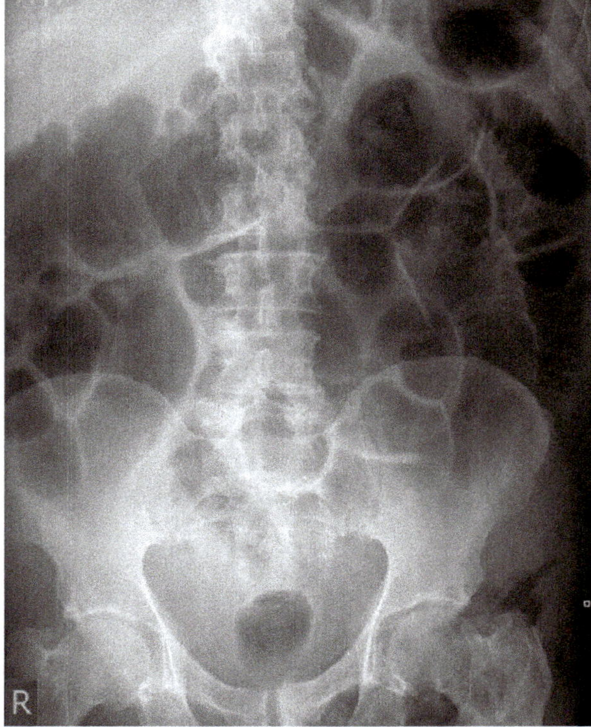

Fig. 8.14.2

Fig. 8.14.3

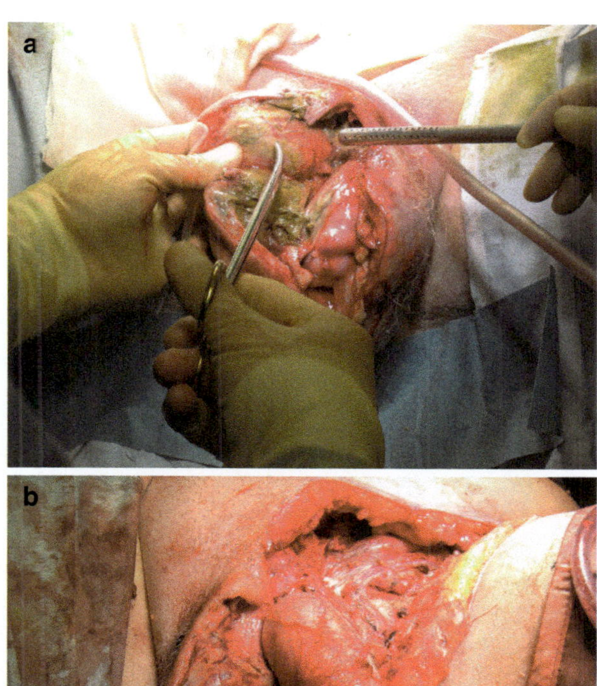

Answers to Case 8.14

1. Figure 8.14.1 shows cellulitis of the genitalia with a necrotic black ulcer at the peno-scrotal junction. On closer inspection, gas bubbles were seen coming from the central purulent area. This is Fournier's gangrene, an infective necrotising fasciitis of the perineal region. Although originally described by Baurienne in the sixteenth century, it gained its eponymous name from the French venereologist Jean-Alfred Fournier who presented five cases in 1883.

   This disease is a synergistic polymicrobial infection usually caused by both aerobic and anaerobic organisms. The most commonly identified pathogens are part of the normal perineal flora and include *Escherichia coli*, Bacteriodes, *Streptococci*, *Staphylococci* and *Clostridia*.
2. Although the diagnosis is made mainly on clinical grounds, radiological studies may reveal air in the soft tissues, as can be seen over the left inguinal region in Fig. 8.14.2.
3. Prompt surgical exploration is mandatory, and can be seen in Fig. 8.14.3a, b. After resuscitation and broad-spectrum antibiotic cover, the anaesthetised patient is placed in the lithotomy position to allow access to all perineal structures.

All necrotic tissue must be debrided until viable tissue is reached. The extent of necrotic tissue is commonly far more widespread than indicated from the cutaneous involvement, and diversion of urine and faeces may be required.

The testes and penile shaft are rarely affected due to their independent blood supply, though testis involvement is a recognised complication and some series report orchidectomy in 20% of patients. When the testes are not involved they can be left covered by an appropriate dressing. Once the infection has resolved they may be covered by a skin graft or inserted into a medical thigh pouch.

After 24–48 h the patient is usually taken back to the operating theatre for further debridement, if required, and a change of dressings. This may need to be repeated several times. Skin grafting may be considered at a later date if secondary intention fails to cover a large defect.

Further Reading

Smith GL, Bunker CB, Dinneen MD. Fournier's gangrene. *Br J Urol.* 1998;81(3): 347–355.

Urodynamics

9

Manit Arya and Rizwan Hamid

Case 9.1

A 45-year-old female complains of frequency and urgency.

1. What does the filling phase show?
2. Is the voiding study normal?
3. Is the subtraction on coughing acceptable?
4. Can this be reported as a normal study?

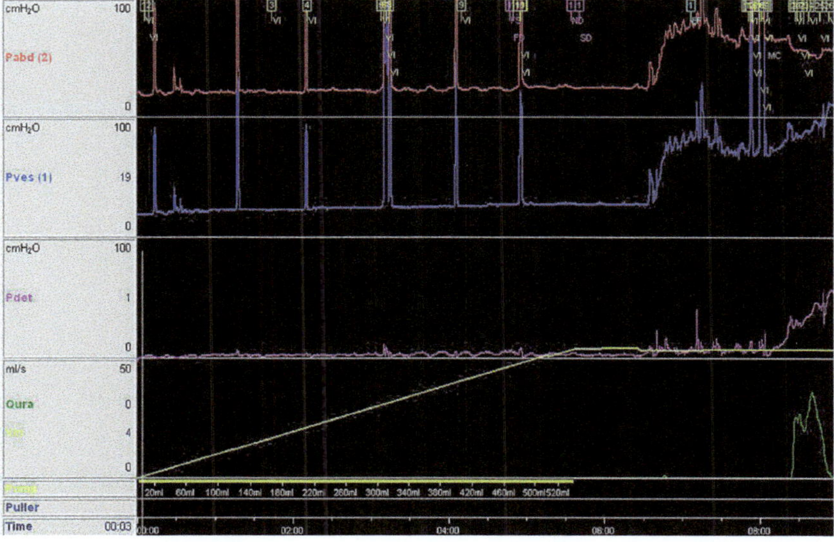

Fig. 9.1.1

S. Bott et al. (eds.), *Images in Urology*,
DOI 10.1007/978-0-85729-769-3_9, © Springer-Verlag London Limited 2012

Answers to Case 9.1

1. Figure 9.1.1 is a urodynamic trace showing 520 ml of fluid was instilled and a straight detrusor pressure rise confirms a stable normal capacity bladder. The cough test was performed regularly (spikes on the bladder and abdominal traces).
2. During voiding there is a flow rate of >25 ml/s at voiding pressure of ≤35 cmH_2O.
3. With each cough action the detrusor line stays steady, confirming good subtraction.
4. Yes, this appears to be a normal study.

Case 9.2

A 55-year-old male complains of frequency, urgency with nocturia and occasional urge incontinence.

1. What does the filling study demonstrate?
2. Is there any leakage during the filling phase?
3. Please describe the voiding phase.

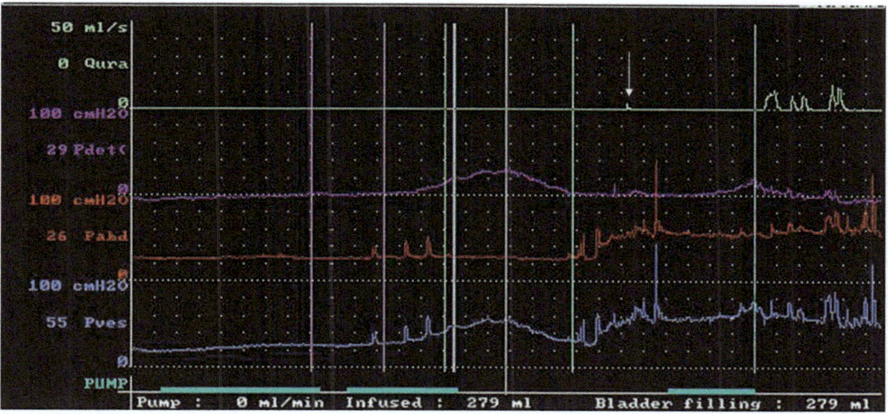

Fig. 9.2.1

Answers to Case 9.2

1. The filling phase in Fig. 9.2.1 demonstrates detrusor overactivity with the detrusor pressure rising to 29 cmH_2O (normal < 15 cmH_2O). This is provoked as it manifests after coughs. Overactivity abates when the pump is stopped (blue bars at the bottom of the image) but there is probably another overactivity phase when the pump is restarted.
2. No leakage is demonstrated. The small spike (arrow) is an artefact.
3. This is a low flow and low pressure voiding trace. The maximum flow rate is about 10 ml/s with a Pdet at Qmax of less than 10 cmH_2O.

Case 9.3

A 48-year-old female presents with symptoms of urgency, frequency and poor flow with a sense of incomplete emptying.

1. Is there any overactivity seen on this trace?
2. Is filling contributing to the abnormality seen on the trace?
3. What is the maximum detrusor pressure during an overactive contraction and is there any leakage?

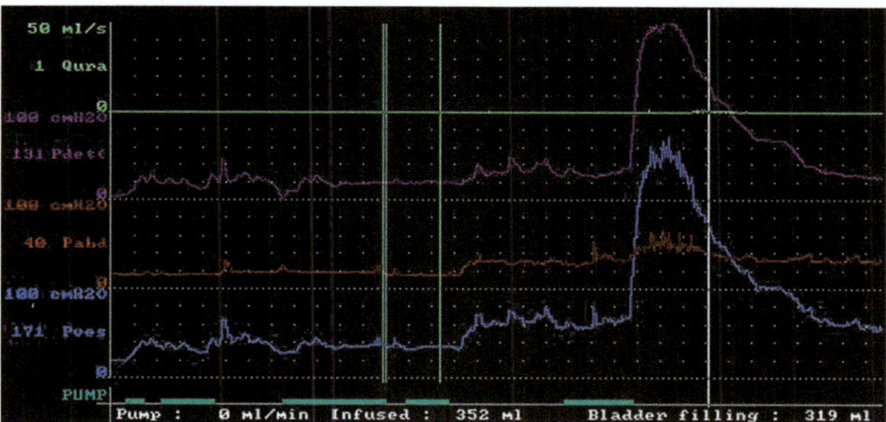

Fig. 9.3.1

Answers to Case 9.3

1. There are multiple phasic contractions consistent with idiopathic overactivity. There is also early overactivity up to a pressure of about 20 cmH_2O.
2. Yes, whenever the pump is switched on it appears to invoke a detrusor contraction. This becomes more marked once the patient is asked to stand up.
3. The maximum detrusor pressure during overactive contraction is more than 100 cmH_2O but there is no leakage demonstrated.

Case 9.4

A 52-year-old lady presents with worsening symptoms of frequency, urgency and incontinence. These are not relieved with anticholinergic medications.

1. What do these traces show?
2. How much fluid was instilled?
3. What is happening on the accompanying video film taken during the filling phase?
4. What can the flow trace signify?

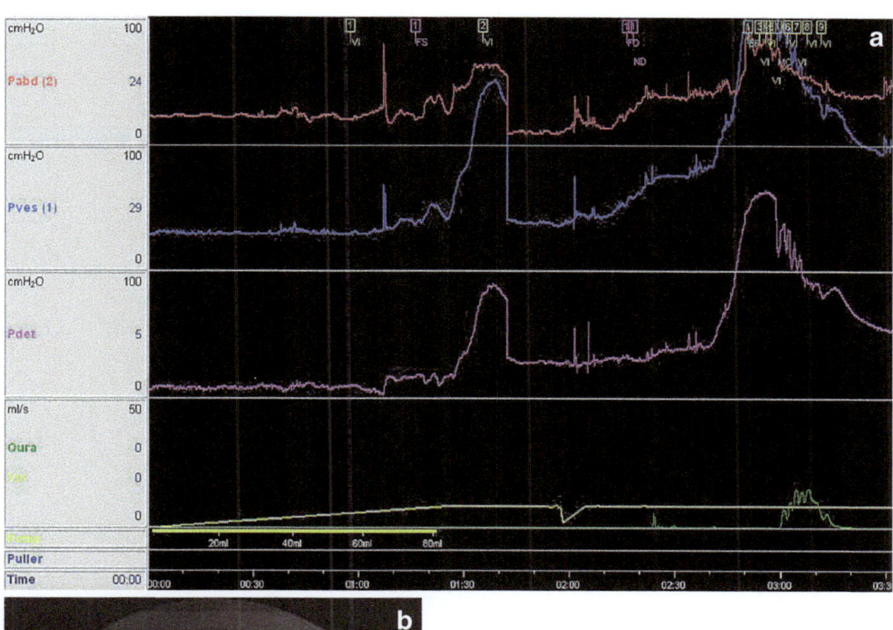

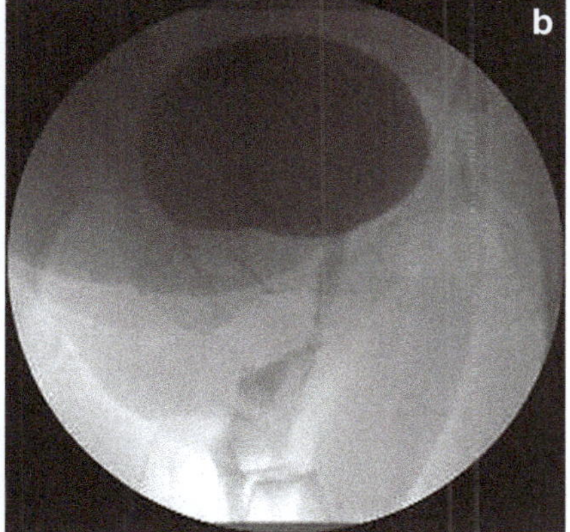

Fig. 9.4.1

Answers to Case 9.4

1. Figure 9.4.1a demonstrates marked detrusor overactivity with pressures rising above 100 cmH_2O.
2. Only 80 ml was infused.
3. Figure 9.4.1b is the video film taken during the filling phase, yet the bladder neck is seen to open with obvious urinary leak. This confirms urge-related incontinence.
4. The flow trace demonstrates a Pdet Qmax of 90 cmH_2O at a flow rate of 12 ml/s. There is no marking for micturition command but there is a mark for end fill (EF). It is difficult to be certain if this is urinary incontinence due to severe detrusor overactivity or this is a voiding trace. Hence, this demonstrates the importance of accurate reporting of the trace by the person performing the urodynamics.

Case 9.5

A 62-year-old man complains of poor urinary flow, hesitancy, a sense of incomplete emptying with frequency and urgency.

1. Is there any detrusor overactivity?
2. What does the voiding phase show?

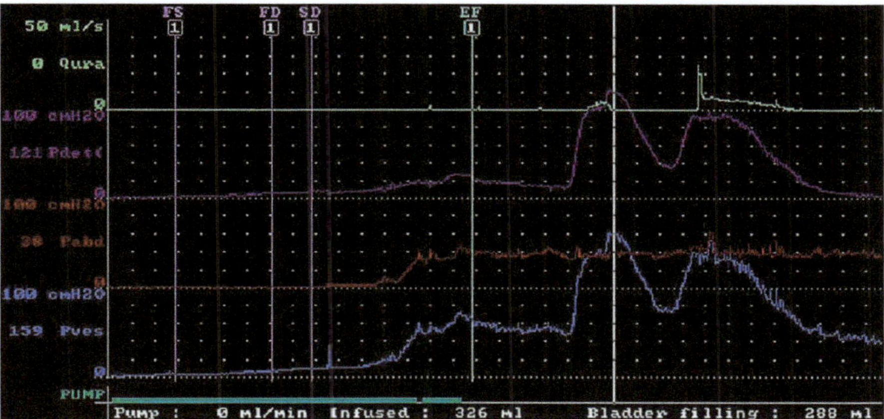

Fig. 9.5.1

Answers to Case 9.5

1. Yes, there is detrusor overactivity in Fig. 9.5.1 on standing with a pressure of around 90 cmH_2O.
2. This reveals severe outlet obstruction with pressures of about 70 cmH_2O but a flow rate <10 ml/s.

Case 9.6

A 68-year-old man complains of poor flow, incomplete emptying along with frequency, urgency and incontinence.

1. Is there any overactivity?
2. Is the compliance normal?
3. Is the voiding phase normal?
4. What type of overactivity is this most likely to be?

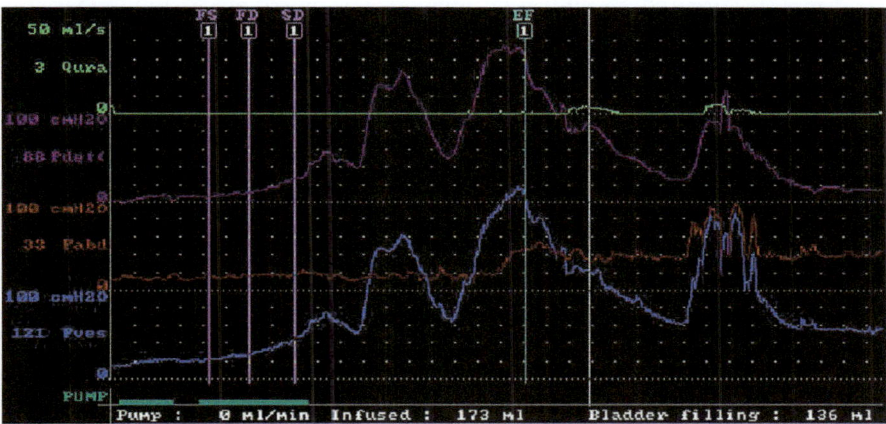

Fig. 9.6.1

Answers to Case 9.6

1. In Fig. 9.6.1 there is severe and early detrusor overactivity with a Pdet around 100 cmH_2O.
2. No, there is an early loss of compliance resulting in an overactive contraction.
3. The voiding phase shows a poor flow (<5 ml/s) and a voiding pressure of over 80 cmH_2O signifying severe obstruction.
4. This is idiopathic detrusor overactivity but is not intrinsic. This means that the detrusor overactivity is most likely secondary to long-term outflow obstruction. It is thought that this type of overactivity is secondary to irreversible changes in the detrusor as a result of outflow obstruction. This might not be fully relieved by outflow surgery e.g., TURP.

Case 9.7

A 27-year-old man sustained a T6 spinal cord injury 18 months ago. He is not on any medication.

1. What is happening in this trace?
2. What type of bladder will demonstrate this tracing?
3. What complication can result from this type of bladder dysfunction?
4. What is the optimal treatment for this type of bladder disorder?

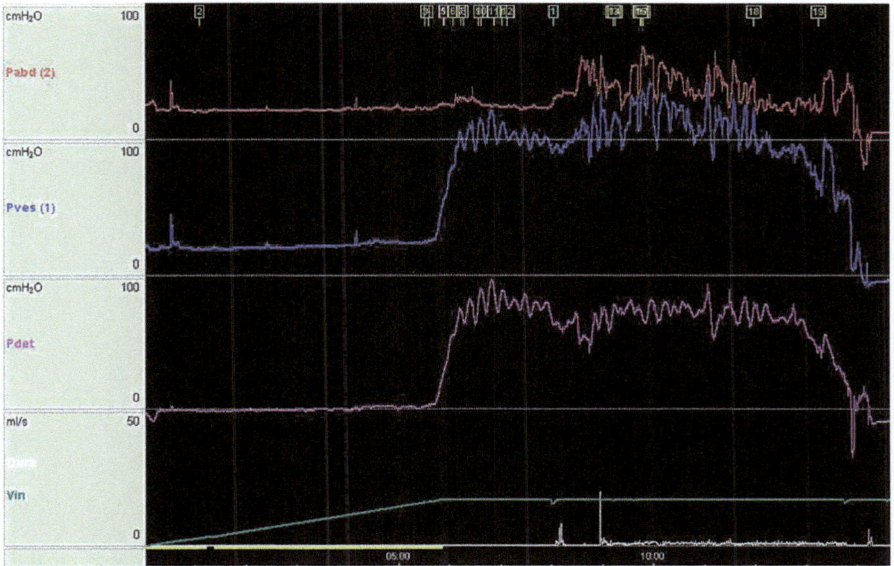

Fig. 9.7.1

Answers to Case 9.7

1. Case 9.7.1 shows high-pressure sustained detrusor overactivity with a pressure rising to around 80 cmH_2O. The contraction is also sustained, lasting for more than 5 min.
2. This is the classical urodynamic traces seen with an upper motor neuron type of spinal cord injury, resulting in high-pressure neurogenic detrusor overactivity, characterised by a 'saw toothed' appearance to the detrusor trace.
3. This can lead to small volume, thick-walled bladder with ureteric reflux and upper tract decompensation. Renal failure may ensue.
4. This patient should be on anti-cholinergic medication and practice intermittent self-catheterisation.

Case 9.8

A 34-year-old woman with T8 level spinal cord injury complains of frequency and urgency.

1. Does this trace show neurogenic detrusor overactivity?
2. Why does the detrusor pressure start to drop?
3. What is the voiding pressure?
4. What is the explanation for the rise of pressure after voiding?

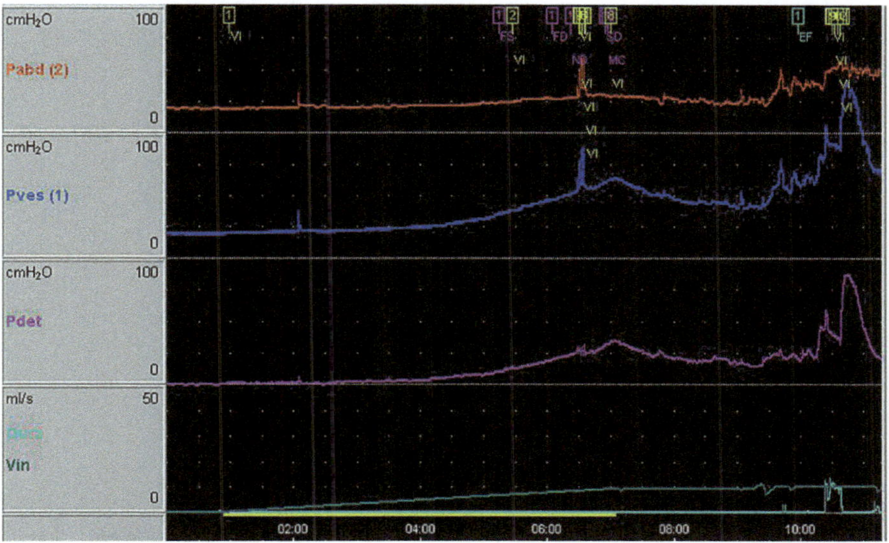

Fig. 9.8.1

Answers to Case 9.8

1. There is no neurogenic detrusor overactivity as the detrusor line rises in a straight line without any non-phasic contractions. However, the rise in detrusor pressure indicates a loss of compliance.
2. The pressure drops when the pump is stopped. Fast filling may show an apparent poor compliance with a rise in pressure during filling, but when the pump is stopped the pressures should decline. A final pressure that remains high once the pump is stopped confirms reduced compliance.
3. The voiding pressure is around 30 cmH_2O.
4. The rise in pressure can sometimes occur in high-pressure bladders called 'after-contraction'. The pressure here is around 90 cmH_2O. The clinical relevance of after contractions is still a matter of speculation.

Case 9.9

A 44-year-old woman with spinal cord injury complains of lower urinary tract symptoms.

1. What does the filling phase demonstrate?
2. What does the accompanying fluoroscopic image show?
3. What category of spinal cord injury will demonstrate this type of bladder dysfunction?

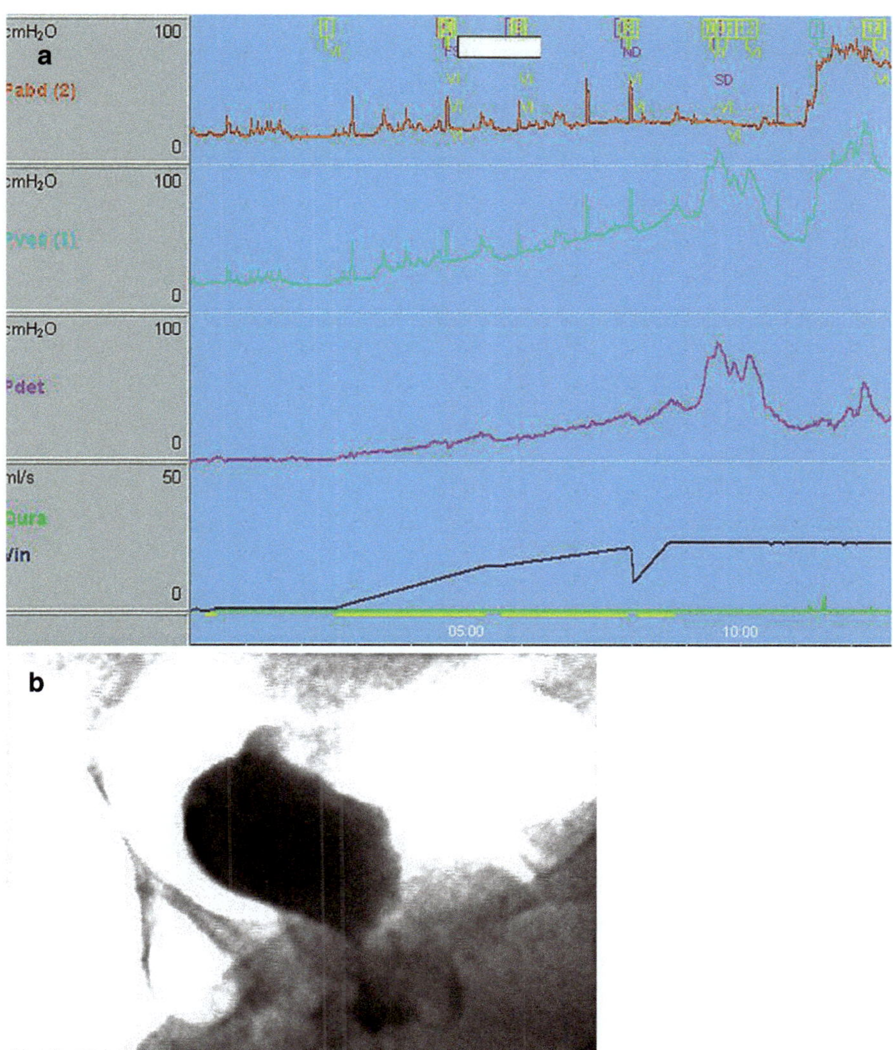

Fig. 9.9.1

Answers to Case 9.9

1. The urodynamic trace (Fig. 9.9.1a) shows initial loss of compliance, with a straight rise in detrusor pressure, followed by phasic detrusor overactivity. There is more phasic detrusor overactivity when the patient stands up. The pressure rises to around 80 cmH_2O.
2. The fluoroscopic image (Fig. 9.9.1b) demonstrates a small capacity bladder and leakage of urine. The bladder outline is trabeculated. The appearances are of neurogenic detrusor overactivity.
3. An upper motor neuron type of spinal cord injury leads to neurogenic detrusor overactivity, reduced compliance and a small capacity trabeculated bladder.

Case 9.10

A 23-year-old man sustained a spinal cord injury at T5 vertebral level 2 years ago. He complains of a sense of incomplete emptying and recurrent urinary tract infections.

1. What does the urodynamic trace show?
2. What does the arrow on the accompanying fluoroscopic image (Fig. 9.10.1b) indicate?
3. Describe the appearances in Fig. 9.10.1c taken from another patient.

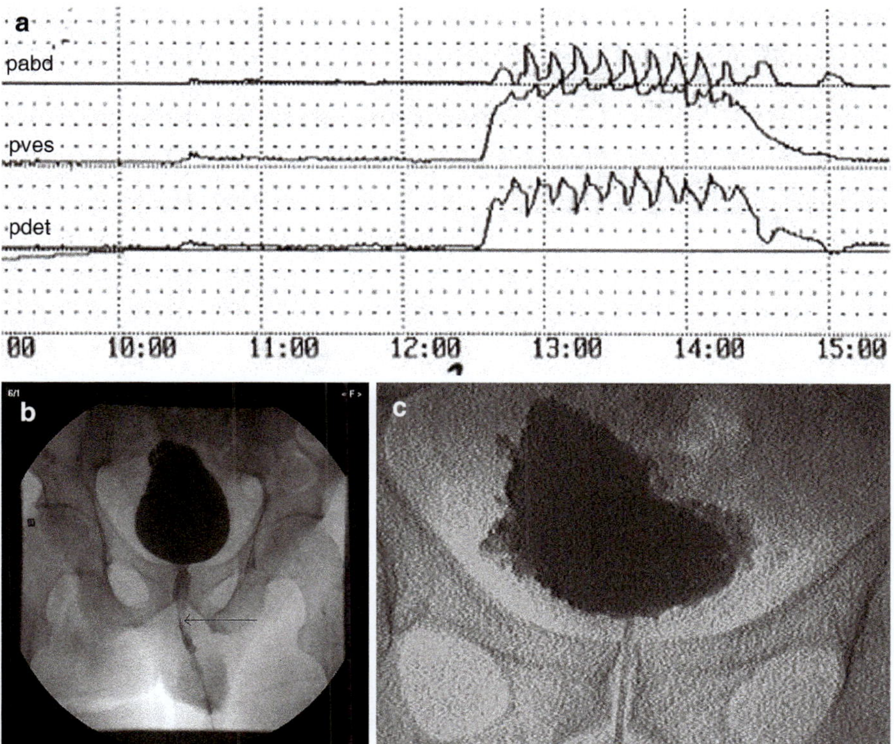

Fig. 9.10.1

Answers to Case 9.10

1. Figure 9.10.1a reveals neurogenic detrusor overactivity with a detrusor sphincter dyssynergia pattern. This is a classical trace for an upper motor neuron bladder demonstrating a dyssynergic voiding pattern with detrusor overactivity.
2. The fluoroscopic image (Fig. 9.10.1b) is marked with an arrow at the external sphincter, there is hold up of urine proximally. This confirms the presence of detrusor sphincter dyssynergia.
3. Figure 9.10.1c has the classical appearance of a neuropathic bladder. It shows a 'Christmas Tree' shape and multiple diverticula. This is also sometimes described as a fir cone bladder.

Case 9.11

A 35-year man presents with frequency and urgency.

1. Is there any detrusor overactivity?
2. Why is there a sudden drop in detrusor pressure, or has the bladder line fallen out?
3. Is the voiding phase normal?

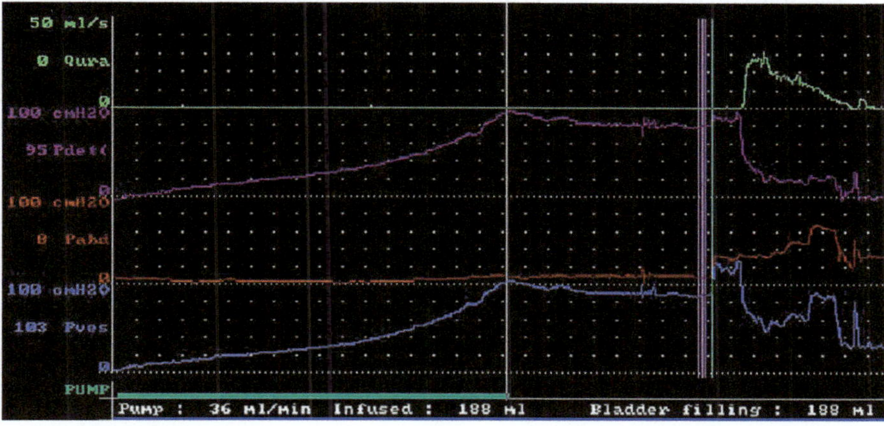

Fig. 9.11.1

Answers to Case 9.11

1. In Fig. 9.11.1 there is no detrusor overactivity, but there is loss of compliance with a steep rise in pressure to 100 cmH_2O.
2. The detrusor pressure drops steeply at the onset of voiding. The lines are in place and the pressure drop is genuine, as there is a cough test at the end of voiding. This situation can happen in a poorly compliant bladder. As demonstrated, there can be a progressive loss of compliance in an undistensible bladder. However, when it starts to empty, the pressure falls rapidly due to the visceroelastic properties of the bladder. This can be the explanation of upper tract obstruction in some cases of high-pressure chronic retention. This is relieved by catheterisation.
3. Yes, there is a good flow rate with a maximum flow of 30 ml/s and a low voiding pressure of 20 cmH_2O.

Case 9.12

A 48-year-old man complains of long standing poor flow and a worsening sense of incomplete emptying.

1. Describe the voiding phase.
2. Describe the findings on the accompanying video fluoroscopic image.
3. Is there any trapping of urine in the prostatic urethra? What is the eponymous name for this diagnostic sign?

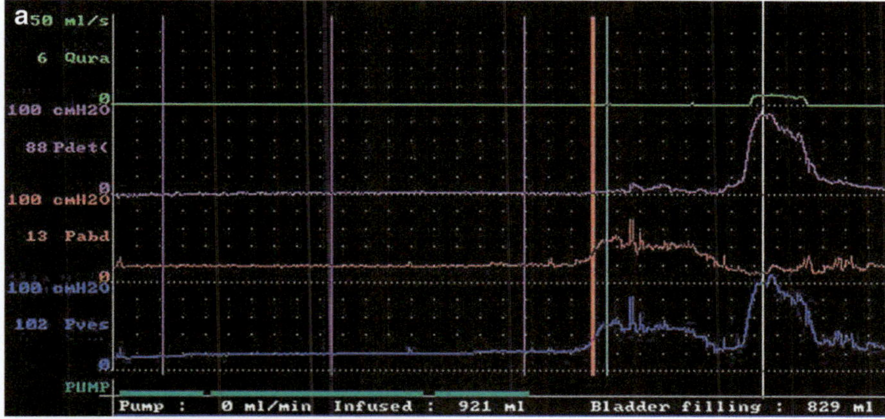

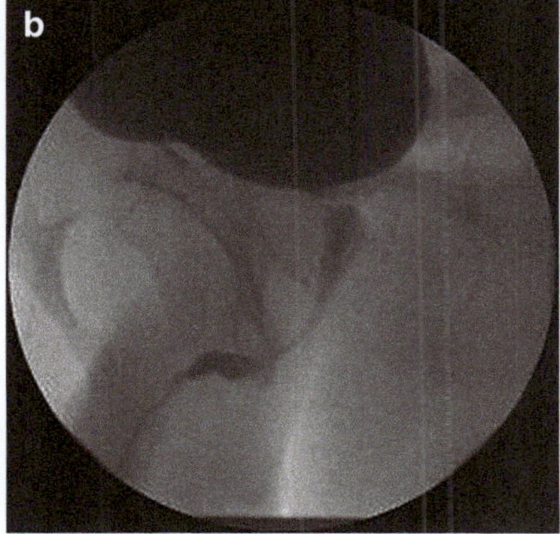

Fig. 9.12.1

Answers to Case 9.12

1. Trace 9.12.1a shows an obstructed voiding pattern, as at a detrusor pressure of 80 cmH_2O the flow rate is reduced at <5 ml/s.
2. The urodynamic traces are highly suggestive of obstructive voiding, and obstruction appears on the fluoroscopic image (Fig. 9.12.1b) to be due to a non-relaxing bladder neck, consistent with bladder neck obstruction.
3. No, to diagnose trapping in prostatic urethra the patient is required to perform a stop test which is not the case in this study. The stop test is performed consciously by the patient on the investigator's instructions during voiding. It will show a sudden interruption on the voiding trace with a corresponding steep rise in the detrusor pressure. This pressure is the isometric pressure and is the measure of the power of detrusor contraction. Trapping of contrast within the prostatic urethra, without any 'milkback', when the urination is consciously interrupted is termed the Whiteside sign.

Case 9.13

A 38-year-old female complains of frequency and poor flow with incomplete voiding.

1. Is there any detrusor overactivity?
2. What is the voiding pressure?
3. What should be the next step in diagnostic work-up?

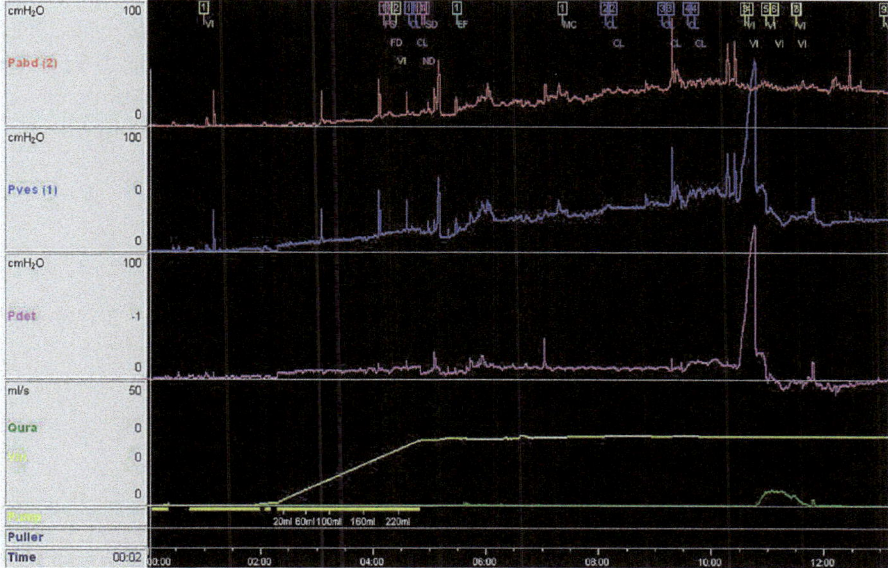

Fig. 9.13.1

Answers to Case 9.13

1. There is no detrusor overactivity in Fig. 9.13.1. Bladder filling is stable with a straight detrusor pressure trace that remains within normal limits.
2. The voiding pressure is around 20 cmH_2O. The very high pressure spike during voiding is an artefact. The exact cause is difficult to ascertain after the study. As there is a very steep rise it is possible that someone has stepped on the bladder line during adjusting the equipment and hence a sharp spike appears on the bladder line. Alternatively, as she tries to initiate a void there is a spontaneous unstable contraction followed by a true detrusor contraction. This highlights the importance of accurate reporting by the person performing the study.
3. Ideally, the investigator should repeat the study at the same setting to have an accurate assessment of the voiding phase. However, if that is not possible then a simple uroflowmetry to measure the free flow rate, with estimation of post-void residue, can be performed later.

Case 9.14

A 55-year-old man presents with obstructive voiding symptoms.

1. Does this trace show any detrusor overactivity?
2. What has happened at point indicated by the red arrow?
3. What does this trace show during the voiding phase?
4. What is P_{iso}?

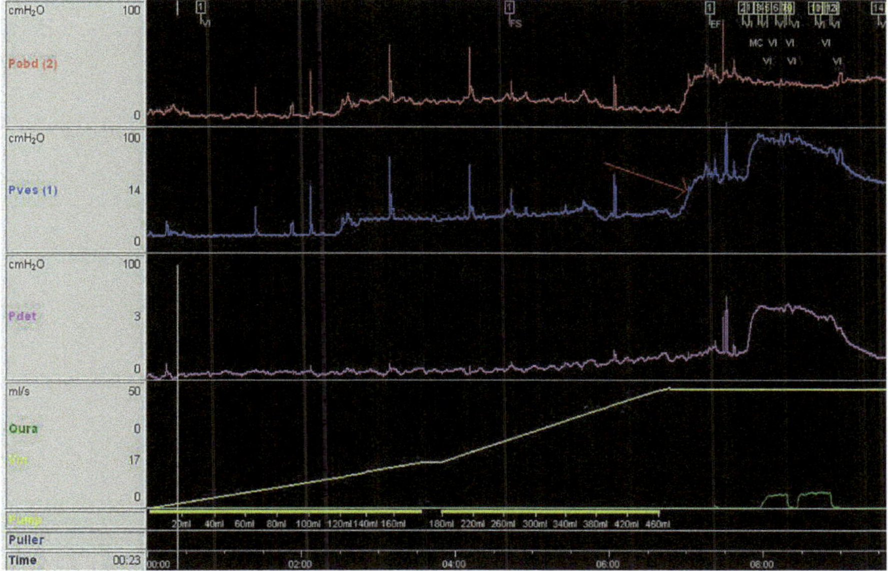

Fig. 9.14.1

Answers to Case 9.14

1. There is no abnormality during the filling phase in this trace (Fig. 9.14.1).
2. The patient has stood up. This accounts for the synchronous rise in vesical and abdominal pressure traces.
3. This shows obstructive voiding. At a raised Pdet at Qmax of 55 cmH_2O, the max flow rate is only 5 ml/s.
4. It denotes isometric contraction of the detrusor muscle against a closed bladder neck. This is evaluated as a stop test during the voiding phase. The patient is asked to hold back and the flow should stop. The detrusor pressure at zero flow is the P_{iso}. It is thought to be a good indicator of detrusor power. In this case the P_{iso} does not rise when the urinary stream is interrupted mid flow.

Case 9.15

A 55-year-old woman presents with obstructive type lower urinary tract symptoms.

1. Describe the voiding study.
2. Is there any detrusor overactivity?

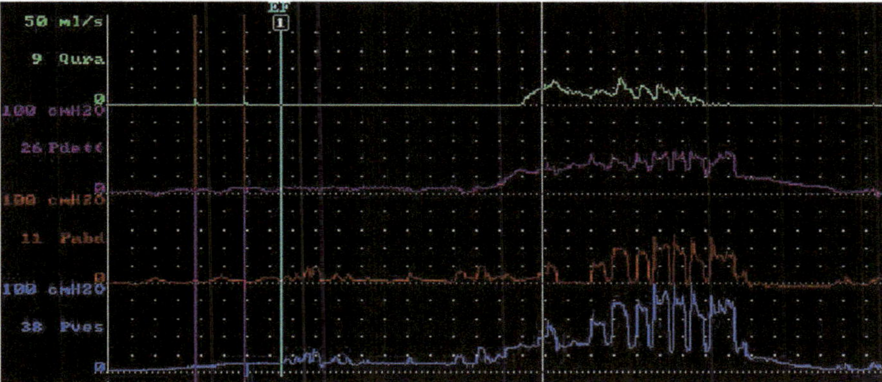

Fig. 9.15.1

Answers to Case 9.15

1. There is prolonged flow with a max flow rate of only 10 ml/s. There is no sustained detrusor contraction. She requires abdominal straining to void. Hence, has mild outlet obstruction with detrusor hypocontractility.
2. No, there is no detrusor overactivity although there is some activity in the rectal line signifying bowel activity.

Case 9.16

A 55-year-old man complains of mixed lower urinary tract symptoms.

1. The computer records a maximum flow rate of 80 ml/s. Is this correct?
2. What is the actual flow rate and voiding pressure?

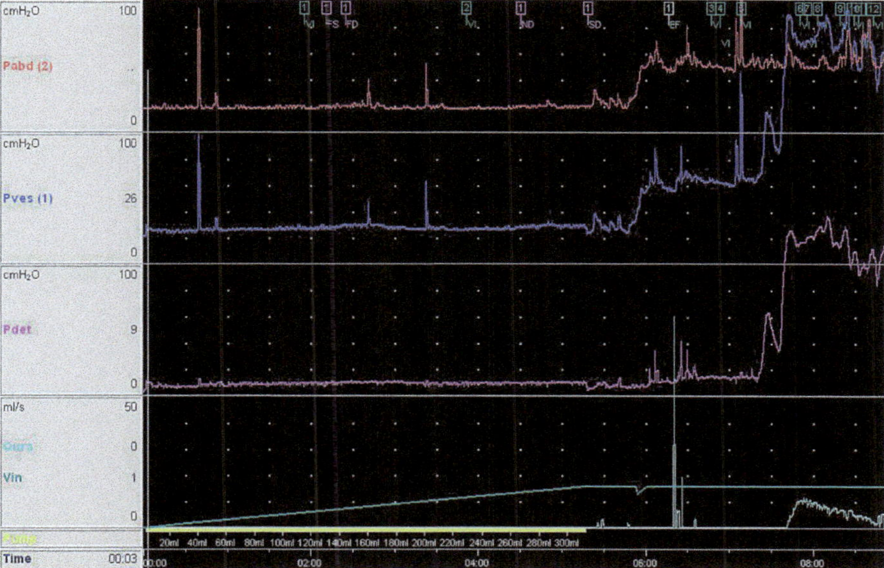

Fig. 9.16.1

Answers to Case 9.16

1. No, the computer reported a peak flow rate of 80 ml/s (Fig. 9.16.1), which is of course wrong. The computer had picked up the spike artefact on the flow rate channel and reported that as Qmax. One must always look at and evaluate the actual traces to confirm the accuracy of the analogue data.
2. The true max flow rate is 10 ml/s at a Pdet at Qmax of around 60 cmH_2O. He is probably obstructed.

Case 9.17

A 35-year-old female complains of frequency and urgency.

1. Is there any detrusor overactivity?
2. Why is there a rise in rectal pressure?
3. What has happened during the voiding study?

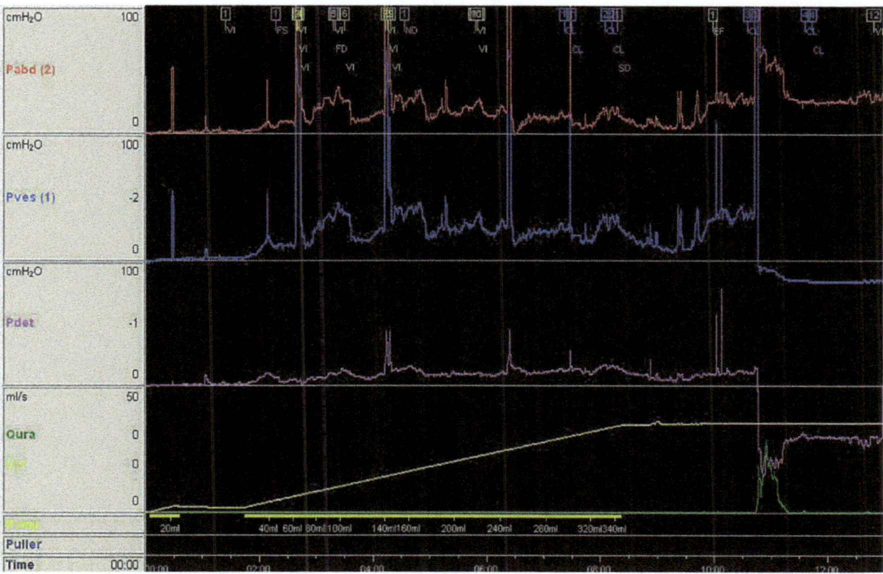

Fig. 9.17.1

Answers to Case 9.17

1. There are phasic contractions consistent with detrusor overactivity in Fig. 9.17.1. The contractions are low-pressure rises at around 15–20 cmH_2O.
2. The rectal pressure rise is due to pelvic contractions. The pressure peaks are identical on coughing.
3. The bladder line had fallen out. The maximum flow rate is about 20 ml/s but no clear comment can be made on obstruction, as no voiding pressure could be recorded before the line fell out. Although the maximal flow rate is normal, it could be associated with high voiding pressures.

Case 9.18

A 35-year-old patient with an indwelling suprapubic catheter, who also undertakes intermittent self-catherisation, undergoes a surveillance urodynamics study.

1. Please describe the study.
2. Is there any abnormal finding on this study?

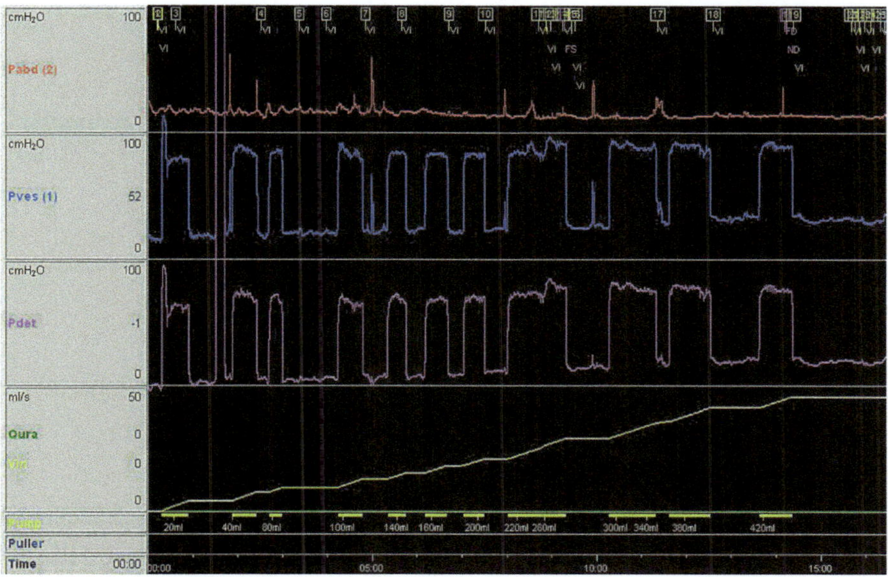

Fig. 9.18.1

Answers to Case 9.18

1. Figure 9.18.1 is a filling study via a catheter. A typical pressure waveform is seen when the bladder is filled through an indwelling catheter. This is performed by adding a three-way tap and connecting the pressure measurement catheter and filling the external line to each of two ports. The thick yellow dashes (at the bottom) show the time when the pump is ON. The steep rise in pressure is therefore the pump pressure plus the bladder pressure. Accurate bladder pressure can be measured by stopping the pump momentarily and carrying out a cough test etc.
2. No, this is a good example of a normal trace with catheter in situ. Surveillance urodynamic studies are important in patients maintained on intermittent self catheterisation (ISC) and/or suprapubic catherisation to ensure that the resting bladder pressure is not greater than 40 cmH_2O, as at this level upper tract drainage will be impeded in patients with neuropathic bladders.

Case 9.19

A 35-year-old lady with lower urinary symptoms also suffers from bowel problems.

1. Is there any abnormality during the filling phase?
2. What is happening in the rectal line during the filling phase?
3. Is the flow signal genuine?

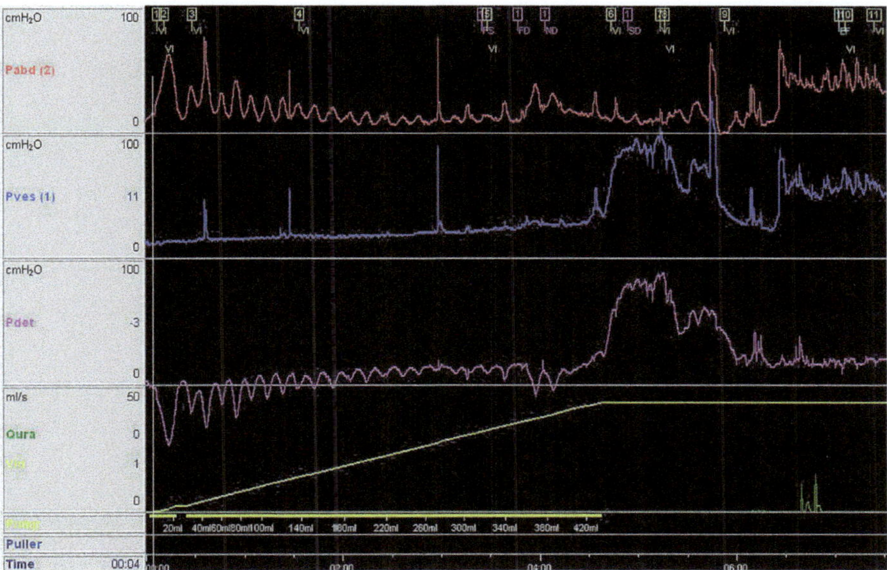

Fig. 9.19.1

Answers to Case 9.19

1. There is evidence of detrusor overactivity. If one concentrates on the detrusor line, one can see a fairly normal pressure rise, with a small phasic contraction at about 360 ml capacity, followed by a severe phasic contraction after filling is stopped at about 430 ml. This is accompanied by a strong desire as marked on the top of tracing. The patient therefore has detrusor overactivity during filling.
2. During the filling phase, the patient had overactive bowel contractions, giving rise to the artefacts seen on the detrusor channel. If in doubt check the bladder channel, and it can be seen that the phasic waveform did not originate from the bladder.
3. No, the low-level signals seen on the flow trace are not normal flow signals. They are most likely an artefact, e.g. when the sensor was knocked or moved.

Case 9.20

A 62-year-old man complains of lower urinary tract symptoms.

1. What do the following two uroflow studies demonstrate?
2. Are these normal studies?

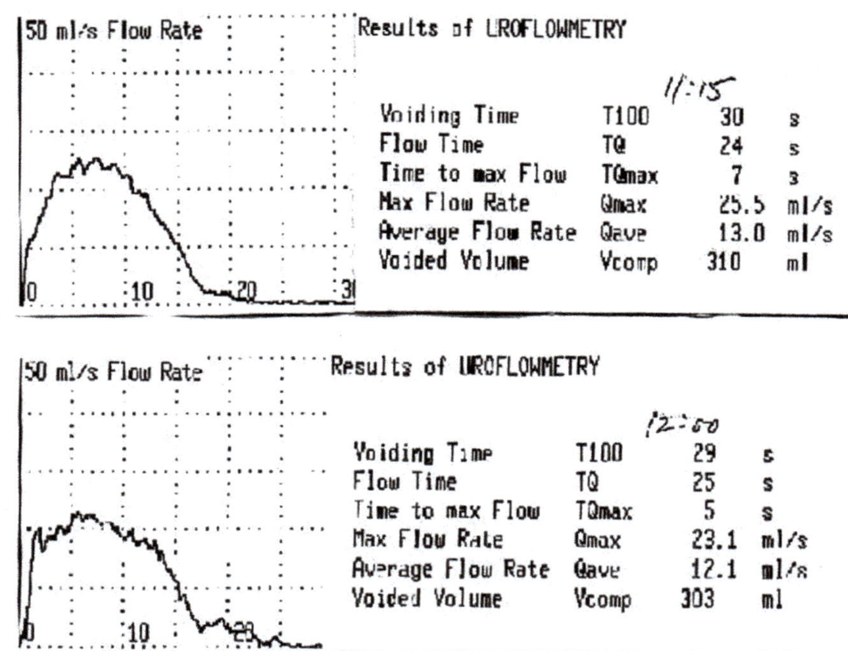

Fig. 9.20.1

Answers to Case 9.20

1. Both curves in Fig. 9.20.1 show a maximum flow rate of >20 ml/s for a voided volume of >300 ml. There is a steep rise in flow rate and the maximum flow rate is achieved within the first third of flow time. The flow time is also <30s in both cases.
2. These flow studies appear normal. The flow parameters are within normal limits and the curves are bell shaped. However, this does not necessarily exclude a urodynamic abnormality. For example, this may be compenstated mild outflow obstruction and the normal flow rates are being achieved only at the expense of high voiding pressures.

Case 9.21

A 37-year-old man complains of long standing lower urinary tract symptoms

1. Describe this flow rate.
2. What is the likely diagnosis?

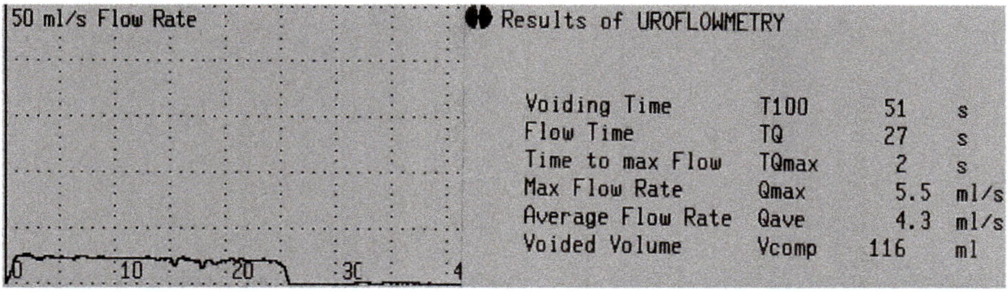

50 ml/s Flow Rate

0 10 20 30 4

Results of UROFLOWMETRY

Voiding Time	T100	51	s
Flow Time	TQ	27	s
Time to max Flow	TQmax	2	s
Max Flow Rate	Qmax	5.5	ml/s
Average Flow Rate	Qave	4.3	ml/s
Voided Volume	Vcomp	116	ml

Fig. 9.21.1

Answers to Case 9.21

1. There seems to be a fixed obstruction as the flow rate goes up and then plateaus. The maximum flow rate is very poor (5.5 ml/s). It has taken more than 20 s to pass only 116 ml.
2. This is the typical flow rate of a patient with urethral stricture.

Case 9.22

A 67-year-old man presented with mild lower urinary tract symptoms.

1. What is this flow pattern?
2. Could this be an artefact?

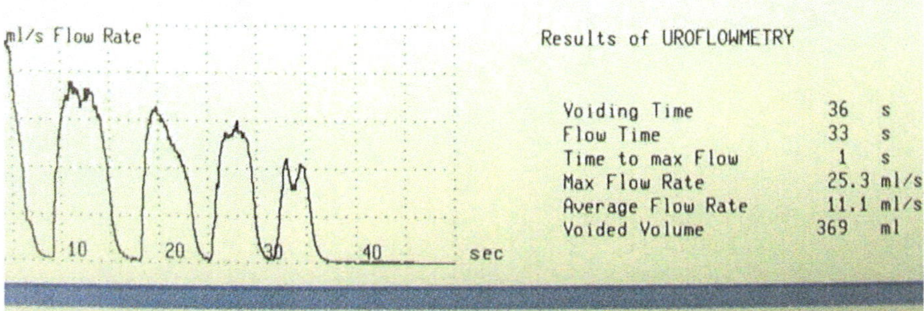

Fig. 9.22.1

Answers to Case 9.22

1. Figure 9.22.1 is a typical flow pattern caused by abdominal straining. The patient may have obstruction or a hypocontractile detrusor.
2. Yes, this pattern can be artefactual, created by the phenomenon of 'pinching'. This entails pinching and letting go of penis. Pinching creates a urinary jet that hits the rotating disc of the flow meter and a high flow rate is momentarily recorded, which rapidly tails off when the pinch is released, resulting in this unusual pattern.

Index

A
Acute bacterial prostatitis, 289, 291
Adenoma
  adrenal cortical, 116, 127
  CT, 124, 125, 128
  MRI sequence, 124, 125
  myelolipoma, 124, 125
Adenomatoid tumour, 304, 305
ADPKD. *See* Autosomal dominant polycystic kidney disease
Adrenal gland
  adrenal metastasis
    contrast-enhanced axial CT, 145
    FDG-PET/CT image, 144, 145
    T2-weighted MR image, 144, 145
  arterial supply and venous drainage, 121, 123
  carcinoma
    FDG-PET/CT image, 140–142
    histological features, 287, 288
    MRI sequence, 140, 142
    phase contrast-enhanced CT image, 140, 142
  ganglioneuromas
    CT image, 134, 136
    occurence, 134, 136
    pathological assessment, 134–136
  hyperaldosteronism
    causes of, 131, 133
    Conn's adenoma and bilateral hyperplasia, 131–133
    diagnosis, 131, 133
    H&E stain, Conn's adenoma, 131–133
  layers of, 121–123
  lipid-poor adrenal cortical adenomas, 126, 127
  lipid-rich adenoma
    adrenal cortical adenomas, 116, 127
    CT, 124, 125, 128
    MRI sequence, 124, 125
    myelolipoma, 124, 125
  myelolipoma
    axial non-contrast CT, 128–130
    complications of, 128, 130
    composition of, 128, 130
    MRI sequence, 128–130
  phaeochromocytoma
    CT and T2-weighted MRI, 137, 139
    histological features, 137–139
    radionucleotide-labelled MIBG, 137–139
  size, 121–123
Adrenal metastasis
  contrast-enhanced axial CT, 145
  FDG-PET/CT image, 144, 145
  T2-weighted MR image, 144, 145
Angiomyolipoma (AML), 56–58
Askin sarcoma, 157, 158
Atypical adenomatous hyperplasia (AAH), 248–250
Atypical small acinar proliferation (ASAP), 248, 250
Autosomal dominant polycystic kidney disease (ADPKD), 45, 47

B
Balanitis xerotica obliterans (BXO), 358–361
Benign prostatic hyperplasia (BPH), 231, 232, 242, 245, 282, 284–286
Benign viral warts, 381
Bladder
  anatomical relationship, 175–177
  calcified mass, 223–224
  cancer, 201, 203
  'cobra head' sign, 199–200
  CT urogram, 185–187
  cystitis, 228–230
  cystitis cystica, 205–206, 209
  cystitis follicularis, 205–206, 209
  detrusor overactivity, 178, 180
  detrusor pressure, 178–180
  E. coli, 225–226

S. Bott et al. (eds.), *Images in Urology*,
DOI 10.1007/978-0-85729-769-3, © Springer-Verlag London Limited 2012

Bladder (*cont.*)
embryology, 175, 177
exstrophy, 190–191
extra-genitourinary associations, 192–193
fistula, 216–219
function of, 178, 180
haematuria, 201–204
haematuria and dysuria, 223–224
Hutch diverticulum, 196–198
innervation of, 181, 182
inverted papilloma, 205–209
KUB X-ray, 223–224
malakoplakia, 205–209
MRI urography, 185–187
pathology, 178–180
PBS, 192–193
PUNLMP, 205–209
PUV, 194–195
rupture, 220–222
stress urinary incontinence, 178, 180
telangiectasia, 181, 182
trabeculation, 181, 182
trauma, 220–222
ultrasound, 183–184
urachal anomalies, 188–189
ureterocoele, 199–200
UTI, 225–226
wall structure, 175–177
Bladder exstrophy, 190–191
Bone scintigram, 270, 273
Brachytherapy, 279, 281
Bulbar urethral stricture, 347–349

C
Carcinoma of the Prostate (CAP), 257, 258, 260
Cavernosography, 377–378
Cobra head sign, 199–200
Computed tomography (CT)
adenoma, 124, 125, 128
fibrosis, 172, 174
ganglioneuromas, 134, 136
inguinal cannal, 330, 331
leiomyosarcoma, 151, 152
lipid-rich adenoma, 124, 125, 128
myelolipoma, 128–130
nodal staging, 326, 328
Congenital adrenal hyperplasia (CAH), 306–308
Conn's adenoma, 131–133
Cryptorchidism, 362–363
Cystic transformation, 309, 310
Cystitis, 228–230
Cystitis cystica, 205–206, 209
Cystitis follicularis, 205–206, 209

D
Detrusor pressure, 389–390
Detrusor sphincter dyssynergia pattern, 403–404
Digital rectal examination (DRE), 234, 236
Digital single lens reflex (DSLR), 16
Dimercaptosuccinic acid (DMSA), 11
Doppler image
hypervascular, 322, 324
intratesticular varicocele, 320, 331
mediastinum testis, 320, 331
Dynamic sentinel lymph node biopsy, 374–376
Dysuria, 223–224

E
Emphysematous pyelonephritis, 43–44
Endometriosis, 84–85
Epididymitis, 298–300
Ewing's sarcoma, 157, 158
Extraprostatic tissue (EPT), 257, 258, 260

F
Fibrosis
aetiological factors, 172, 174
CT and nephrostogram image, 172, 174
idiopathic RPF, 172–174
RPF complication, 172–174
Fibrous septa, 295, 297
Fistula, 216–219
Fournier's gangrene, 382–384

G
Ganglioneuromas
CT image, 134, 136
occurence, 134, 136
pathological assessment, 134–136
Genitourinary tuberculosis, 342, 343
Gleason sum score, 254–256
Glomerular filtration rate (GFR), 8, 11
Gonococcal urethritis, 350–351
Granulomatous prostatitis, 292, 391

H
Haematuria, 201–204, 223–224
High–grade prostatic intra-epithelial neoplasia (HGPIN), 237, 239, 248, 249
Histopathological image
aim, 13
governance and storage, 18–19

operative surgical specimen
bivalved orchidectomy, 15
examination and fixation, 13
hesitant cut, 14
nephrectomy, 14
ureterectomy, carcinoma, 15
Wegener's granulomatosis, 16
photography technique, 18
tissue and photography, 17–18
uses, 13
Horseshoe kidney, 94–96
Hutch diverticulum, 196–198
Hydrocele
anechoic fluid collection, 315, 317
inflammatory debris, 315–317
treatment, 315, 317–319
tunica vaginal, 315–317
Hyperaldosteronism
causes of, 131, 133
Conn's adenoma and bilateral hyperplasia, 131–133
diagnosis, 131, 133
H&E stain, Conn's adenoma, 131–133
Hypertrophic column of Bertin, 97–98
Hypospadias, 362–363

I
Immunohistochemistry, 237, 239
Inferior vena cava leiomyosarcoma. *See* Leiomyosarcoma
Inverted papilloma:, 205–209

K
Kidneys and ureters
aetiology, 43–44
angiomyolipoma, 56–58
autosomal dominant polycystic kidney disease, 45, 47
cortico-medullary phase, 25–27
CT KUB, 25–27
CT protocols, 25–27
CT urogram, 25–27
emphysematous pyelonephritis, 43–44
endometriosis, 84–85
grading system, 28, 31
horseshoe kidney, 94–96
hyperechoic cortex, 21–24
hypertrophic column of Bertin, 97–98
imaging modality, 25–27
intermittent flank pain, 59–60
macroscopic haematuria, 51–52
multicystic dysplastic kidney, 89–90
nephrocalcinosis, 73–76
nephrographic phase, 25–27
non-specific chronic back pain, 56–58
oncocytoma, 59–60
orientation, 21–24
papillary necrosis, 33–35
pelvicutereic obstruction, 33–35
post-renal transplant complications, 117–118
primary megaureter, 102–103
pyeloureteritis cystica, 38–39
radiolucent stones, 77–79
renal artery aneurysm, 106–108
renal cystic lesions, 45–47
renal infarction, 104–105
renal lymphoma, 70–72
retrocaval, 102–103
staghorn calculus, 82–83
transitional cell carcinoma, 53–55
tuberculosis, 40–42
ureteric calculus, 77–79
von Hippel Lindau (VHL) disease, 45–47
XGP, 33–37

L
Leiomyosarcoma
central low attenuation area significance, 151, 152
CT image, 151, 152
gender predilection, 153, 154
hydronephrosis, 153, 154
inferior vena cava, 153, 154
metastasis frequency, 151, 152
venous leiomyosarcomata, 153, 154
Lichen sclerosis. *See* Balanitis xerotica obliterans (BXO)
Lower urinary tract symptoms
detrusor overactivity, 421–422
flow rate, 415–416, 425–426
flow signal, 421–422
obstruction/ hypocontractile detrusor, 427–428
overactive bowel contractions, 421–422
pinching, 427–428
spike artefact, 415–416
urethral stricture, 425–426
uroflow study, 423–424
Lymphoedema, 364–365
Lymphoma
chronic lymphocytic leukaemia, 167, 169
retroperitoneal adenopathy, 167, 169

M
Magnetic resonance imaging (MRI)
adenoma, 124, 125
adrenal gland, 140, 142

Magnetic resonance imaging (MRI) (*cont.*)
bladder, 185–187
importance, 302, 303
lipid-rich adenoma, 124, 125
myelolipoma, 128–130
phaeochromocytoma, 137, 139
prostate, 240, 241
abnormality, 240, 241
central gland, 242, 245
CT, 231, 232
diffuse abnormal low signal, 292, 293
image, feature, 234, 236
low signal, 254–256, 257, 260
marked improvement, 289–291
prostatic mass, 277, 278
rectoprostatic angle, 257, 260
right posterior PZ, 251, 253
staging, 234, 236
T2 and diffusion weighted, 257, 259, 261
testes and adnexae, 302, 303
undescended testis, 302, 303
urological disorder, 8, 10
uses of, 302, 303
Malakoplakia, 205–209
Malignant peripheral nerve sheath tumour (MPNST), 159, 160
Marked hyperaemia, 298–300
Meatal stenosis, 358, 360
Mercaptoacetyltriglycine (MAG), 11
Metaiodobenzylguanidine (MIBG), 137–139
Micturating cystourethrogram (MCUG), 194–195
MPNST. *See* Malignant peripheral nerve sheath tumour
Multicystic dysplastic kidney, 89–90
Myelolipoma
axial non-contrast CT, 128–130
complications of, 128, 130
composition of, 128, 130
MRI sequence, 128–130

N
Nephrocalcinosis, 73–76
Nocturia and occasional urge incontinence
detrusor overactivity, 387–388
leakage, 387–388
voiding phase, 387–388
Non-seminomatous germ cell tumour (NSGCT), 326, 328, 329
axial CT, 163, 164
metastasis, 16, 163
orchidectomy relapse rate, 163, 164
post-chemotherapy, 163, 164

O
Oncocytoma, 59–60
Orchiectomy specimen
transverse section, 330, 332
white fibrous mas, 330, 332

P
Papillary necrosis, 33–35
Papillary Urothelial Neoplasm of Low Malignant Potential (PUNLMP), 205–209
Paraganglioma
benign pathology, 155, 156
malignancy, 155, 156
organs of Zuckerkandl, 155, 156
radionuclide tracer, 155, 156
sign and symptoms, 155, 156
Pelvicutereic obstruction, 33–35
Penile Doppler study, 379–380
Penis
arteriography, 379–380
benign viral warts, 381
Bowenoid papulosis, 366, 368
bulbar urethral stricture, 347–349
cancers
risk factors, 370, 372
staging of, 370, 372
subtypes, 370–373
cavernosography, 377–378
cryptorchidism, 362–363
dynamic sentinel lymph node biopsy, 374–376
Fournier's gangrene, 382–384
fractured, 355–357
surgical exploration, 355–357
tunical rupture, 355–357
urethral distraction injury, 355–357
glans resurfacing, 358–361
hypospadias, 362–363
intra-epithelial neoplasia (IN)
keratin production, 366, 368
treatment, 366, 368
lichen sclerosis, 358–361
lymphoedema, 364–365
meatal stenosis, 358, 360
palpable lymph nodes, 374–376
penile Doppler study, 379–380
Peyronie's disease, 377–378
reduced maximum flow rate, 347–349
trauma
antegrade urethrogram, 352–354
diastasis, 352, 354
management and investigation, 352, 354

pubic ramus fracture, 352, 354
transection, 352–354
urethrography, 347–349
epithelial irregularity, 350–351
gonococcal urethritis, 350–351
urethroplasty, 347–349
Zoon's balanitis, 366, 368
Peyronie's disease, 377–378
Phaeochromocytoma
CT and T2-weighted MRI, 137, 139
histological features, 137–139
radionucleotide-labelled MIBG, 137–139
Picture archiving and Communication Systems (PACS), 2
Posterior urethral values (PUV), 194–195
Primary megaureter, 102–103
Primitive neuroectodermal tumour (PNET)
coronal and axial CT, 157, 158
Ewing's sarcoma and Askin sarcoma, 157, 158
prognostic factor, 157, 158
Prostate
AAH, 248, 249
abnormal intermediate signal, 282–284
acinus, 237, 239
acute bacterial prostatitis, 289, 291
adenocarcinoma cell, 270, 272, 273
advanced disease, 274, 276
ASAP, 248, 250
basal cell, 237, 239
biopsy core, 251, 253
bone metastases and lymphadenopathy, 266, 267
bone scintigram, 270, 273
bone turnover, 270, 273
brachytherapy, 279, 281
CAP, 257, 258, 260
clinical stage
T4N1 M1b, 266, 267
T4N1 M1c, 268, 269
compare with normal gland, 248, 249
cystic huperplastic nodule, 242, 243, 245
differential diagnosis, 240, 241, 262, 264
EPT, 257, 258, 260
extensive retroperitoneal lymphadenopathy, 274–276
extraprostatic extension, 257, 260
fat–suppressed T1 weighted, 268, 269
Gleason grading system
glandular micro–architecture, 254, 256
pattern, 254, 256
granulomatous prostatitis, 292, 293
H, E and IH preparation, 248–250
hip, explanation, 266, 267
histological feature, 287, 288
hyperplasia
morphology, 242–245
nodular, 246, 247
immunohistochemical technique, 270, 272, 273
immunohistochemistry, 236, 238
invasive cancer, 233, 253
leiomyosarcoma, 285, 286
magnetic resonance imaging (MRI)
abnormality, 240, 241
central gland, 242, 245
CT, 231, 232
diffuse abnormal low signal, 292, 293
image, feature, 234, 236
low signal, 254–256, 257, 260
marked improvement, 289–291
prostatic mass, 277, 278
rectoprostatic angle, 257, 260
right posterior PZ, 251, 253
staging, 234, 236
T2 and diffusion weighted, 257, 259, 261
microscopic feature, 237, 239
necrosis, 246, 247
non–adenocarcinoma, 285, 286
non–caseating granuloma, 292, 293
pathological and clinical significance, 248, 249
pelvic node, 279–281
PET CT image, 282–284
positive surgical margin, 257, 258, 260
post–mortem coronal section, 274–276
prostatic adenocarcinoma, 277, 278
radical prostatectomy (RP)
coronal macroscopic section, 251–253
specimen, 298–300
radical radiotherapy, 279, 281
radiological feature, 266, 267
radiological staging, 251, 253
right external iliac node, 277, 278
right side of, 234–236
sagittal T2 and T1 weighted, 270, 271, 273
significant pathology, 266, 267
stroma, 237, 239
structure
axial and coronal high–resolution T2–weighted image, 231, 232
axial CT image, 231, 232
surgical resection specimen, 242, 243, 245
T2c prostate cancer, 254–256
transrectal ultrasound (TRUS)
abnormality, 240, 241
biopsy, 236, 236, 287, 288

Prostate (*cont.*)
echogenicity, 254, 256, 257, 260
irregular cavity, 287, 288
thinned PZ, 242, 243, 245
tumour stage, 262–264
T2 signal
low, 257, 260, 279, 281
TUR defect, 268, 269
ultrasound image, 234, 236
utricle cysts, 240, 241
well differentiated carcinoma, 248, 249
zones of, 231, 232
Prostatic adenocarcinoma, 277, 278
Prune belly syndrome (PBS), 192–193
Pyeloureteritis cystica, 38–39

R

Radical prostatectomy (RP)
coronal macroscopic section, 251–253
specimen, 298–300
Radical radiotherapy, 49, 51
Radiological image
computed tomography (CT), 3
contrast media
chemotoxic effect, 10
limitation, 9
MRI, 11
signal–noise ratio, 8
ultrasound, 10–11
contrast nephropathy, 10
hazards
effective radiation dose, 12
stochastic effect, 12
X-ray interact, 11
hounsfield or CT Unit, 3
magnetic resonance imaging (MRI)
physics, 7
signal, 8
T2 weighted, 9
urological disorder, 8, 10
nuclear medicine, 11
plain, 2
tissue-energy interaction, 1
ultrasound
grey–scale, 7
moving interface, 6
urological disorder, 6
window level and width
renal–specific protocol and CT technique, 4–5
screen setting, 3
urological disorder, 5
X–rays
PACS, 2
production, 2
Radiological staging, 251, 253
Radiolucent stones, 77–79
Renal artery aneurysm, 106–108
Renal cystic lesions
Bosniak classification, 48, 50
malignancy, 48, 50
nephrectomy specimen, 28–31
USS and CT findings, 53–55
Renal infarction, 104–105
Renal lymphoma, 70–72
Renal-specific protocol and CT technique, 4–5
Renal trauma, 28, 31
Resistive index (RI), 7
Retrocaval ureter, 102–103
Retroperitoneum
de-differentiated liposarcoma
anatomical structure, 149, 150
CT scan, 149, 150
resection recurrence rate, 149, 150
symptoms, 149, 150
fibrosis
aetiological factors, 172, 174
CT and nephrostogram image, 172, 174
idiopathic RPF, 172–174
RPF complication, 172–174
leiomyosarcoma
central low attenuation area significance, 151, 152
CT image, 151, 152
gender predilection, 153, 154
hydronephrosis, 153, 154
inferior vena cava, 153, 154
metastasis frequency, 151, 152
venous leiomyosarcomata, 153, 154
liposarcoma
characteristics, 147, 148
de-differentiation risk, 147, 148
radiological appearance, 147, 148
treatment modality, 147, 148
lymphoma
chronic lymphocytic leukaemia, 167, 169
retroperitoneal adenopathy, 167, 169
metastatic lymphadenopathy
differential diagnosis, 170, 171
histology, 170, 171
metastatic non-seminomatous germ cell tumour
α–FP and β–HCG, 165, 166
lymph node mass, 165, 166

NSGCT
axial CT, 163, 164
orchidectomy relapse rate, 163, 164
post-chemotherapy, 163, 164
paraganglioma
benign pathology, 155, 156
malignancy, 155, 156
organs of Zuckerkandl, 155, 156
radionuclide tracer, 155, 156
sign and symptoms, 155, 156
plexiform neurofibroma
malignant transformation risk, 159, 160
MPNST, 159, 160
NF-1, 159, 160
PNET
coronal and axial CT, 157, 158
Ewing's sarcoma and Askin sarcoma, 157, 158
prognostic factor, 157, 158
tuberculosis
CT-guided aspiration/biopsy, 161, 162
diagnosis, 161, 162
psoas abscess, 161, 162

S
Sonography
anechoic dilated structure, 320, 331
detection, 302, 303
epididymis, 295, 297–300
homogenous reflectivity, 295–297
inguinal region, 302, 303
mediastinum testis, 295, 297
tunica albuginea, 295, 297
Sperm granulomata, 336, 337
Spinal cord injury
detrusor sphincter dyssynergia pattern, 403–404
filling phase, 401–402
fluoroscopic image, 401–402
neurogenic detrusor overactivity, 401–402
Squamous cell cancer (SCC), 370–372
Staghorn calculus, 82–83

T
Testes and adnexae
acute focal testiclar infarction, 312, 314
adenomatoid tumour, 304, 305
anatomy
fibrous septa, 295, 297
tunica albuginea, 295, 297
tunica vaginalis, 295, 297
bi–valved orchidectomy specimen, 298, 300
blood supply, 295, 297
CAH, 306–308
CT
inguinal cannal, 330, 331
nodal staging, 326, 328
cystic dysplasia, 309, 311
cystic transformation, 309, 310
Doppler image
hypervascular, 322, 324
intratesticular varicocele, 320, 331
mediastinum testis, 320, 331
preserved vascularity, 340, 341
vascularity, 332, 335
epididymal tail
abnormality, 304, 305
heterogeneous, 298–300
epididymitis, 298–300
extratesticular collection, 340, 341
fibrcaseous tissue, 342, 343
florid recent infarction, 312–314
genitourinary tuberculosis, 342, 343
haematological malignancy, 322–324
H and E section, 302, 303
heterogeneous testicular, 326, 328
hydrocele
anechoic fluid collection, 315, 317
inflammatory debris, 315–317
treatment, 315, 317–319
tunica vaginal, 315–317
intratesticular varicocele, 320, 321
lack of vascularity, 298–300
marked hyperaemia, 298–300
mediastinum testis, 306, 307
MRI
importance, 302, 303
undescended testis, 302, 303
uses of, 302, 303
multiple punctate echogenic foci, 338, 339
multitude condition, 338, 339
NSGCT, 326, 328, 329
orchiectomy specimen
abnormality, 309–311
bivalved, replacemaent, 326–328
epididymis, 312–314, 322–324
risk management, 342, 343
risk of condition, 342, 343
transverse section, 330, 332
white fibrous mas, 330, 332
poor vascularity, 326, 328
sonography
anechoic dilated structure, 320, 331
detection, 302, 303
epididymis, 295, 297–300
homogenous reflectivity, 295–297

Testes and adnexae (*cont.*)
inguinal region, 302, 303
mediastinum testis, 295, 297
tunica albuginea, 295, 297
spermatic cord, tumour, 330, 331
sperm granulomata, 336, 337
surgical exploration, 340, 341
symphysis, 322–324
testicular cancer, 302, 303
testicular lymphoma, 322–324
testicular microlithiasis, 338, 339
TGCT, 333, 335
tunica albuginea, 295–297, 340, 341, 344
UDT, 302, 303
ultrasound technique
undescended testis, 302, 303
upper pole, 336, 337, 340–343
Testicular appendages, 295, 297
Testicular cerm cell tumor (TGCT), 333, 335
Testicular microlithiasis, 338, 339
Tissue–energy interaction, 1, 3
Transitional cell carcinoma (TCC), 53–55, 203–204, 214
Tuberculosis, 40–42
CT-guided aspiration/biopsy, 161, 162
diagnosis, 161, 162
psoas abscess, 161, 162
Tumour stage, 262–264
Tunica albuginea, 295–297, 340, 341, 344
Tunica vaginalis, 295, 297
TUR defect, 268, 269

U
Ultrasound technique, 302, 303
Undescended right testis (UDT), 302, 303
Ureteric calculus, 77–79
Ureterocoele, 199–200
Urethral stricture, 425–426
Urinary tract infection (UTI), 225–226
Urodynamics
frequency and urgency
anticholinergic medications, 391–392
cough action, 385–386
detrusor overactivity, 393–396, 405–406
detrusor pressure, 405–406
filling phase, 385–386
nocturia and occasional urge incontinence, 387–388
obstruction, 395–396
overactive contraction, 395–396
rectal pressure, 417–418
T8 level spinal cord, 399–400
urge-related incontinence, 390–391
voiding phase, 393–394
voiding study, 385–386
incomplete emptying
detrusor pressure, 389–390
filling, 389–390
fluoroscopic image, 407–408
overactivity, 389–390
prostatic urethra trapping, 407–408
voiding phase, 407–408
incomplete voiding, 409–410
indwelling suprapubic catheter, 419–420
lower urinary tract symptoms, 413–414
detrusor overactivity, 421–422
flow rate, 415–416, 425–426
flow signal, 421–422
obstruction/hypocontractile detrusor, 427–428
overactive bowel contractions, 421–422
pinching, 427–428
spike artefact, 415–416
urethral stricture, 425–426
uroflow study, 423–424
obstructive voiding symptoms, 411–412
spinal cord injury, 396–397
detrusor sphincter dyssynergia pattern, 403–404
filling phase, 401–402
fluoroscopic image, 401–402
neurogenic detrusor overactivity, 401–402
Urological disorder
computed tomography, 5
MRI, 8, 10
ultrasound, 6

V
Von Hippel Lindau (VHL) disease, 45–47

X
Xanthogranulomatous pyelonephritis (XGP), 33–37

Z
Zoon's balanitis, 366, 368

CPI Antony Rowe
Chippenham, UK
2017-11-03 10:13